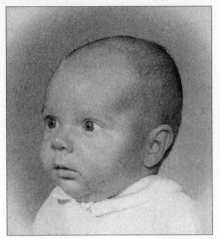

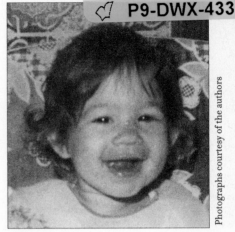

# About the Authors

ROBERT W. SEARS, MD, FAAP, is a board-certified pediatrician in private practice with his father, Dr. Bill Sears, in Dana Point, California. "Dr. Bob," as his little patients like to call him, received his medical degree in 1995 from Georgetown University and completed his pediatric training at Children's Hospital Los Angeles in 1998. He is a co-author of six books so far in the Sears Parenting Library, including *The Healthiest Kid in the Neighborhood*, *Father's First Steps*, *The Baby Book*, *The Premature Baby Book*, and *The Baby Sleep Book*. His latest and first solo work, *The Vaccine Book: Making the Right Decision for Your Child*, highlights his passion for providing America's parents with a fair and objective look at childhood vaccines. Dr. Bob is also passionate about combining mainstream medicine with a more natural and holistic approach to pediatric care in his office and his writing. He is a medical consultant for HAPPY**BABY** Organic Baby Food and is an Advisory Board Member for Kaplan University Department of Health Sciences. Dr. Bob has appeared on *The Early Show*, *The Ellen DeGeneres Show*, CNN, and the *Dr. Phil* show. He is the proud father of three boys, ages sixteen, thirteen and seven. In his spare time Dr. Bob enjoys surfing the California waves, mountain biking, playing bass guitar with his teenage son guitarist, trying to keep up with his youngest son, reading, speaking at parenting conferences throughout the United States, and is the chief editor and writer for www.AskDrSears.com. He lives with his wife and kids in Dana Point, California.

HAPPY**BABY** is the leading brand of premium organic baby foods in the US, founded by Shazi Visram. The socially responsible business is dedicated to providing optimal organic nutrition for infants and toddlers and their 30 products are sold in over 5,000 stores nationwide. As the company and its many offerings have grown over the years, the mission has evolved to also provide education and awareness to parents so they can make informed decisions about raising their children in a safe, healthy, and toxin-free environment. Shazi lives in New York and is expecting her first baby. AMY MARLOW, MPH, RD, CDN is HAPPY**BABY**'s nutrition adviser. She is a registered dietitian and a published health writer who speaks on many nutrition and health topics in New York City, where she lives with her husband and two young children. Please visit www.happybabyfood.com for more information.

HAPPY**BABY**™

## Also by Robert W. Sears, MD, FAAP

*The Vaccine Book*
*The Baby Book*
*The Baby Sleep Book*
*The Premature Baby Book*
*The Healthiest Kid in the Neighborhood*
*Father's First Steps: 25 Things Every New Dad Should Know*
*The Autism Book (2010)*

# HAPPY**BABY**™

## The Organic Guide
## to Baby's First 24 Months

By the Founders of HAPPY**BABY**,

### Robert W. Sears, MD, FAAP,

and

### Amy Marlow, MPH, RD, CDN

HARPER

NEW YORK · LONDON · TORONTO · SYDNEY

HARPER

HarperCollins books may be purchased for educational, business, or sales promotional use. For information please write: Special Markets Department, HarperCollins Publishers, 10 East 53rd Street, New York, NY 10022.

*Designed by Jennifer Ann Daddio/Bookmark Design & Media Inc.*

Library of Congress Cataloging-in-Publication Data is available upon request.

ISBN 978-0-06-171136-7

11 12 13   DIX/QWF   10 9 8 7 6 5 4 3 2

*To my dear wife, Cheryl, for sharing my passion for*
*raising our kids healthy and green, and for being*
*willing to do more than her fair share of the work*
*that this lifestyle demands!*

—DR. BOB


*To my own happy babies, Noah and Alana,*
*and to Josh, my homemade baby food making,*
*plastic avoiding, let's-find-a-way-to-*
*recycle-that husband extraordinaire.*

—AMY

# Contents

## Part Three

# The Green and Happy Home

## Part Four

# More Happy Habits

# Introduction

Congratulations on being blessed with life's most precious gift—a brand-new baby! You have begun a new and exciting phase of your life and are ready to embrace the challenges and rewards to come. Having a baby can throw many aspects of your world into chaos, but it also brings some things into focus. Looking at your tiny vulnerable child probably makes you want to do all in your power to keep her safe and healthy. But as a parent today, you might feel overwhelmed by all the potential dangers lurking in our world which can get in the way of raising a happy baby. Toxic plastics, dangerous toys, mysterious illnesses—we have good reason to be concerned, and good reason to make Baby's health our number-one priority.

We wrote this book because we want to share with you our way to make the daunting task of protecting Baby a little simpler. Here's how: go green. Call it green, call it eco-friendly: whatever you call it, we're talking about healthy choices that are not only good for the planet, but also good for Baby's health. This "Organic Guide" will help you be a greener parent. From breast milk and organic first foods to all-natural baby toys and cleaning supplies, we'll help you navigate Baby's first two years.

And really, we're not just talking about Baby. Much of our advice will help you make changes for yourself and your spouse as well. We know that you want to live a long, healthy life. You don't want to just be a mother, but a healthy, active, energetic, and positive Mama. We'll help you get there—chapter 2 is devoted to your health and well being! Even better, how about being an active grandparent someday, free of chronic illnesses, physically fit, and energetic. Plus, by adopting a healthy eco-friendly lifestyle when Baby is young you're teaching her how to grow up to be an eco-friendly parent herself—another way your actions will make the planet better for your grandchildren and future generations.

We know that many parents decide to simply ignore many of the issues we'll discuss in this book. Rather than taking steps to avoid chemicals, they choose to accept them as an inevitable part of our modern society; their babies will have some exposure to the toxins in our environment and that's that. Because these parents do not notice the effects of these so-called toxins on their own health, they figure Baby will be just fine. Ignorance is bliss, right? Except that babies, as we will discuss, are much more susceptible to toxins than we are and most products approved by the Food and Drug Administration are actually approved for adults without babies in mind.

Well, we know that you are reading this book because you do want to take steps to improve your baby's, and your whole family's, quality of life. You do want to make the effort. We want to help. As a pediatrician, author, speaker, and father (Dr. Bob), and as a mom and dietitian (Amy), we have the joy of working with parents and children in our professional lives. We also have the responsibility of committing to these changes in our own lives and making sure this passion rubs off on our own children. We created this guide so that every parent across America would have the tools they need to change themselves, their children, and their world for the better.

We realize that after reading just a few pages about going green you may feel in over your head. You are not alone. Many new parents feel this way. But it doesn't have to be so hard. True, some of the green lifestyle choices that we'll discuss will take some getting used to. But on the other hand, going green is often as simple as choosing an organic apple instead of a conventional one. Or recycling a food package, or spraying an all-natural solution on your kitchen counter instead of a blend of toxic chemicals. Let's make a deal: if you promise to read this whole book, we promise to make going green doable. Becoming a more health-conscious parent will take effort, but we will organize and prioritize it for you in a way that will allow you to succeed in this most important endeavor. Your children, and their planet, are worth it!

Robert W. Sears, MD, FAAP
and
Amy Marlow, MPH, RD, CDN

## PART ONE

# The Happy (and Green!) Family

# 1

# The Healthy Baby

## Looking at Baby Through a Green Lens

When it comes to keeping a new baby healthy and happy, all parents want to do their best. But figuring it all out, well, that can get a little perplexing. With new ideas, research, and products cropping up almost every day, parents find themselves overwhelmed and still asking the basic questions: What do I feed her and when? How can I protect her at home and away? What toys are safe? Am I doing all that I should be doing?

In this chapter we're proposing that you can help make sense of it all when you actually broaden your vision to include not only Baby but also her planet—when you start looking at Baby through a "green" lens, so to speak. Many of the behaviors and lifestyle choices that are eco-friendly are good for your health, too. If you strive to be a green parent you'll not only minimize your impact on natural resources and protect and preserve the planet, but also minimize your and Baby's exposure to toxic substances. We think it's one of the best ways to protect Baby and keep her healthy today and for years to come.

This chapter is meant to give you some background information about how taking steps to protect the planet will also benefit Baby. The rest of the book is meant to provide you with the how-to information you need to actually take those steps. In this chapter, we'll introduce you to what it means to go green, why it is so important, how various aspects of a green lifestyle will benefit Baby's health, and we'll suggest a good place to start: your kitchen.

# Getting Started: Different Shades of Green

We want to help you find a green approach that works for you and your family. As you read, keep in mind that you don't have to change over every facet of your lifestyle at once and there's no right or wrong way to go about it. That's why we'll provide you with different "shades of green" throughout the book—the "palest green" kinds of changes that you can make if you're just getting started, habits and behaviors that are "a little greener," and then the lifestyle choices that represent "the deepest shade of green" for Mamas who are ready to take bigger steps. The idea is for you to pick the shade of green that you're ready to be, and once you're comfortable, to move on to a deeper shade. Even small steps toward a greener life will benefit Baby. And the one thing that is certain is that you should start your family's greening as soon as possible—whether you're reading this while pregnant or if Baby has already arrived.

## BEFORE BABY IS CONCEIVED
## AND DURING PREGNANCY

In 2004, a small and shocking study by the Environmental Working Group found that, on average, the ten newborn babies they tested had two hundred industrial chemicals in their umbilical cord blood. Pesticides, chemicals from consumer products, by-products of industry and waste incineration—the list went on and on.[1] All were chemicals that Mama was exposed to and that were able to cross through the placenta and into Baby. Mama's exposure to some of these chemicals happened before she was even pregnant. We know that many environmental toxins are stored in fatty tissues and can build up over time.

In terms of the health effects of these exposures in the womb, we know that they can have long-lasting consequences. For example, when Mamas use household chemicals frequently during pregnancy, their children have a higher chance of wheezing by the time they reach preschool. Baby is most vulnerable to the effects of hazardous exposures during the first trimester, when the brain and other organs are forming. Serious exposures during this time period can lead to birth defects, low birth weight, and even miscarriage. Later in pregnancy, when blood and nutrients are exchanged directly between Mama and Baby through the umbilical cord, toxic chemicals can get into Baby's body and begin to accumulate (as did the 287 chemicals scientists found in babies' cord blood samples).

If you're a pregnant Mama, adopting green habits will reduce your exposure to toxins and provide obvious benefits to Baby's health. Plus, changing your lifestyle now may be easier than waiting until Baby arrives, when you'll be taking on all the new responsibilities and your to-do list may seem more overwhelming.

## AT BIRTH AND BEYOND

More likely than not, you're reading this book after Baby has already arrived, and maybe you even have older children at home. As you read on, you may start to feel that for all the months or years leading up to this point you've been ruining the fragile planet or exposing your child to chemicals without knowing it. Check your guilt at the door, Mama. If this stuff is new to you and you're just starting to adopt a more green lifestyle, don't waste time feeling guilty or nervous about what you have or haven't done up until this point. You can't go back and do things differently, but what you can do now is to do better. Start today! Pick something small, for example, buying the organic applesauce instead of the conventional. Or bring an old tote bag to the store instead of using its plastic bags. Walk to the library instead of driving. Choose a safer fish from the list on page 212 instead of the tuna steak (which likely contains mercury) you planned to buy for dinner tonight.

No matter when you start adopting green habits, you don't have to do it all at once. Most of this stuff is not all-or-nothing. We like a phase-in approach that takes things one step—or one shade of green—at a time. As with many changes in life, sometimes seemingly big changes aren't so hard to do after all, and sometimes even small changes can have a big impact.

## For the One-Thing-at-a-Time Mama

If you're committed to making some meaningful changes at home and in the way you care for Baby but need a stepwise approach, our advice is to pick things that have the highest potential impact on Baby's health and do those first. Here are some examples of how you can take baby steps toward a green lifestyle:

- *Organic foods:* For the palest green change, switch to organic versions of the foods that are most likely to have residues of pesticides and other chemicals. There's a list on page 194. Then incorporate other organic foods as you are able to.
- *Safe cooking, storing, and serving:* First, stop microwaving Baby's food in plastic. Then go greener by making the switch to BPA-free and phthalate-free plastics or other materials in the kitchen. Info on bottles and cups is in chapter 3. Healthy tableware is discussed in chapter 7.
- *Green cleaning:* First, stop buying the harshest chemical cleaners altogether (a list is on pages 312–13). Next, switch to green, nontoxic cleaning products for your everyday cleaning. And if you're ready for the deepest shade of green, take a closer look at your cleaning routine and use more homemade natural cleaning aids instead of purchasing cleaning products. Lots of green cleaning tips are found in chapter 9.

### For the Once-I-Start-There's-No-Stopping-Me Mama

Sometimes the switch to a healthier or greener lifestyle comes in waves and takes over your consciousness. When we started trying to make more eco-conscious choices for our families, we saw green everywhere we looked. The chemicals in the cleaning supply closet, the chemicals in the medicine cabinet, the plastics in the kitchen, the amount of garbage we created, the number of paper towel rolls we went through—the list went on and on! If you want to do everything in one fell swoop, that's great. But don't throw out all the nonorganic food in your pantry and start from scratch—that's wasteful! And don't go so green-crazy that you alienate the people you love. The tips we provide will help you go green without going nuts.

## The Meaning of Green

In general, the aim of a green lifestyle is to have as little negative impact as possible on the well-being of the planet by doing the following four things:

1. Protecting the planet (and Baby) from toxins
2. Reducing the amount of stuff your family throws out by avoiding consumption, and recycling and repurposing the things you no longer need
3. Reducing your family's use of nonrenewable natural resources
4. Paying it forward: buying from green companies to bolster the positive impacts of their green practices and teaching the next generation how to live a sustainable life

Maybe you already do some of these things. Or maybe you're just getting started with your transition to a more eco-conscious lifestyle. No matter how green you are at the moment, the actionable and practical advice in this book will help you raise a healthy baby by incorporating green habits into your life. We'll be giving you a lot of suggestions for how to make choices, adopt behaviors, and select products that will help you and your family be green. But first, we think it's helpful to understand what's behind all that advice—the whys of being green. So, allow us to guide you on a tour of all things eco. Information like this is sometimes inspiring, sometimes overwhelming, but it's all good for you to take along in your journey toward a greener lifestyle and a healthy baby.

## 1. PROTECTING BOTH BABY AND THE PLANET FROM TOXINS

We come in contact with chemicals every single day—some occur naturally, others are synthetic. Many are toxic, meaning they are poisonous to humans or wildlife. Just to give you an idea of the scope of this issue: The state of California publishes a list of toxic chemicals that are known to cause birth defects, cancer, or developmental problems, as part the state's Safe Drinking Water and Toxic Enforcement Act (Proposition 65). As of September 2008, the list included 775 chemicals![2]

### Why Toxins Are a Concern

Chances are you and Baby come in contact with toxins every day, maybe in products in the bathroom, in Baby's toys, in the foods that you feed her, or even in the plate that she's eating from. You may breathe in toxins in the air or drink them down from your water supply. Chemicals from industry and our homes can also pollute waterways, soil, animal habitats, and the air, putting at risk not only our health, but the health of animals, aquatic life, and their habitats. Chemicals used outside the home, such as pesticides in the garden or harsh chemicals used for cleaning or home improvement projects, can be washed away by rainfall, and this polluted runoff gets into rivers and streams that head to the oceans, affecting aquatic life and the whole food chain.

Some industrial chemicals are persistent organic pollutants, meaning they are virtually impossible to get rid of once they are released into the environment. A prime example is polychlorinated biphenyls or PCBs. They were banned in 1977, but more than thirty years later they still show up in fish caught from polluted rivers and lakes and in

# POSSIBLE HEALTH EFFECTS OF TOXIC EXPOSURES

Believe us when we tell you that we don't mean to scare you or cause panic with this grim picture, but learning some of the facts about toxic exposures will help you make choices that will protect Baby as she grows. So here we go:

| | |
|---|---|
| Asthma and lung disease | Toxic chemicals released into the air as pollution—indoors and outside—irritate the lungs and can contribute to asthma. Here are some examples of why this is a concern. See chapters 8 and 9 for tips on keeping Baby's air at home as safe as possible.<br><br>• For children with asthma, air pollution can make their condition worse and increase their risk of other lung problems like bronchitis.[4]<br>• Children who live on farms where pesticides and herbicides are sprayed have an elevated risk of asthma.[5]<br>• Volatile organic compounds (VOCs) found in certain cleaning supplies, craft supplies, air fresheners, and other household chemicals vaporize into the air and are potent lung irritants.[6]<br>• Children who live close to high-traffic areas are at an increased risk for developing asthma, likely due to the effects of inhaling smog—the mixture of car exhaust, sunlight, and other compounds in the air.[7] |
| Autism | Autism, or autism spectrum disorder, is a developmental disorder that is a syndrome of social, language, behavioral, and sensory symptoms. The prevalence of autism has risen sharply in the past decade with only a portion of the increase being attributable to improvements in diagnosis and reporting of the disease. We know it's on the rise, but we don't know what causes it. Experts agree that there is likely a strong genetic component, evidenced by twin studies that show a 70 to 90 percent chance of identical twins having a similar autism diagnosis as opposed to fraternal twins, who have only a 5 to 10 percent chance.[8,9] |

We suspect that it's not genes alone that cause the condition. A growing field of study is focusing on possible environmental triggers that may increase a child's risk of developing autism. Studies have found that when pregnant women live or work very close to areas that have been sprayed with certain pesticides, especially during the first trimester, their children have an increased incidence of autism.[10] Another exposure that may be linked to autism is a Mama's exposure to the rubella (German measles) virus during pregnancy.[11] Researchers don't know if environmental triggers may only contribute to the condition if a child is exposed at a particularly susceptible stage of development or if perhaps it only affects children who already have the genetic tendency toward the disease.

One substance that is being investigated as a potential environmental trigger for autism is mercury. Though studies haven't determined the way mercury might trigger autism, researchers have shown that some autistic kids seem to metabolize mercury (and other metals) differently than kids who do not have autism. Parents and health advocates have expressed concern that the mercury-containing vaccine preservative Thimerosal may be a trigger that causes autism, although to date no cause-and-effect relationship has been proven.[12] Regardless, the preservative was removed from vaccines in the year 2002 (except for most flu shots), so that's not something you need to worry about for your baby. Mercury itself still remains on the list of potential environmental triggers, though, and concern over the safety of vaccines is still on the minds of parents.

The main source of mercury exposures in babies, children, and Mamas is from dietary sources. When mercury is released into the environment as a by-product of industrial processes, it ends up in our oceans, rivers, and lakes, and can accumulate in fish. In chapters 4 and 6 we'll share advice for avoiding fish sources of mercury.

| Reproductive development | Many of the toxic chemicals found in consumer products are known to be endocrine disrupters, meaning that they interfere with Baby's hormones—hormones like estrogen and testosterone, which influence Baby's reproductive development. Endocrine disrupters may affect Baby when she's still in the womb because they cross into Baby through Mama's placenta. They also accumulate in breast milk. |

Effects of the exposure to these chemicals could include early puberty, reproductive problems like infertility, abnormalities in reproductive development, hormone-related cancers, and developmental problems. Plastics tend to be the most common sources of exposures to these chemicals. Throughout the book we'll give you specific ways to avoid these unsafe plastics. Here's a brief sneak preview:

- Bisphenol A, or BPA, is found in plastics made from polycarbonate. This clear, hard plastic is labeled with the number 7 or PC. Although the FDA has decided BPA doesn't pose a clear enough danger to remove it from the marketplace, many people aren't convinced. It's a known endocrine disrupter, and studies show that it can leach from plastics into foods and beverages.[13]
- Certain chemicals called plasticizers are added to plastics to make them flexible and to beauty products to make them perform better. They are found in many products, among them toys and other products made with polyvinyl chloride, or PVC. One type of plasticizer of particular concern is phthalates. They've been linked to reproductive problems in baby boys, including small penis size.[14] Since PVCs cross the placenta, prenatal exposure is a big concern. Luckily, it's easier than ever to avoid them: in July 2008 the United States Congress agreed to ban 3 kinds of phthalates, and as of January 1, 2009, stores such as Wal-Mart, Toys "R" Us, and Babies "R" Us won't be selling products known to have phthalates in them.

| Intellectual development and behavior | Baby's brain more than doubles in size during the first year, so it's particularly vulnerable to the effects of certain toxins. The National Academy of Sciences estimates that 1 in 4 developmental behavioral problems in children may be linked to either genetic or environmental factors like exposures to lead, mercury, and pesticides.[15] Here are just a few examples of ways we know that toxic chemicals could harm Baby's brain: |

- The chemical flame retardants called PBDEs cause permanent brain changes that lead to behavior problems like hyperactivity.[16]

| | |
|---|---|
| | • Babies born to Mamas who were exposed to polychlorinated biphenyls (PCBs) during pregnancy could have delays in motor skill development and memory problems.[17]<br>• Lead exposure is one of the more common toxic exposures of childhood. This metal, found in contaminated soil and dust, causes behavior problems, learning disabilities, and memory deficits.<br>• Exposure to mercury, found most often in contaminated fish, can impair Baby's central nervous system development and lead to learning disabilities. |
| Cancer | There are hundreds of known and suspected carcinogens, or substances that cause cancer. Many of the chemicals already discussed above fall into this category. Here are some examples of probable or known carcinogens and where they're found:<br><br>• Parabens: These endocrine disrupters are found in beauty supplies. Look for them on the ingredients label.<br>• Perchloroethylene: The common dry-cleaning solvent, also known as perc.<br>• Certain pesticides, including the banned organochlorine pesticides like DDT and chlordane.<br>• Formaldehyde: This embalming fluid is also found in some particleboard furniture, certain plywood, chemical sealants, and even beauty products and hair treatments.<br>• Perfluorochemicals (PFCs): This group of chemicals includes PFOA (perfluorooctanic acid), found in the lining of microwave popcorn bags, in stain-protection treatments like Scotchgard, and in nonstick cookware made with Teflon.<br>• Bisphenol A (BPA): This chemical, found in certain plastics including some baby bottles, is an endocrine disrupter and possible carcinogen. |

food grown in polluted soil. These chemicals present a serious threat to human and animal health.

Although most chemicals that we find in our homes are regulated in some way and approved for use, it doesn't mean they are safe for Baby. Organizations like the Food and Drug Administration and the Consumer Product Safety Commission do not always design their guidance with babies in mind. Policies often are based on what is known about the potential harm a chemical may do in adults, but we don't always know what constitutes a safe level of exposure for the most vulnerable populations like the unborn children, young babies, and toddlers, who are in critical stages of development.

What we do know is that many toxins accumulate in fatty tissues and babies' bodies tend to have more body fat than adults'. Since babies are so much smaller than adults, chemicals tend to show up in higher concentrations in their tiny bodies. Not to mention that most babies put everything they see in their mouths, so they may have more exposures than the adults and older children in the home. As a result of all of these factors, babies are at greater risk for chemical exposures than adults. Just one example: an Environmental Working Group study recently found that a group of toddlers and preschoolers had three times more PBDE—a type of chemical flame retardant found in many consumer products—in their blood than their mothers.[3]

### What's a Green Parent to Do About Exposures to Toxins?

Much of the advice we'll give you throughout the rest of the book will focus on ways to reduce Baby's exposure to potentially dangerous chemicals. Here are some examples of ways to reduce the chances of Baby ingesting and breathing in toxins, as well as ways you can avoid sending these toxins out into the environment:

- Choose BPA-free and phthalate-free plastics in the kitchen (chapters 3, 5, and 7).
- Feed yourself and Baby with organic, all-natural foods (chapters 4, 5, and 6).
- Dispose of Baby's unused prescription medications safely.

- For Baby's furniture, choose wood that hasn't been treated with harmful solvents like formaldehyde, and avoid furniture and accessories painted with lead-based paint (chapter 8).
- Steer clear of toys and bibs made with polyvinyl chloride, or PVC (chapter 8).
- Dress Baby in clothes made from organic fibers that haven't been treated with chemical flame retardants (chapter 8).

## 2. REDUCING THE AMOUNT OF STUFF YOUR FAMILY THROWS OUT BY AVOIDING CONSUMPTION, AND RECYCLING AND REPURPOSING THE THINGS YOU NO LONGER NEED

Think about how much of what you buy ends up in the garbage. In 2006, Americans generated 250 million tons of trash, more than half of it from our homes. About 3.6 million tons were the 18 billion disposable diapers we threw away that year. Containers and packaging accounted for almost one third of our garbage—80 million tons of pizza boxes, plastic food and beverage containers, cereal boxes, shoe boxes, snack bags . . . and most of this ended up in a landfill and not at a recycling facility. Although Americans are recycling more than ever before, only about one-third of our garbage is getting recycled or composted.[18]

### Why It's a Concern

To put it simply, the more stuff we throw away, the more energy our society has to spend to deal with this old stuff and create new stuff to replace it. Landfills or incinerators have to hold or manage this garbage, which leads to air and water pollution. Some trash, like Styrofoam coffee cups and plastic grocery bags, is so lightweight that taking up space in a landfill is actually the least of the concerns. Worse, these items blow out of trash cans and off landfills to pollute waterways and choke wildlife. Depending on what's in the trash that we throw out, landfills can be a source of pollution and toxins that get into the water supply and soil, and accumulate in animals and plants. One out of every five sites identified by the Superfund program for being toxic waste sites are former municipal landfills.[19] And incinerating trash isn't much better: it produces dangerous emissions like dioxins (which are linked to cancer) and heavy metals like lead and mercury (which can cause birth defects and developmental delays).

Recycling helps matters. First, it reduces the volume of garbage in landfills, which means less trash is breaking down and polluting the surrounding environment. When recycled materials are used to create new products, it lowers industry's fuel usage because the recycled materials have already undergone refining and processing and are that much closer to being the end product. The EPA estimates that the recycling that Americans did in 2006 saved the equivalent of more than 10 billion gallons of gasoline that would have been required to dispose of the garbage, get virgin materials, and produce new products from scratch. They also estimate that by recycling 7 million tons of metal in 2007 Americans reduced emissions by 25 million metric tons of carbon dioxide equivalents.[18]

## What's a Green Parent to Do About Consumption and Household Waste?

Although you'll probably find that your consumption increases dramatically once Baby is in the picture, you can still take steps to reduce, reuse, and recycle in order to minimize household waste and your drain on natural resources. We'll give numerous examples in the rest of the book. Here is a preview:

- Make more of your own baby food to avoid packaging waste (chapter 5).
- Consider cloth diapers and use fewer disposable wipes (chapter 8).
- When buying packaged foods for Baby, choose glass or recyclable plastic over materials that aren't recyclable (chapters 6 and 7).
- Buy less baby stuff—reevaluate what you really need. Does the baby who isn't even walking yet need more than one pair of

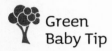
. . . . . . . . . . . . . . . . . . . .

Even small changes can make a big difference. Consider this: if every Mama of a baby in the United States used one fewer diaper wipe today, that would be more than four million wipes kept out of landfills!

shoes? Does your son need another toy truck? Don't you have enough sippy cups? (chapter 8).

- Don't throw out outgrown clothes and toys. Instead, donate them to families in need, use as rags, or make quilts or doll clothes out of them.
- Use more durable goods instead of disposable ones, for example, dish towels instead of paper towels, real plates instead of paper ones (chapter 9).

A NOTE FROM DR. BOB

## Just Say No to Bags

One way that I've begun reducing my consumption of resources that has nothing to do with being a doctor is to stop using plastic or paper grocery bags. I carry several reusable cloth bags in my car. Of course, I usually forget to bring them into the store (despite the reminder sign at the store entrance). I just walk right back out to my car and grab them before I get into the checkout line. It's a pain, but it actually makes me feel good. I've even started saying no to any bag at all when I'm buying just an item or two from anywhere. When I stop by a sandwich shop, I politely ask them not to put my wrapped sandwich into a bag. I'm going to eat the sandwich anyway! Why do I need a bag? When I stop by a pharmacy or drugstore to buy one medication, they always try to put it into a bag. Why is that? When I take the medication out of the bag and say, "I don't need a bag," they look at me weirdly, probably thinking, "But you *have* to have a bag! You can't just carry a single item in your hand without it being in a bag!" By just saying no to bags we can help reduce a large amount of waste.

## 3. REDUCING YOUR USE OF NONRENEWABLE NATURAL RESOURCES

We depend on natural resources, including fossil fuels, metals, woods, water, and plants for survival and for the comforts of modern daily life. The way we use these resources will impact not only the health of the planet and our communities, but Baby's health as well.

Some natural resources are called nonrenewable because once you use them up, you can't get more (or they take hundreds of years to re-generate). These include oil, natural gas, and coal. Oil, of course, is everywhere: it's in the gasoline in your car, we use it to heat our homes, and it's an ingredient in thousands of industrial products from plastic bags to diapers. Coal is burned to make most of the electricity we use. Natural gas may be used to heat your home and your hot water. Other natural resources may technically be renewable, but when used in a nonsustainable way they may as well be in the nonrenewable category. These include freshwater (see sidebar), certain woods, and certain metals.

Families can cut back on energy use in two ways: by conserving energy and by being more energy efficient. When you conserve, you simply use less. You cut back on some of the activities that require energy, like driving and keeping more lights on in the house than you really need. Being more energy-efficient means that you still do the things you used to do, but you do them in a way that requires less energy.

### Why Energy Conservation and Energy Efficiency Is Important

Using natural resources is inevitable, of course, unless you want to raise Baby in a cave somewhere. But reducing your family's use of natu-ral resources is important for ensuring that we have a supply for Baby's future. It's also important because our use of certain energy sources can impact human and animal health right now. Burning fossil fuels like oil and coal creates air and water pollution. Smog, soot, and dust—by-products of fuel combustion—are inhaled and can irritate Baby's

# A NATURAL RESOURCE AT RISK:
# OUR WATER SUPPLY

Once Baby is about six months old, you'll start serving her water in a cup so she can develop her cup-drinking skills. If Baby is formula-fed, it's likely that she's exposed to tap water all the time. All the more reason to give more thought to your tap water—to the amount that's available and the safety of the supply.

Your tap water comes either from a groundwater well or from a surface water reservoir. For about half of all Americans, their tap water is groundwater. This water originated as rain, which seeped into the ground, was naturally filtered by the earth as it flowed to its resting place in an underground aquifer, and then eventually was pumped up into your house. The other half of the country gets its drinking water from surface water reservoirs. This water must be treated (filtered, purified, etc.) before it gets to your home or business. Here are some water facts to get you thinking about water waste and pollution, and what we can do about it:

- U.S. households use between seventy and a hundred gallons of water per person each day.
- Americans are not using groundwater in a sustainable way, meaning we're using it up faster than it is replenished. The U.S. government predicts that by 2012 there could be water shortages in thirty-six states.[20]
- Millions of gallons of water are wasted every year. An open faucet sends about five gallons down the drain every two minutes.
- One leaky faucet that is dripping one drip per second will waste five gallons a day. That's more than two thousand gallons a year! In fact, leaky pipes alone can account for up to ten gallons a day of a family's household water use.
- A large proportion of our country's energy use goes to dealing with water. According to the California Energy Commission, almost 20 percent of that state's electricity and 30 percent of its natural gas go to treat, pump, heat, cool, and dispose of water.[21]
- The U.S. drinking water supply is already more polluted than we once thought. A 2005 study found more than 260 contaminants in municipal drinking water supplies around the country.[22]
- Common water pollution sources: agriculture and construction runoff, leaking underground fuel or chemical storage tanks, urban sprawl, and industry.

- At home, you can take steps to minimize water pollution by properly disposing of hazardous materials like automotive oil, paints, pool chemicals, and gardening chemicals. Ask your local sanitation department, public works department, or environmental health department about how to get rid of these materials in your community. There may be special pickup days or drop-off sites.
- Before feeding your tap water to Baby you should have it tested, just to be sure it's safe. See page 100 for details on testing your water and finding alternatives to tap water, if needed.

lungs. Sulfur oxides and nitrogen oxides released into the air when fuels are burned fall into our waterways as acid rain and contribute to algal blooms in coastal waterways. Carbon dioxide ($CO_2$) and other greenhouse gases enter the atmosphere and contribute to global climate change.

## What's a Green Parent to Do About Nonrenewable Resources?

Every day as you raise Baby you have opportunities to use less electricity, less oil, and less water. Here are some ideas to get you started. You'll find more ideas in chapter 9 and sprinkled throughout the rest of the book.

- Don't let the water run when bathing Baby or brushing her teeth.
- If you can walk somewhere to run your errands, put Baby in a stroller and head out for a fossil-fuel-free shopping trip.
- Dress Baby appropriately for the season instead of jacking up the heat or the air conditioning so high. In the winter, put a sweater on her during the day and footie pajamas at night. In the summer, dress her in light organic cotton onesies to help keep her cool.
- Wash most of Baby's clothes in cold water, and if you're in the market for a new washer or dryer, buy the most energy-efficient one you can afford.

- If your toddler tends to open and close your refrigerator all day, install a fridge lock to reduce energy waste.

## 4. PAYING IT FORWARD: SUPPORTING SUSTAINABILITY THROUGH BUYING FROM GREEN COMPANIES AND TEACHING THE NEXT GENERATION A SUSTAINABLE WAY OF LIVING

Part of the green movement is to make the green way of life sustainable by supporting companies and organizations that are already doing

## GLOBAL WARMING AND CARBON FOOTPRINTS IN A NUTSHELL

Our society's use of fossil fuels and our modern industrial processes contribute to global climate change, also referred to as global warming. Here's how it works: When we burn oil or coal, carbon dioxide and other gases are released into the air. These gases are called greenhouse gases because they trap heat and keep it within our atmosphere the same way a greenhouse itself traps light and heat inside. Over the past hundred years, the rise in industry and fossil fuel use has led to the release of more and more carbon dioxide and other greenhouse gases into the atmosphere. As a result, the earth's temperature is actually rising faster than it ever has before—too fast for wildlife and humans to adapt. Scientists believe that global climate change is leading to melting ice caps, rising water levels, lost animal habitats, less biodiversity in our oceans, lower farming yields, and extreme weather that puts human and animal life at risk.

The amount of carbon dioxide that an industry's or individual's actions generate is sometimes quantified as a "carbon footprint" and is usually measured in the number of pounds of $CO_2$ that are released into the air as a result of a particular process or action. For example, every gallon of gas burned by a car releases about twenty pounds of carbon dioxide. It's estimated that the average American household emits more than forty-one thousand pounds of $CO_2$ each year.[23] Conservation and improved efficiency can help reduce our carbon emissions. For example, adjusting your thermostat just two degrees cooler in the winter and two degrees warmer in the summer can reduce your home's carbon dioxide emissions by two thousand pounds a year.

their part and by teaching the next generation how to make earth-friendly choices. "Paying it forward" in this way will help the positive effects of your green lifestyle continue even after you're gone. Perhaps it's a bit premature to teach Baby about her carbon footprint, but even before age two she observes your habits and absorbs your opinions, so it's never too early (or late) to start showing Baby how to tread lightly on the planet and make healthy choices.

What's a Green Parent to Do?
- Support companies that are using recycled materials for packaging or for the products themselves (chapters 7, 8, and 9).
- When you're separating your recyclables and your other garbage, or finding new uses for things you would otherwise throw out, explain what you're doing to Baby. Soon enough she'll be old enough to really understand.
- When you treat yourself to coffee, tea, or chocolate, look for Fair Trade Certified or Rainforest Alliance Certified products.
- For Baby's room, look for furniture made with wood that's certified by the Forest Stewardship Council (FSC) to be sustainable and harvested in a way that promotes healthy forest management (chapter 8).
- Buy in-season foods from local and organic farmers. Taking Baby to the farmer's market will help foster her appreciation for fresh produce and will help to teach her where her food comes from (chapter 6).

# Start in the Kitchen! Green Feeding Basics

You're going to find a lot of great tips in this book—practical ways to go green in your home and to raise Baby in a greener way. Sometimes, though, getting started is the hardest part. We wrote this book because our own green journeys seemed to start in the same place: the kitchen. We didn't decide to make just any baby food—we decided to make *organic* baby food. And of all the aspects of Baby's health, what she eats is perhaps one of the things most within your control, so it's a great place to focus your efforts. We call it green feeding, and it includes aspects of all four of the green living behaviors outlined above. It involves:

1. Reducing Baby's exposures to toxins by choosing all-natural organic foods and preparing and serving them in a healthy way
2. Minimizing your family's kitchen waste by choosing grocery products wisely and recycling food containers and packaging
3. Reducing your family's strain on natural resources by being conservation-minded at the grocery store and when you're cooking, serving, and cleaning up
4. Buying from organic farms and producers, local food producers, and other responsible food companies

## 1. GREEN FEEDING REDUCES BABY'S (AND THE PLANET'S) EXPOSURE TO TOXINS

The foundation of green feeding is organic food. Organic food is grown or produced without the use of artificial chemicals and in a way that preserves the earth. Organic farms don't use synthetic pesticides, chemical fertilizers, or genetically modified seeds or other genetically modified organisms (GMOs). Organically raised animals are not given growth hormones or antibiotics, and they are fed with organic feed that is free of animal by-products. Organic farmers believe that it takes healthy soil and healthy animals to create healthy food, so their farming practices are sustainable and their animal practices are as humane as possible.

It used to be that you had to go to a health food store or natural supermarket to find organic produce, meats, and other foods. It was the hippie "earthy-crunchy" Mamas who sought out these kinds of products. Today, all that has changed. Big-box stores sell organic products, and large and small food producers alike offer organic options. You've probably seen more and more articles and advertisements about organic foods in the media in the past few years. We know that all of this media attention brings out the skeptic in some people. We have a few friends who firmly believed that organic food was just a marketing ploy until we bombarded them with scientific evidence that it is actually better for us, our kids, and the planet. So, despite the hallmarks of trendiness, don't mistake organic foods for a passing fad. Clean, healthy foods will never go out of style. Serving Baby organic foods is similar to baby-proofing the house. It's something you do to keep Baby safe and well during the years when she's most vulnerable.

In chapters 6 and 7 we'll give you tips on choosing organic foods for Baby. First, here's some scientific nitty-gritty about why to do so:

## Pesticides

This may strike you as a "Well, duh!" statement, but it's worth stating anyway: young children who eat organically grown foods are exposed to fewer pesticides than children who do not. In one particular study, the children who ate conventional fruits and vegetables over three days had about nine times more pesticide metabolites present in their urine than the children who ate organically during the same time period. What's even more troubling is that the pesticide levels in the conventional group exceeded the safe guidelines set by the Environmental Protection Agency (EPA).[24]

This certainly doesn't sound like a good thing, but how bad is it? Although in the United States foods and pesticides must meet certain standards for safety, these standards are based on adults, not babies and children, so we can't be sure that pesticides are safe for children at all. Plus, we don't fully understand the risks of everyday exposures to pesticides from the foods that we eat because there aren't good studies on the long-term health effects of being exposed to pesticides from infancy through adulthood.

What we do know about pesticides and health isn't reassuring:

- Many chemical pesticides kill brain cells and cause cancer when tested in laboratories.[25]
- Pregnant women who are exposed to pesticide spraying have increased risk of having a baby with a birth defect.[26]

- Farmers who work with pesticides have reported various ailments related to their exposures, including headaches, nausea, cancer, and serious neurological effects.[27]
- Some pesticides, particularly organochlorine insecticides, are known to cause cancer.[28]

Eating organic and all-natural foods is particularly important for Baby because babies are more vulnerable to the effects of pesticides and chemicals in our food supply than adults. For one thing, they eat more food, pound for pound, than we adults do, so Baby's relative dose of these and other chemicals is going to be higher. Also, babies tend to eat the same foods over and over, increasing their exposure to any chemicals in their chosen foods. And finally, as we mentioned above, pesticides and other environmental chemicals are stored mostly in fat, something babies and young children have plenty of.

### Artificial Hormones and Antibiotics

Before we tell you everything you ever (or never?) wanted to know about hormones and antibiotics, you can sneak a peak at our conclusion: the synthetic hormones and antibiotics used in conventional farms aren't good for the environment or for Baby. Organically raised animals aren't treated with these chemicals.

Animals raised on organic farms and sold at the market aren't permitted to be treated with synthetic hormones or antibiotics. Cattle raised on conventional farms, on the other hand, are often treated with one of six different hormones used to increase milk or meat production, including:

- Natural and synthetic forms of estrogen and progesterone, both linked with increased risks of certain cancers.
- A genetically modified hormone called recombinant bovine growth hormone (rBGH) or recombinant bovine somatotropin (rBST). Farmers use this hormone to increase milk production. One effect of this treatment is that the milk from these cows is

higher in another hormone called IGF-1 (insulin-like growth factor). Some people find that concerning because high levels of IGF-1 have been linked to cancer.

The hormones given to cattle can cause health problems for the animals themselves, leading many experts to question their safety for human consumption. This is especially worrisome for the most vulnerable consumers—pregnant and lactating women, babies, and young children. Some of the health problems in animals and other wildlife caused by these chemicals are:

- Cows given synthetic hormones tend to have more foot problems, reduction in fertility, and higher rates of mastitis (requiring them to be treated with more antibiotics than untreated cows).[29]
- Fish that live downstream from a large Nebraska cattle feedlot (where hormones were used) had significant reproductive problems.[30]

European governments have banned the import of meat from the United States and Canada due to the use of hormones. The use of hormones remains controversial, though. According to the Food and Drug Administration (FDA), the milk from cows given hormones isn't any different from the milk of other cows. They've also found that the hormones in milk don't have any actual hormonal effects in the people who drink the milk or eat the beef from treated cows. The World Trade Organization agrees and ruled that Europe's ban on American meat is unjustified because the WTO believes the scientific evidence doesn't support the notion that hormones in meat pose any risk for humans. Whom should we believe? In scientific matters, things are rarely black and white. In our opinion, the studies that show potential harm raise enough questions in our mind to make us recommend against feeding these foods to your family.

Hormones aren't the only concern. Cows, chickens, and other food

# The "Safety" of Chemicals

If pesticides, chemicals, and hormones are so bad for babies, why does the government allow them? That's a great question. Some people would use the very fact that the government *does* allow them as proof of their safety. After all, if these chemicals were really that dangerous, they would be banned, right? Wrong. Banning all nonorganic imported food and forcing all U.S. farmers to go 100 percent organic would be a very expensive undertaking. It would have huge political and economic ramifications on the world farming economy. The government decided that as long as we keep the poison to a minimum, it's better to leave "well enough" alone. But don't think that the government allows pesticides and hormones to be used because they have been proven safe. There is no research showing these things are safe. What the research shows is that at minimal levels, these chemicals don't cause enough harm to warrant banning them. That's like saying it's OK to feed children a cancer-causing food, as long as only a very small percentage of the children actually come down with cancer. The government has to make this decision based on what's best for the domestic and world economy, not based on what is safer for individual people. I'm not saying that's a wrong decision; I'm saying that *you* have the power to decide what's best for your individual child and your family by going organic. If more and more people do so, that will force a gradual (and economically manageable) shift toward worldwide organic farming that our planet, and its children, need.

animals raised on conventional farms are given antibiotics at an alarming rate. Almost 70 percent of the antibiotics used in the United States are given to farm animals.[31] Sometimes antibiotics are given to treat infections. But farmers also use antibiotics to prevent illness and boost animal growth. This kind of antibiotic use is problematic because it can lead to antibiotic resistance. What happens is that the strongest bacteria in the animals' systems survive the antibiotic treatment, either because the dose of the antibiotic is too low or the treatment is stopped too soon. These strong bugs multiply and pass their drug-resistant genes on to their offspring. The next time an animal or human gets infected with those bacteria, the original drug doesn't work anymore.

The bottom line is that there are many unknowns about the health effects of hormones and antibiotics in our food supply. That's why we recommend choosing organic foods instead. In matters of baby and toddler health, we believe in following the precautionary principle, which basically means that until there is conclusive scientific understanding, it's wise to proceed with caution and avoid foods made from animals that were treated with synthetic hormones and antibiotics.

## Chemical Pollution

Organic farming usually generates less pollution than conventional farming because the farmers use natural fertilizers instead of chemical fertilizers or sewage sludge. In contrast, the chemicals used in conventional farming seep into surrounding ecosystems. Conventional fertilizers send nitrates and phosphates into rivers and streams, threatening the health of wildlife. Large factory farms are significant sources of nitrate pollution, which can contaminate drinking water. Excess nitrogen from chemical fertilizers and from excessive amounts of animal waste also feeds algae blooms in the ocean. The algae steal all the oxygen from other plants and aquatic life, which leads to "dead zones" where nothing can survive. As we mentioned above, conventional cattle farms send synthetic hormones and antibiotics into the surrounding groundwater and animal habitats, possibly threatening the health of humans and fish farther downstream. When you buy organic foods you are helping to change this system.

## More Ways to Reduce Toxic Exposure in the Kitchen: Green Cooking, Serving, and Storing

Serving Baby organic foods is the best way to reduce her exposure to certain chemicals that can be found in the food supply. Other aspects of green feeding have to do with how you cook, serve, and store Baby's meals in order to minimize her contact with chemicals that may be found in pots and pans, bowls and plates, etc. In chapters 3, 5, and 7 we'll give you all kinds of tips on choosing safe cookware and tableware for Baby.

## 2. GREEN FEEDING INVOLVES MINIMIZING KITCHEN WASTE

About 30 percent of Americans' household waste is packaging, much of it food-related.[18] We also waste a shocking amount of food; the average America household throws about a pound of food into the trash each day. Being really green in the kitchen means not just thinking about the foods you give Baby, but also choosing packaging wisely and taking other steps to reduce the amount of food-related waste that goes into your family's garbage cans. You'll find tips in chapter 7, but here are some ideas to get you started:

- Buy more whole foods instead of packaged, processed ones. For example, a pint of strawberries instead of a box of individually wrapped strawberry fruit leathers.
- Buy foods packaged in recycled materials, such as recycled paperboard.
- Choose food packages that are recyclable over those that are not. For example, cardboard egg cartons are usually recyclable, but the Styrofoam ones are not.
- Learn about your community's recycling policies so you know how to handle recyclable items. For example, most recycling centers require food containers to be clean and the tops to be removed from bottles and containers.
- Start a compost pile in your yard to make use of certain food scraps.

## 3. GREEN FEEDING INVOLVES REDUCING STRAIN ON NATURAL RESOURCES

When you choose organic foods, you support farms that use a variety of methods to conserve resources. Organic farms use less fossil fuel than conventional farms since they don't use nitrogen fertilizers or pesticides (both made with fossil fuels). A recent two-decade study of corn farms found that the organic ones used 30 percent less fuel and yet they produced the same crop yield. The same study showed that the soil on organic corn and soy farms conserved more water, probably due to crop rotation and other methods for preserving the health of the soil.[32] Buying locally grown and produced organic foods saves even more energy because the food doesn't have to travel as many miles in planes and trucks.

The food itself is just the beginning. Other green feeding behaviors help reduce your strain on natural resources. For example, when you switch away from plastics in the kitchen and use more glass and stainless steel for feeding Baby, you're not only protecting her health, but you also reduce the amount of fossil fuels that go into producing your household items.

## 4. GREEN FEEDING IS A WAY TO "PAY IT FORWARD"

Green feeding is sustainable in so many ways. First and foremost, organic farms use sustainable practices to preserve the land for future generations, and to promote fair treatment of workers and humane treatment of animals. Crop rotation helps prevent the soil from becoming depleted of nutrients. Using cover crops provides natural pest control and helps prevent soil erosion. Animals on organic farms are given access to pastures instead of being kept inside all the time. Grass-fed cows on sustainable farms require far less fossil fuel inputs than livestock fed with grain—50 percent less by some estimates.

Second, other green lifestyle changes we've introduced you to in this chapter, such as minimizing food and packaging waste and recycling in your kitchen, help preserve the planet for your children and grandchildren.

Perhaps most important is this: feeding Baby organic and all-natural foods lays the foundation for health for many years to come. Not only does this provide valuable nutrients and minimize her exposure to potential toxins, but it also fosters her personal preference for healthy and fresh-tasting foods. For more on this, flip ahead to chapter 5.

## GREEN FEEDING BONUS: ORGANIC FOODS ARE NUTRITIONALLY SUPERCHARGED AND EXTRA YUMMY

Not only do organically grown foods provide you with the benefit of ingesting fewer pesticides, hormones, and antibiotics, and provide the planet with numerous benefits as well, they may even be more nutritious! Compared with conventional produce, many organic crops have higher levels of beneficial disease-fighting phytochemicals like flavonoids, antioxidants, and phenolic compounds, which are powerful anti-inflammatory compounds that may protect Baby against allergies, cancer, and other ailments.[33,34] Meanwhile, the nutrient content of conventionally grown fruits and vegetables has actually dropped over the last fifty to sixty years.[35]

**Organic fruits and vegetables have more of these nutrients than conventional produce**

| |
| --- |
| phenolic compounds |
| vitamin C |
| lycopene |
| iron |
| magnesium |
| phosphorus |

**Conventional fruits and vegetables have
fewer of these nutrients than they used to**

| |
| --- |
| protein |
| calcium |
| vitamin C |
| riboflavin |
| phosphorus |

Organic supporters aren't surprised that the quality of the product has deteriorated as conventional farms churn out higher and higher volumes of food. How do farming methods affect the nutrient content?

- When plants grow bigger, faster, the plant's ability to draw nutrients from the sun or soil is reduced.
- Conventional farming may deplete the soil of its nutrients over time, so there's actually less to draw from over the years.
- Plants develop phytochemicals to protect themselves against pests, infection, and other threats. When synthetic pesticides and herbicides are used, they do this work for the plant, so it doesn't need to build up its natural defenses. As a result, these healthy compounds are not as plentiful in the final conventional product. Organic methods, on the other hand, force the plants to fend for themselves, stimulating the production of these phytochemicals. This means more disease-fighting and cancer-preventing phytonutrients for us!

It's not just plant foods that become more nutritious through organic farming methods. Organically raised cows, particularly if they are also grass fed, produce meat that is lower in saturated fat and higher in conjugated linoleic acid (CLA) than conventionally raised, grain-fed

# A Lesson in Beef

I do a lot of speaking on nutrition, and one of my PowerPoint slides reads, "Beef. It's what's for . . . colon cancer and heart disease." The line usually gets a good laugh. Sadly, regular non-organic, non-grass-fed beef is really bad if you overdo it. The unhealthy saturated animal fats are a big risk factor for these two health conditions, especially for men. During one talk that I was giving in Colorado many years ago, before I had learned that organic grass-fed beef *is* a different story and is healthy, an audience member (who happened to raise organic grass-fed cattle) pointed out my ignorance. I was actually thrilled to hear there was a type of beef I could feel better about eating. I had stayed away from beef for many years because colon cancer runs in my family. Now beef is what's for dinner at my house on occasion. Not the lazy, sit-around-all-day-and-get-fat conventional beef, but the stroll-around-in-green-pastures-to-stay-lean-and-healthy organic beef.

cows.[36] CLA is a fat that acts as an antioxidant in the body. It has been shown to have anticancer properties, support immune function, and may even help reduce body fat in overweight people. Organic beef and milk are also higher in essential omega-3 fats.[37]

And if these health benefits aren't enough for you, consider that organic foods may even taste better than conventional foods. You can do a taste test for yourself, but there are actually studies that confirm that organic apples and strawberries, for example, are tastier than the conventional ones.[38] Even though Baby doesn't seem like a gourmet at this early age, taste is truly important to consider. Eating should be a pleasurable experience. When a food tastes good, Baby will want to eat it again, so you can start fostering a preference for healthy foods by giving Baby fresh and delicious unadulterated foods from the first time she takes a bite.

## Taking It Home . . .

This chapter was an introduction to why you, and everybody else, should be going green. But you've probably just had (or are about to have) a new baby. Who has time to worry about all these other details? We hope that the very fact that you've brought a brand-new life into this world has prompted you to want to help preserve the planet for your child. Plus, you are now asking the planet to help support another life. You can return the favor by supporting the planet. We know this was a lot of information, and it's only chapter 1! The good news is, you don't have to remember very much at all! We promised you earlier in this chapter that we would make going green doable for you, and we will hold to that promise. All you need to get from this chapter is an understanding of why you should go green. If you've come to that conclusion, then forget about the why. Let's move on to the how. That's what the rest of this book is all about.

..............................................................................................

## 2

# The Happy Mama

### How to Take Good Care of the Caretaker
### (That Means You)

We are thrilled that you have decided to take a closer look at your family's lifestyle through a green lens. You have embarked on a journey into better health, and there are many steps along the way. But we want to pause for a moment, set aside the rest of the family and household, and focus on your general health and mind-set for a chapter. You've heard the saying "If Mama ain't happy, ain't nobody happy!" Well, this also holds true for going green. If Mama isn't healthy and green, no one in the family will be. In this chapter we want to show you two steps that you can take right away to improve your postpartum health and peace of mind so you can find the energy to make green changes. Once you are on the right track for yourself, you will be empowered to move on to the rest of the household.

The way we see it, there are three main areas you as a new Mama need to pay close attention to right now: exercise, stress reduction, and proper nutrition (Oh! And your baby! But we'll save that for the rest of the book). The exercise and stress reduction is mostly for your benefit (although Baby does benefit from your relaxed and positive demeanor), to keep your mind and body healthy for the challenges that will follow.

Good nutrition benefits both you and Baby, not only now through your breast milk, but as Baby grows and develops healthy eating habits by taking after your own eating habits. In this chapter we will introduce you to the first two ideas, the ones that require you to take time to focus on yourself, even as you embark upon one of the most selfless roles of your life, being a mother. Successfully implementing exercise and stress reduction will give your body the foundation it needs for you to move on to what this book is all about—nontoxic, organic living for the whole family. Proper nutrition will be presented in chapter 4.

Today we know so much about health, and we ask so much of our young mothers: Eat this but don't eat that. Stay active but don't overdo it. Avoid chemical exposures as best you can. Don't get too stressed. Are we expecting too much? Maybe, maybe not. The advice "you can never be too careful" certainly rings true for bringing a baby into the world. But exactly how cautious do you need to be? You certainly don't want your attempts to be a perfect mother to cause you more stress and worry than they're worth.

We are going to show you how to bounce back from the birthing process, get active and motivated, and ease away the stress that is already starting to build up. So instead of worrying about how much there is to do to become a green family—and how much you don't know yet—let's just take a deep breath and focus on you and your mind-body health.

## Bouncing Back: Postpartum Fitness

Think of postpartum exercise as your sanity and wardrobe protection plan. Mentally, exercise can elevate your mood and may even help you be more alert and able to focus. The physical benefits of exercise are undisputed. Being active is one of the best ways to get back to your prepregnancy weight and shape (so you can get back into those prepregnancy jeans). Mamas who are more active, even those who just walk for an hour a day, are less likely to hold onto extra baby weight than the Mamas who are not active.[1]

If that's not motivating enough, consider that the benefits of fitness extend to your child. Most important, Baby will have a healthy parent, one with enough energy and strength to keep up with her as she grows. By being active you also share an important value with your child. Although she will be oblivious at first, soon Baby will take notice of her Mama's dedication to keeping herself healthy, and she too will grow up with an appreciation for exercise and a healthy lifestyle. Starting as young as age three, our own kids learned the concept of exercise being good for the body from watching their parents be active over the course of their lifetimes.

We can't tell you when your body will be ready to start exercising after childbirth. Most women can begin easy, leisurely walks and light stretching once they are home from the hospital. After about four to six weeks you'll be ready for more intense exercise. Ask your obstetrician or midwife about exercise at your first postpartum visit. Once you get the OK, start moving!

One specific exercise to start soon after childbirth (we're talking hours or days here, not weeks) is the Kegel exercise for strengthening your pelvic floor. This exercise will help you reduce your future risk of urinary incontinence and also helps to strengthen the deepest part of your core, the foundation for your abdominal muscles. If you had a vaginal delivery this exercise might feel a bit odd at first, as if you can't quite contract the muscles the way you used to. Keep at it—doing this exercise will help tighten and strengthen those muscles as you heal.

### MYTH OR FACT?

*If you are breast-feeding your baby you shouldn't exercise or try to lose weight.*

Myth! Breast-feeding Mamas are encouraged to exercise so they can reap the benefits we've discussed here. Many studies have shown that moderate exercise, although it expends calories, does not harm your milk production or endanger your

# HOW TO DO A KEGEL EXERCISE

- First, make sure you're squeezing the right muscles. Next time you urinate, isolate the pelvic floor muscles by squeezing in order to stop the flow of urine. (Don't regularly do Kegels while urinating, though, because this could lead to incomplete bladder emptying and urinary tract infections.) Or, insert a clean finger into your vagina and try to squeeze the muscles around it. These are the muscles you want to contract when doing a Kegel.
- While seated comfortably, squeeze your pelvic floor muscles as tightly as you can, keeping your abdomen and buttocks relaxed. Then fully relax the muscles. You just did your first Kegel.
- Practice makes perfect. Hold each squeeze for five to ten seconds, and then fully relax and rest for a moment before doing another. Vary the exercise occasionally by doing ten to twenty fast short pulses or by contracting the muscles very slowly and releasing even more slowly.
- Do at least three sets of ten Kegels each day. Choose a set time each day to practice this exercise. For example, every time you're waiting at a red light in the car or during commercial breaks while watching TV.

baby.[2-5] Exercising as a strategy for slow and steady weight loss (i.e., about one pound per week) is perfectly safe for nursing women. For your comfort, you may want to plan for your workouts to be right after a feeding so your breasts are not too full or engorged. Speaking of which, be sure you have a good supportive bra for your workouts. Look for one without underwires.

Once you're ready to be more active, start gradually and think small. Don't have a gym membership? You don't need one. Here's a list of easy ways to get moving without creating a formal exercise routine:

- Running errands = exercise! If there is a grocery or drugstore in walking distance of your home, take advantage of this built-in opportunity for exercise and walk there to pick up diapers or other gear. Or drive to a village or town where you can do some

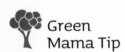

## Green Mama Tip

If you plan to exercise outdoors, check your local news for an air quality report during the weather forecast, especially in the warm weather months. If you live in a high-traffic, high-smog area or the forecast is for poor air quality, choose indoor activities and keep your windows closed. Smog contains airborne polycyclic aromatic hydrocarbons (PAHs) and other compounds known to be harmful to babies, and it's not so great for Mamas either.

simultaneous walking and shopping. In a pinch, the local mall works as a walking course, too.

- Sneak in mini exercise sessions with Baby throughout the day. Try these simple exercises:

  - While you're down on the floor, giving Baby some tummy time on her play mat, do ten push-ups. Or better yet, lay her face-up on the floor and do push-ups over her, pausing at the bottom each time to give her a kiss. Do this a few times during the day and you're going to build some nice chest and arm muscles.

  - Sit Baby in a bouncy seat and do some simple stretching while you sing or talk to her. It's especially good to stretch your chest, back, and shoulder muscles because these can become tight and sore from being in a feeding and rocking position all the time.

  - Do bridges with Baby on your lap (for babies old enough to sit up). Lie on your back with knees bent, feet on the floor. Place Baby, seated, on your hips, holding her hands or trunk to stabilize her. Then push your feet into the floor and lift your buttocks several inches off the ground for a simple bridge exercise. Hold for a few seconds, and then slowly lower your hips until your back is again flat on the floor. Do this fifteen times, a few times a day for a stronger behind. Baby will love the ride.

  - When Baby won't let you sit down, don't just pace aimlessly around the house with her in your arms. Do some walking lunges to strengthen and tone your lower body. Just be sure to hold onto something for balance. Or better yet, put Baby in a baby carrier or sling so her weight is more evenly distributed while you do this exercise.

- While you're out for a walk with the stroller, add little bursts of speed to maximize calorie burn and shake up your metabolism. Seek out the hills in your neighborhood to give your legs and behind a more challenging workout.
- Let the TV be your trainer. Most cable systems offer at least one exercise channel featuring a vast array of programming. You can record yoga classes, aerobics programs, or other fitness classes and turn them on when you have time for a workout. Or try exercise DVDs. Find them online, at your local library, or create a lending library with your friends so you can all switch DVDs when your own gets boring or is no longer challenging.

## BUT WHO HAS THE TIME!

We know you're busy. Whether you are a dedicated exerciser or new to working out, having children can make it difficult to find the time to exercise. But the trick here is not to view exercise as another burdensome task on your to-do list. Instead, look at it as a way to treat yourself to something that will make you look and feel good. Plus, you can do many activities with your baby or older child, so you don't have to choose between your own needs and the desire to be with your children. Here are some tips for staying motivated and fitting exercise in:

- *Exercise in the morning.* By getting active early in the day you reduce the chance that unforeseen obligations will prevent you from working out later. Right after breakfast, put Baby in the stroller and head outside for some fresh air. Or do an exercise DVD while Baby takes her first nap of the day.
- *Find an exercise buddy.* Instead of meeting a friend for coffee or at a local library or bookstore, meet her for a brisk walk or an exercise class. It's probably easier to find the motivation to be social than to exercise.

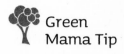

## Green Mama Tip

Stay hydrated during exercise by keeping a bottle of water close by. But don't buy disposable water bottles, which just waste plastic. Instead, fill up a reusable bottle made from BPA-free plastic, aluminum, or stainless steel. Check out the offerings from CamelBak (www.camelbak.com), Nalgene (www.nalgenechoice .com), Klean Kanteen (www .kleankanteen.com), and Sigg (www.sigg.com).

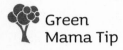

- *Make an appointment.* You would never skip a meeting at work or a doctor appointment. Make the same true for exercise by actually putting it on your calendar. You can also take turns with your significant other. One of you has baby duty while the other gets to head out for a jog or go to the gym. By planning in advance and having a set schedule, you may rarely skip a day.
- *Have your gear ready to go.* On the days when you're home with Baby, get dressed in comfortable clothes so you're ready for an impromptu power walk or in-house exercise session. Half the battle is just getting dressed and out the door, so anything you can do to help that process along will serve you well.
- *Exercise* with *your baby.* Besides the ideas listed above, you can look for group fitness classes in your community where Baby is welcome to join in the fun, like Stroller Strides workouts or "mommy-baby" yoga classes. Or purchase a jogging stroller so Baby can join you on your morning jogs.

Most important, find something that you enjoy because you'll be more likely to stick to it. The goal is to be active in a moderate-intensity activity for at least thirty minutes every day of the week.

## Stress, Relaxation, and the New Mama

Ah! Being pregnant was wonderful. Everyone was excited for you, and it was so much fun imagining life with Baby and picking out adorable tiny baby things. Then all of a sudden, Baby is real, and she's coming home. For most of us, this big life change brings stress and anxiety along with all those cute little socks. It's one of our first acts of motherly multitasking: feeling both overjoyed and overwhelmed . . . at the same time!

Some of your new-Mama stress is the same as before you conceived: job pressures, the demands of managing your household and your relationships, and the juggling to balance them all. Now Baby brings new stressors. You're probably overtired, juggling visitors and well-wishers, trying to decipher the cries of a hungry or tired or bored baby,

## Too Tired Not to Exercise

You may think you don't have the energy to exercise, but the reality is that exercising actually *gives* you more energy. When I see a new mom in my office with a baby who is a few months old, I like to guess whether or not they have started regularly exercising. A mom who seems tired, worn out, and stressed is much less likely to have begun a postpartum exercise routine. I like to ask, so I can offer encouragement when needed. Being active gives you more mental energy and physical stamina, as well as a more positive attitude and self-image. It's not about weight, it's about health and quality of life. You will definitely *feel* the increased day-to-day energy after just a few weeks.

and maybe worrying about whether or not you can even handle all this responsibility. You may also feel pressure regarding your choices for raising her (aka meddling parents and in-laws), worries about money, and stress due to the changes you've had to make in your living arrangements and lifestyle to accommodate the little one.

Consider yourself lucky if none of this sounds familiar. We'd venture to say that most new Mamas have felt some kind of stress. Unfortunately, the stress won't affect just you; it can affect your baby and your relationships if you don't find healthy ways to cope. (As if you needed one more thing to worry about!)

When you're stressed, your body responds with a reaction called fight or flight—your blood pressure rises, your heart races, and your palms sweat. If the stress becomes chronic and these kinds of effects are maintained over time, your body will suffer. Equally important is to realize that stress can affect your young baby. Baby will pick up on your mood and mirror your anxiety through her behavior. More important, as your baby grows into a child, if you continue to handle your stress in unhealthy ways, such as turning to food or other addictions or losing your temper, your child might learn that this is how she should handle her challenges as well. On the flip side, taking everything in stride creates a calm home environment and teaches your child valuable coping skills.

Fortunately, nature has provided you with a built-in natural anti-anxiety medication/personal therapist to help you cope with having a new baby. Breast-feeding actually helps your body handle stress. We know that the first week or two of breast-feeding can be a challenge, but once it settles into an easy routine, it will help relax you. Studies have shown that when you breast-feed, your body releases relaxing hormones. Your body's reaction to stress is blunted, leaving you feeling more calm. And breast-feeding has also been shown to have a positive effect on a woman's mood.[6]

## AM I STRESSED?

Recognizing stress is an important step in managing it, so pause for a minute now to think about whether you have felt worried, anxious, or restless lately. You may have already found ways to manage stress effectively. But if not, you might already be feeling its effects.

Do you clench your jaw or teeth often, feel as though your heart races on a regular basis, or have trouble sleeping because you can't quiet your mind? Do you get stomachaches because of nerves, snap at people too quickly, or have tension headaches or migraines? Even more serious symptoms of stress include feeling the need for alcohol or tobacco to calm you down, exhibiting road rage or other violent behaviors, and hyperventilation or panic attacks. Any of these sound familiar? If so, your stress may be getting out of control, and it's time to take action.

## HOW TO COPE

Is all this information stressing you out? Well, there's good news: even if you are finding life with your baby to be stressful, it doesn't mean you

## The Worried Mama

Most of my job as a pediatrician is to make sure a baby is healthy. But I know that if a new mom is stressed and worried, this will affect her enjoyment of parenting and may affect the baby's behavior. I like to explore how every new mom is coping. If I see a mom sit calmly in my office, relaxing with her baby in her arms, looking like she doesn't have a care in the world, I don't worry. But if a mom seems tense, shows unusual worry over insignificant matters (such as, "What's that tiny little dot on my baby's skin?"), and doesn't have that relaxed pose, I know this mom isn't in the land of postpartum bliss. If you find yourself overly worried about minor details, are always concerned about your baby's day-to-day well-being, and don't ever find yourself just sitting there basking in your baby's radiance, then take stock of your stress. This section will show you how to relax. And I hope you aren't now saying to yourself, "Great! Now I'm even *more* stressed over the idea that my stress may be making my baby stressed."

or she has to suffer consequences of that stress. You just need to have the skills and tools to take control. Here are some ideas:

### Manipulate Your Mind

- *Eliminate the negative and think positively.* If you tend to see the glass as half empty, you may not be able to change your temperament, but you can actually learn how to think more positively in order to protect yourself from the effects of stress. Try it: Next time you have a thought that is pessimistic, such as "I'm going to be a terrible mother," try to recognize that you are thinking negatively. Then come up with a more positive thought to replace it, for example, "I may be scared, but I'm going to love this baby and do my best."

- *Journaling.* Another way to rid yourself of negative toxic thoughts is to get them out of your head and onto a piece of paper. Keep a journal by your bed, and write down all your thoughts and fears before you go to sleep. Hopefully, they will stay on the paper, and your mind will be quiet so you can get some rest.

- *Mantras.* In yoga and other meditative practices, a mantra is a word or phrase that you repeat to yourself as a way to block out mental chatter and quiet the mind. It's also supposed to help you actualize your best intentions. Choose a word or phrase that embodies a feeling you want to have ("I am calm and strong") or a thought that relieves your stress ("This too shall pass"), and repeat it whenever you feel stressed. One mom shared these words with us:

"For me, in the early weeks after my second baby was born, when life seemed always on the verge of spiraling out of control, I used to repeat: 'One day at a time. I just have to get through one day at a time.' Through the two-year-old's temper tantrums and the infant's screams, this simple thought, repeated over and over, brought me so much comfort."

- *Laugh it off.* Let's face it, when Baby's diaper leaked on the dress your mother-in-law gave you, it was kind of funny! Try to make light of stressful situations. If that doesn't come naturally to you, pick up some parenting humor books at your local library or share your stories with friends or your partner so you can laugh together about the craziness of parenthood. It may even help Baby's health: after laughing through a funny movie, moms in one study made breast milk that was rich in melatonin, a "feel good" hormone, and their babies actually experienced relief from their eczema symptoms as a result.[7]

- *Prayer.* If you are religious, prayer can be very relaxing. It's a way to share your worries with someone who is always there to listen, and let Him (or Her!) take your worries off your hands.

## Tap into the Mind-Body Connection

Sometimes you need to focus on the body in order to change the mind. Relaxing actually triggers a physical response in your body that reverses some of the effects of the flight-or-fight reaction to stress, bringing blood pressure and heart rate back to normal. It's called the relaxation response. These exercises will help to induce it:

- *Regular exercise.* Don't be stressed about making sure your exercise is vigorous and calorie burning! The most important thing is to make sure you exercise regularly. Even light exercise is beneficial and relaxing, such as walking, swimming, and casual bike riding.

- *Yoga.* The perfect example of an activity that has positive mental effects in addition to the physical benefits is yoga. Yoga requires you to be mindful and live in the moment, leaving little room in your brain for negative or stressful thoughts. A regular yoga practice can help to quiet your mind, relax the body, and may even decrease the risk of certain health conditions. Many yoga studios offer special classes for Mama and baby. Not having to find a babysitter makes the activity all the more stress-relieving!

- *Massage.* Who knew that a spa treatment could be so beneficial? One study of pregnant women with depression found that massage therapy increased circulation of the feel-good hormones dopamine and serotonin, and led to lower rates of premature birth and low birth weight.[8] Just because your baby is already born doesn't mean that some good old-fashioned relaxing isn't an important item on the to-do list. If it's too hard (or expensive) to go to a massage professional, enlist your husband or partner to help. Exchange foot massages or shoulder rubs as a way to relax and connect.

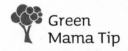

### Green Mama Tip

Salon spa treatments feel wonderful and help you unwind, but some beauty products contain toxic chemicals, so it's important to choose wisely.

Check out greenspanet work.org to find spas in your area that operate in an eco-conscious and health-conscious way. And check out chapter 4 for information about how to green your beauty routine.

- *Progressive muscle relaxation.* This is a technique that reduces muscle tension in order to tell the brain that you're relaxing. It's simple: you tense and then release the major muscle groups until the body is fully relaxed. While you do this exercise, be sure not to hold your breath, grit your teeth, or tighten your face or jaw. Breathe normally and try to tense only the muscle that is supposed to be engaged. If you have any pulled or strained muscles or other injuries, consult with an expert before trying this technique.
- Sit comfortably in a chair, or recline on the couch or in bed. (This is a great one to do if you're having trouble falling asleep at night.)
- Tense each of the following muscles for ten seconds, release the muscle, and relax for another ten seconds before moving to the next body part.
  - *Hands and arms:* Clench hands into fists and relax. Then open hands as widely as possible and relax again.
  - *Arms:* Flex your biceps.
  - *Shoulders:* Shrug them up to your ears (and then drop to release).
  - *Neck:* Tuck your chin into your chest.
  - *Eyes and forehead:* Open your eyes widely and relax. Then close eyes tightly and relax again. Make sure you relax the forehead and nose, too.
  - *Mouth:* Open your mouth as widely as possible.
  - *Abdominals:* Exhale and pull in the abdominal muscles while pressing your lower back into the chair or bed.
  - *Hips and buttocks:* Press your buttocks together tightly.
  - *Thighs:* Clench the thighs, extending your feet a few inches off the floor (if sitting) or bed (if lying down).
  - *Lower legs:* Flex your feet, each toe pulling back equally, and then relax. Then point your foot and curl toes under and relax.
- *Focusing on your breath.* This helps you block out stressful or upsetting thoughts and sends a signal to your brain that you

# NATURE'S BABY GIFT TO YOU

The next time you want some peace and relaxation, venture into the great outdoors. Connecting with nature, even for just a few minutes, is a great way to infuse a sense of calm in the midst of a crazy day. And it doesn't matter where you live—nature is free and accessible for every Mama, and even the most urban of city dwellers can find a tree or two. Plus, connecting with nature can help you remember one reason you're trying to be more green: because the earth's beauty and resources are worth protecting and preserving.

- Pause for a few minutes to look at a tree, a flower patch, a rolling hillside, a stream. Take some slow, deep breaths as you bring your focus to what you're seeing. The stillness and focus will serve as a quick meditation.
- Sit on a park bench and close your eyes for a minute to listen to the sounds of leaves rustling or birds chirping.
- Spend time in your garden or plant flowers in your yard. Baby can watch from a nearby blanket or stroller.
- If it's cold and wintry where you live, admire the unique shapes of dangling icicles and the perfection of untouched patches of snow.
- If you're lucky enough to be close to the ocean, sit and listen to the waves.
- Set up a bird feeder within view of one of your windows so you can watch birds come and go. Baby will delight in the busy birdie activity.

are relaxing. All you do is sit in a quiet place and pay attention to your inhalations and exhalations. Breathe in, breathe out. Don't try to control the breath; rather, notice the easy flow, in and out. Do this for several minutes.

- *Deep breathing.* This provides deeper relaxation than the mindful breathing exercise above, but you can still do it anywhere and at any time. Follow these steps whenever you feel tense:
  - Place one hand on your abdomen and one on your chest.
  - Inhale slowly and deeply, filling the abdomen with air, the middle chest, and then the upper chest. You will feel

your hands rise as the air enters. If done correctly, your shoulders should be still, not rising up toward your ears.

- Even more slowly, exhale this breath, starting at the top of your lungs and moving down the body until the air from the abdomen is exhaled.
- Repeat this for several minutes.
- Don't ever overdo it. If you feel uncomfortable or light-headed, immediately return to normal breathing.

### MORE PATHS TO MAMA ZEN

- *Ask for help.* Friends and family may be able to help relieve you of some burdens. All you have to do is admit that you can't (or don't want to) do it all, and ask for help. Is your older child too much to handle some days? Ask someone to watch him for an hour or two. Do you feel obligated to throw your annual Fourth of July party even though you're exhausted? Make it potluck so you're not doing all the work. People who love you *want* to help. Let them.
- *Create a new-Mama network.* A strong social network can help us get through anything, even life with a newborn. Form a supportive network of other new Mamas to share and swap ideas, toys, clothes, recipes, even babysitters. When you hang out with others who are going through similar experiences, you'll find shoulders to lean on and practical help with your challenges. Most of all, you'll be reminded that you're not going through this alone. What a relief!
- *Live in the moment.* It's very tempting to count the hours until bedtime or wish away your baby's early days ("I just want her to be able to walk already!"). But being present in what you're doing will help you find peace in your day-to-day life. So pause for a moment now and then to take it all in. Look into Baby's eyes, breathe in the delicious scent of her freshly washed body, enjoy the beautiful colors of the baby food you've cooked for her. These moments are so fleeting in the great scheme of things. Try to notice and enjoy them.

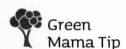 Green Mama Tip

Swapping baby toys, clothes, and gear isn't just a way to connect socially with other Mamas. It's also a great way to reduce waste and conserve resources. If none of your friends wants your outgrown gear, look for local organizations that take donations.

A NOTE FROM DR. BOB

# Network Mothering

I see all kinds of new moms in my office. Some are completely relaxed and comfortable in their new role, but some appear very overwhelmed, which is completely understandable. I don't know how you moms do it! We men definitely aren't wired for a twenty-four-hour job. But some moms who may need support might not want to admit it or feel motivated to seek it out. Well, caring for a baby doesn't necessarily get easier over the months. It changes, yes, but not always for the easier. For some of my patients, I see the day-to-day demands of caring for a baby leave them drained, stressed, and eventually depressed. Motherhood should be a blessing and help you thrive as a woman. Here is what I recommend to any new mom who seems to be stressed and drained—get networked. The best support group you can have is other new moms. Call up everyone from your prenatal class and organize a weekly get-together. You can bet that most of the other moms will jump at the chance for such support. Another good resource is La Leche League, an international group of moms who have monthly meetings to offer breast-feeding education and support. Search their Web site, www.llli.org, to find a group in your area. The "Green Resources" section on page 385 lists more parenting support groups for you.

- *Learn something.* If you have baby-related questions or challenges that you can't seem to figure out, don't convince yourself that ignorance is bliss. The opposite is true: the more informed you are about how to manage your challenges, the less anxiety you will have. So read a book (look, you're already doing something

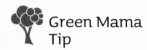

### Green Mama Tip

. . . . . . . . . . . . . . . . . . . . .

When you meet your Mama friends at the local coffee shop for a chat, bring your own mug. In 2006, Starbucks coffee customers did this more than seventeen million times, keeping 674,000 pounds of paper from going to the landfill.[9]

positive!), talk to your pediatrician about your concerns, or talk to a friend or relative who has already been there, done that.

- *Honor your need for sleep.* If Baby is still waking up at night for feeding (or for soothing), you're probably fairly sleep-deprived. Take advantage of any opportunity you have for a power nap or extra rest. It can be very tempting to spend Baby's naptime doing things that you've been neglecting, like cleaning or cooking, but resist this urge and just lie down for a quick snooze instead. Your body and mind will thank you.

- *Honor your limitations.* This falls into the easier-said-than-done category, but it is simple: if you are overextended and have too many obligations, remember that your first responsibility is to yourself and your baby, and just say no.

- *Find personal solutions.* Perhaps you unwind by watching your favorite sitcom or window-shopping. Or maybe visiting a local dog park to watch the pups calms your spirits. If you've found something that works for you (and it's not a risky behavior like getting drunk or drag racing, for example), do it routinely!

## The Baby Blues and Postpartum Depression

Many Mamas experience the baby blues and feel stressed out by the overwhelming responsibility of motherhood. Did you know that certain foods may help calm you down and make you feel happier? Components of foods influence the levels of neurotransmitters in the brain, which in turn stimulate emotions and moods.

- *Omega-3 fats.* Not only are these fats crucial for your breast-fed baby's brain and eye health, they may also be helpful for preventing or managing mild depression. The research is mixed, with some studies showing a benefit to eating foods rich in these fats or taking supplements, while other studies show no effect.[11] Find good food sources: cold-water fish like wild salmon, tuna (but not if you're breast-feeding—too much mercury), halibut, herring; walnuts, soybeans and tofu,

# Can You Be Too Attached to Your Baby?

Babies are very dependent creatures, and for good reason. All that time spent in your arms, snuggled close during sleep, gazing face-to-face, feeling your touch during feedings and massages, hearing your soothing voice, and smelling your scent, all help enhance baby's neurological development. Virtually every research study done on child development and behavior shows that the more physically and emotionally attached an infant is in the first year, the faster its intellectual and motor development, and the more independent and emotionally healthy it will be as an older child and adult. Studies have even demonstrated higher IQ points in such babies, compared to what I call playpen babies—those that are more often set down to play alone and soothe themselves.[10] The research is very clear on this. So, to answer my opening question, no! You can't be too attached. In fact, babies are supposed to be attached. Wear your baby around the house in an infant carrier or sling, snuggle with her, enjoy quiet interaction during feeding times (whether breast or bottle), lie down with her for a nap. These practices strengthen the bond between Mama and baby. The closeness will not only soothe her, but believe me, those calm moments with your child will bring you peace, too.

kale, collard greens, and Brussels sprouts. Or you can take a supplement—fish or flaxseed oil or capsules.

- *Serotonin boosters.* Certain foods have a calming effect because they increase your brain's level of serotonin. High carbohydrate meals like a pasta dinner raise serotonin. So does chocolate. Chocolate can raise your endorphin levels, making you feel happy. Dark chocolate has the added bonus of having high antioxidant levels. It's almost as if you could say dark chocolate is good for you! So if you're craving a sweet treat, reach for a square of good-quality dark chocolate.

## WHEN IT'S MORE THAN JUST STRESS: POSTPARTUM DEPRESSION

The birth of your baby set into motion extreme physical, hormonal, and lifestyle changes, so it's normal to feel out of sorts, to cry more than usual, and to feel nervous or overwhelmed afterward. For most women these "baby blues" go away within a couple of weeks after Baby's birth. But for 10 to 15 percent of women these feelings deepen into true sadness and a detached feeling that continues for weeks or months after the birth or that surfaces sometime later during Baby's first year. This is called postpartum depression (PPD). You may be experiencing postpartum depression if any of the following is true:

- You feel hopeless, guilty, or worthless
- You have no appetite or find yourself overeating in binges
- You have little interest in your baby or your friends or family
- You are overly worried about minor details and problems concerning your baby
- You have trouble sleeping, even when Baby sleeps
- You are sleeping more than usual
- You often cry for no apparent reason
- You have thoughts of harming yourself or Baby
- You are unable to do everyday tasks including caring for Baby
- You just don't enjoy life as much as you did in the past

It can be scary and sad to realize that you are experiencing depression, but luckily there are treatment options, including individual or group talk therapy and medication that can help you feel better. Your primary care physician, obstetrician, or midwife can help you get treatment so you can feel like yourself again.

Another effective treatment and prevention for PPD is regular exercise. If you haven't begun this yet, start right away with a brisk morning walk. Research has shown that this is an effective treatment for the blues. This helps you start each day with a more positive attitude and outlook. Bring Baby along in a jogging stroller, wear Baby in a sling, or enlist Dad's help so you can enjoy a walk alone.

If you were in therapy for depression before you became pregnant or during pregnancy, don't stop that treatment now. If you were taking medications, you may have been advised to gradually taper off them before you conceived or immediately following conception. You may be able to resume taking these medications now. Talk to your obstetrician or midwife about your options. Bear in mind that if you're nursing, all medications need to be evaluated carefully for their safety. There are some antidepressant medications that have been researched and shown to be safe during breast-feeding. Natural remedies for depression may or may not be safe during nursing. If you use an herbal therapy to treat your depression, talk to your herbalist and obstetrician or midwife to determine the best course of action while you're nursing.

## Taking It Home . . .

We hope you've gotten some insight into how well you are adjusting to life with Baby and identified any areas that you could get started on to help ensure a healthy transition into motherhood. What does this have to do with going green? In general, a healthy mind and body are important foundations on which to build a positive and proactive outlook on life. Throughout the rest of this book we are going to ask you to make some changes in your family life and habits. We want you to have the energy to do it. Baby is going to suck much of that energy out of you. But you can keep replenishing with daily exercise and relaxation techniques. You will *feel* the extra energy and motivation these activities provide. Nutrition is also a very important aspect of this lifestyle, and in chapter 4 we will provide you with everything you need to know about postpartum and breast-feeding nutrition for new moms.

## PART TWO

# The Happy (and Well-Fed!) Baby

# 3

# *Really* Homemade Baby Food

## Babies, Breast Milk, and Bottle-Feeding

Breast-feeding is your first real opportunity to feed Baby in a green way. It's the ultimate example of how green living and good health intersect. What could be more earth-friendly: it creates almost no waste, it doesn't require the acquisition of a lot of stuff, and it's certainly all natural. And talk about eating locally! Health wise, when we talk about the best nutrition for promoting good health in new babies, nothing can come close to breast milk.

**American Academy of Pediatrics Recommendations**[1]

| | |
|---|---|
| Birth to 6 months | Exclusive breast-feeding. This means that Baby gets no other liquid or food except breast milk until she starts on solid foods. |
| 6 months to 1 year | Baby continues on breast milk with solid foods as a supplement. |
| 1 year and beyond | Breast-feeding may continue as long as it's what Mama and Baby want to do. Food starts to play a more significant role in Baby's nutrition at this time. |

We believe that breast-feeding is best for Baby. Infant formula provides adequate nutrition, but it's just not the same. The closer you follow the recommendations of breast-feeding experts and adopt the "best practices" we discuss in this chapter, the greater your chances of breast-feeding success—meaning that you will have the supply and the skills to do it for as long as you want, and the greater the benefit to you and Baby. We should add, though, at the risk of sounding wishy-washy, that just like other aspects of parenting, breast-feeding is not necessarily an all-or-nothing proposition. Mamas may find compromises and combinations of feeding methods that work for them and their families. We provide helpful information about formula feeding later in this chapter for Mamas supplementing with infant formula.

# Miracle Milk

When you think about it, it's amazing that a woman's body can make the only food her new baby needs to grow. Breast milk is perfectly designed for Baby's needs and protection, with these powerful ingredients and benefits:

| Ingredient | What It Does for Baby |
|---|---|
| Immunity factors and antibodies | Help protect Baby against infections, particularly respiratory, ear, and stomach bugs |
| Oligosaccharides—prebiotics | Encourage the growth of lactobacillus bacterium, a probiotic, or "friendly," bacterium that protects the gut lining from infection |
| Bifidobacteria—probiotics | Helpful bacteria that protect Baby's gut against diarrhea illnesses and other nasty infections |

| Omega-3 fatty acids, specifically docosahexaenoic acid (DHA) | Promote eye and brain development |
| --- | --- |
| Whey | Easily digestible protein source |
| Highly absorbable iron | Allows baby to use almost 50 percent of the iron (compared with 10% iron absorption from infant formula) leaving little to stay unabsorbed in the intestines[2] |
| Flavor compounds from some of the foods that Mama eats | Provide Baby with hints of tastes to come, helps promote interest in foods |

Most of the benefits that Baby receives from breast-feeding are from the ingredients of the milk itself. But Baby also greatly benefits from the overall experience of feeding right from the breast. The months Baby spends using his jaw muscles, tongue, and lips to drain milk from the breasts are thought to help the position of Baby's teeth, gums, and palate form correctly. Breast-feeding also exercises the jaw muscles and joints, which may protect against TMJ disease (sore jaw joints) later on in life.

Compared to formula-fed babies, breast-fed babies (especially those babies who are breast-fed exclusively from birth until starting solid foods around six months of age) receive the following benefits:

- Decreased risk of developing eczema, allergies and asthma[3-5]
- Fewer ear infections[6]
- Fewer stomach illnesses, less constipation, and less painful reflux of acid from their stomachs (gastroesophageal reflux disease, or GERD)[7-10]
- Protection against the effects of secondhand smoke[11]
- Lower risk of becoming overweight and developing type 2 diabetes[12-14]

## Colostrum First!

A baby's intestines undergo some changes during the first few days after birth in order to prepare for digestion of breast milk. The first milk that you produce is different from the "mature milk" that will come later. The first milk is called colostrum, and it has several factors that help initiate these intestinal changes and help Baby's intestines mature quickly. If a foreign substance, such as formula, is introduced during the first few days of life (before colostrum has done its job), we don't exactly know what permanent effects that might have on the intestines. I worry that such a practice may contribute to allergies and digestive problems later on. I know that in *some* instances a supplement may be needed, but this decision shouldn't be made lightly; some doctors or nurses may advise you that you need to feed your baby formula during the early days without giving it a second thought. It's best to keep Baby's little tummy pure and natural if you can.

- Tendency to form secure attachments with their Mamas, encouraged by the skin-to-skin contact and physical closeness and comfort
- Ability to become kids who can handle stressful situations better than those who were not breast-fed [15]

And since it's perfectly OK to think about yourself sometimes, consider the benefits of breastfeeding for the Mama:

- Contracts the uterus to help it return to its original size after childbirth

- Seems to help Mamas return to their prepregnancy weight [16]
- May ease depression after childbirth [17]
- Helps protect against breast and ovarian cancers [18,19]

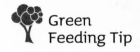

**Green Feeding Tip**

Breast-feeding is an eco-friendly choice compared with formula feeding because it requires no fuel for production or transport, it creates no container waste, and breast milk is a sustainable resource!

Besides the health benefits for Mama and Baby, breast-feeding also affords Mama some financial and logistical benefits. It can mean more money in your pocket—a year's supply of infant formula can run you around nine hundred dollars. Breast milk, though valuable as gold, is free! (And you'll have more money to spend on organic food.) And many families find that breast-feeding is actually more convenient—there are no bottles to prepare or wash and nothing to pack when you're away from home. You always have Baby's next meal available at a moment's notice.

## MYTH OR FACT?

*With all the environmental chemicals in our bodies that can get into breast milk, maybe it's actually safer to feed Baby infant formula.*

Myth! While it is true that when Mama is exposed to certain chemicals and medications they can enter her milk, the benefits of breast milk and breast-feeding far outweigh the risks of these tiny exposures. Plus, a breast-feeding Mama can take preventive measures by avoiding certain exposures in order to minimize the presence of chemicals in her milk. Finally, as we learned from the recent scare involving poisonous chemicals in infant formula made in China, you never know what toxins may exist in manufactured formula.

Mamas and babies are most successful with breast-feeding when they follow certain best practices. This doesn't mean there's one right way to feed, though. Babies differ in their feeding patterns, their temperaments, and their development, so sometimes you'll need to adapt to Baby's individual needs and learn to go with the flow (no pun intended!). Adapting to Baby's needs and your personal circumstances will be easier if you get off to a good start, establish an adequate milk supply, and help Baby learn how to nurse effectively. The how-to info we have for you here will help you do just that.

A NOTE FROM DR. BOB

## Getting Started with Breast-Feeding Is a Piece of Cake, Right?

Every new mom-to-be envisions quietly nursing her newborn baby in a softly lit room, with quiet music playing in the background and birds singing outside the window, without a care in the world. It's supposed to be easy, right? Babies should automatically know how to latch on perfectly and calmly nurse to their heart's content. Wouldn't that be nice.

Now let's talk reality. In my experience with many hundreds of new moms, the first few days of breast-feeding a first baby almost never go perfectly. Babies *are* born knowing how to open their mouth and suck, but it's that darn latching-on process that many just don't get right away. Plus, there's usually nothing calm and quiet about a suckling newborn. They squirm, snort, pull away from the breast, and get annoyed because your milk hasn't come in yet.

If you find yourself getting frustrated, take a step back and realize that this is how most newborns behave with nursing at first. Hang in there. Once your milk starts flowing, around day three or four, baby will taste that reward and get a lot more serious about nursing and will settle into that nice routine you imagined.

# Milk-Making 101

Not to turn this into a biology class, but it's actually very helpful to have a basic understanding of how the body makes milk because then you will see how certain feeding practices will promote milk production. This knowledge may also help you avoid any bad advice from others that might inadvertently sabotage your efforts.

In general, breast milk is produced on an on-demand basis. When Baby (or a breast pump) sucks on the breast, a letdown reflex is activated, which causes vessels in the breast to contract and send milk toward the nipple. This reflex may also occur when you hear your baby cry. When letdown occurs, you may feel a sensation like pins and needles in your breasts, and then as your milk starts to flow, Baby will switch from quick little sucks to slow and steady sucking and swallowing. Milk continues to flow during the feeding as Baby continues to suck. The breast is drained as Baby fills his belly, but it never is completely empty. You may even have more than one letdown per feeding. In between feedings, the milk ducts in the breast begin to refill to get ready for the next letdown. With few exceptions, the body is able to supply as much milk as Baby needs, as long as the breast tissues are stimulated enough.

The milk that comes out at the beginning of the feeding, called the foremilk, is sweet and a bit watery, great for quenching Baby's thirst. As this milk is drained, toward the end of a feeding, the fattier hindmilk becomes available, helping to satisfy Baby and make him feel full.

Most Mamas who are exclusively breast-feeding make about twenty to thirty ounces of milk per day by the time Baby is about a month old. The amount of milk that Baby gets at each feeding may influence how many feedings Baby needs in twenty-four hours, and this will vary from woman to woman. Some of the variation may be due to how much milk Mama's breasts are able to store at one time. Some breasts, big or small, are able to store a lot of milk in between feedings, so Baby may get more milk at each feeding and be able to go longer between feedings. Don't worry—breasts that store less milk at a time will still satisfy Baby, but he may become hungry again sooner.

# Baby's Very First "Meal"

As soon as Baby is born your body launches into milk-making mode. The best way to start is to let Baby nurse right after birth, or at least within the first hour, while Baby is awake and alert.

Baby's first feedings are known as colostrum, a nutrient- and immunity-filled milk with a rich golden color. You won't make very much at first, but that's perfect, because Baby doesn't need very much. Frequent nursing during Baby's first days helps him get all the colostrum, and it helps your body ramp up its milk production. Around day three or four your mature milk will start to come in, and you'll have much more milk to give. The more Baby nurses, the better your supply will become.

## Tips for Establishing Success in Breast-Feeding from Right After Birth

- *Frequent feedings.* Feed Baby every two or three hours around the clock—at least eight times in every twenty-four-hour period. Ten or twelve times is even better. Baby will let you know when he needs to eat (see below for details) but if he seems hungry fewer than eight times in twenty-four hours you should just go ahead and feed him at least every three hours. This will help bring in your milk supply, prevent jaundice in your baby, and it may even make your milk more nutritious: the more frequently you feed your baby, the higher the fat content in your milk, and high-calorie fat-filled milk is what Baby needs to grow and thrive.
- *Rooming in.* When Baby stays in the hospital room with his Mama, it's more likely that you'll feed early and often during the first few days. If you've decided to have your baby stay in the nursery at night, ask the nurses how they'll determine feeding times—whether by the clock or whether they will bring him to you whenever he seems hungry.

# Your Baby May Get Dehydrated . . . Not

A very common misconception about newborns is that they need to take in a lot of milk in the first few days. If they don't, they will get dehydrated. This simply isn't true. Here's where we can take a lesson from Mother Nature by understanding how a mom's milk comes in. Since moms don't make much milk in the first few days, it stands to reason that babies therefore don't need much milk during these days. If they did, the human species would have died out long ago. God or nature or evolution designed it this way. Babies are born with a lot of extra water to keep them hydrated for the first few days. They pee off about three-quarters of a pound of their weight in water during this time. They nurse for colostrum, and they start to get hungry. This makes them nurse more, which helps mom's milk come in. By day three or four, when Baby really starts to get hungry (and a little annoyed!), voilà! Mom's milk comes in and everyone's happy.

But nurses and doctors used to be trained that babies need to take in a lot of milk during the first few days, so they must be given formula until mom's milk comes in. They would tell you that your baby would become dehydrated if you didn't supplement. Now doctors and nurses are trained with the truth, but word hasn't gotten around to everyone yet. In thirteen years of being a doctor, I have never once seen a newborn get dehydrated in the first five days of life (unless there was a medical problem, such as prematurity or a traumatic birth). So, don't let anyone bully you into supplementing. Just be patient; your milk will arrive!

- *At first, wake a sleepy baby.* Until Baby is a few weeks old, if he is too sleepy to feed eight to ten times in twenty-four hours, wake him up for feedings. Or, if he falls asleep while feeding, gently wake him so she gets a full feeding. Tickle his feet or his back, get him undressed, change his diaper, or speak to him softly. As a last resort, gently dab a cool damp washcloth on his forehead and cheeks. Once your milk has come in and breast-feeding is well established and Baby is growing well, you can let him sleep as long as he wants.

- *Pump, if necessary.* If you have to be separated from Baby at birth because one or both of you need medical attention, make sure the doctors and nurses know that you want to breast-feed as soon as it is possible. If it's going to be more than a couple of hours, ask for a breast pump so you can start expressing milk to bring in your supply and to capture the colostrum.

- *Ask for help.* After childbirth your body will need to recover and rest. If you've had a C-section, your surgery recovery will take several weeks. Breast-feeding, like so many aspects of being a new parent, takes time and it takes energy. So it's helpful to have people lined up to assist you at home—to cook and clean, to change diapers, and to hold Baby while you rest. Try to have your partner or a family member stay with you for as long as possible. If it's financially possible, you may even consider hiring a postpartum doula or a private nurse who has experience with breast-feeding Mamas to help you during your first couple of weeks at home.

## BREAST-FED BABIES AND JAUNDICE

Babies are born with more red blood cells than they need, and their bodies gradually break down these extra cells and get rid of them. One of the by-products of this process is bilirubin, a yellow pigment that is processed by the liver, sent into the intestines, and excreted in Baby's stool. If it takes Baby a long time to pass her first several stools, the bilirubin stays in her intestines long enough to get reabsorbed into the

# ESPECIALLY FOR C-SECTION MAMAS

A C-section is major surgery, and the first few days of recovery can be difficult. However, there's no reason to think it will prevent you from breast-feeding. Spinal or epidural anesthesia won't numb your upper body, so as soon as it's feasible you should be able to put Baby to breast. Baby may be a little groggy from the anesthesia, but breast-feeding is perfectly safe even right after the delivery. Plus, if you feed Baby before your anesthesia wears off, you'll get a relaxed and pain-free feeding in before your incision site starts to hurt. Most Mamas can feed right away, either right after the delivery or in the recovery room. You will need assistance holding and positioning the baby—a nurse or your partner can help.

For the first several days, while your body is healing, position the baby so she's not putting pressure on your incision site. A side-lying position where Mama and Baby lie in bed facing each other is good, as is the football, or clutch, hold where you are sitting up in bed, supported by plenty of pillows, and Baby's body is held on the side of yours. Ask for a lactation consultant to come to your room to assist you.

Many Mamas are concerned about taking pain medication when nursing. Though it's always best to avoid unnecessary medications while nursing, you don't want your pain to sabotage your efforts to feed effectively. The best thing to do about pain is to manage it. Ask for a medication that's compatible with breast-feeding; there are several safe options.

bloodstream. This circulating bilirubin causes jaundice, a yellowing of Baby's eyes and skin.

This kind of jaundice is fairly common in newborns, and especially in breast-fed babies because they don't pass as many stools as formula-fed babies. Jaundice in newborns is usually harmless and goes away on its own as baby passes her first stools. Doctors monitor baby's skin color carefully, and may test the blood's bilirubin levels because extremely high levels place a baby at risk for brain damage. Luckily, this is rare.

The best way to avoid jaundice is to feed Baby early and often during the first few days. Eight to ten feedings a day is the target for a minimum number of feedings for preventing jaundice, and ten to twelve feedings is even more effective. Colostrum, your first milk, is a natural laxative and can help Baby make those dirty diapers that the doctors

## Successful Breast-Feeding Begins Before Birth

Take steps to help breast-feeding go smoothly, even before Baby is born.

*Take a class.* Learn a little so you're not going into the experience blind. Most communities have breast-feeding classes given by lactation consultants or health educators. Sign up for one and bring your partner along if at all possible.

*Tell people.* Talk to your partner, family, and obstetrician or midwife about your plans to breast-feed, especially if there's a chance that a person may not be fully supportive.

*Make a plan.* You may have heard of birthing plans—a list of intentions surrounding the delivery of your baby. Write your breast-feeding preferences into your birth plan. It may help you communicate with your nurses and nursery staff. It may also help you remember what you had intended to do, if you're exhausted from labor, recovering from surgery, or if things don't go exactly as you planned with the birth. Here are some ideas for what to include:

- I would like to nurse my baby as soon as I can after birth.
- I want my baby to stay in my room and be able to nurse as often as we would like.
- If my baby has to be separated from me after birth (if either she or I need additional medical treatment), I would like every effort to be made to breast-feed as soon as is medically possible. In the meantime, I wish to express milk using a breast pump, and I want the first milk that goes into my baby to be my pumped colostrum.
- I don't want my baby to have a pacifier or bottle nipple during our hospital/birthing center stay because I want her to learn how to suck properly at the breast first. If supplemental feeding is required for any reason, I want to use a supplemental nursing system (SNS) or a feeding dropper instead of a bottle.

and nurses like to see. Sometimes Mamas are told that supplementing with formula is a good way to bring down bilirubin levels. However, in the majority of jaundice cases, simply breast-feeding often will be sufficient.

If Baby's pediatrician truly feels that supplementing with formula is the medically prudent course of action to help with your baby's jaundice, it doesn't have to negatively impact your breast-feeding. You can continue to nurse and/or use a pump to bring in your milk supply. You can feed Baby his infant formula using a feeding syringe or supplemental nursing system (an apparatus that sends milk or formula through a tiny tube that is attached to Mama's breast so Baby can suck at the breast while getting the supplemental nourishment) instead of a bottle nipple to avoid interfering with Baby's breast-feeding learning process.

## Baby's Latch

When Baby is positioned properly he can achieve a proper latch more effectively. Without a good latch, Baby's sucking is inefficient, which can tire out Baby and shorten his feedings—not ideal for your milk supply or Baby's nutrition and growth. A bad latch may also hurt your nipples. Three common feeding positions are the cradle hold, the clutch hold, and the side-lying position.

- *Cradle hold:* Cradle Baby in your arm, his head and neck resting in the crook of your arm and her body supported by your forearm and hand. Turn his whole body so that he is facing you tummy to tummy. Then bring him straight toward your breast. Tuck his bottom arm under yours so nothing is between Baby and breast. You shouldn't have to crouch or lean forward too much, which will strain your back and neck. Instead, elevate your legs by resting your feet on a footrest, and lay Baby on a pillow to bring him up to the level of your breasts and close to your body.
- *Clutch hold:* This position is good for Mamas recovering from a C-section and for tiny or premature babies. It is also called the football hold because you tuck Baby under your arm as you would carry a football. To nurse on your right breast, for example, sit in a chair or sofa with a pillow or armrest supporting your right arm. Hold Baby facing toward your body

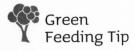

along your right side with his head resting in your right hand
and body resting on your forearm. Pull your Baby in toward the
breast and hold him close to you as he latches on. You can use
the pillow or armrest to help support his weight. Extra pillows
behind you may help you feel comfortable in this position, too.

- *Side-lying position:* This is another good position for C-section
Mamas and for nighttime feedings when you'd rather lie in bed
than sit up in a chair. Lie on one side, with pillows supporting
your back and head and neck. You can also put a pillow between
your knees to reduce hip strain. Baby will lie facing your breast,
resting in your arm. Line his mouth up with your nipple and
bring him close to you to latch on. He shouldn't have to strain
to reach you, and you shouldn't need to bend. Elevate Baby on a
pillow if need be.

Once in position, some babies seem to know just what to do, while
others need a little coaxing and education. You want Baby's mouth to
close around your whole areola—the dark area around your nipple—not
clamp down on the nipple itself (Ouch!). Baby's tongue will be scooped
under the nipple as he sucks. His nose, lips, and chin should be close to
the breast. If Baby needs help figuring out what to do, stroke his lower
lip a bit to get him to open his mouth. Once open, you can gently hold
his head to guide him straight onto the breast.

## When to Feed

Feed Baby on demand, especially during the early weeks and months.
This means that you let Baby decide when to eat, not the clock. The only
caveat to this statement is if your newborn is feeding fewer than eight
times in a twenty-four-hour period, he needs to be encouraged to eat
more. Also, if Baby's growth is a concern, his pediatrician may recommend feeding at least every two hours whether or not Baby seems to
want to eat.

If you're the type who likes to follow a plan or schedule, you may

# The Lower Lip Flip

One of the easiest tricks I've found as a pediatrician when a mom says Baby's latch hurts is to show Mom or Dad how to slide a finger in between Baby's chin and mom's breast and gently pull down on the lower lip and chin without breaking the suction. This pulls the lip away from the nipple and down onto the breast tissue and often immediately results in a more comfortable latch. I call this the lower lip flip.

A funny story that I can't resist telling is about one mom who came to me complaining that her newborn's latch-on was still painful. "I'm flicking her lower lip every time I latch her on just like you told me to in the hospital, but it still hurts," she reported. "Can you say that again?" I asked. "I flick her lower lip right after she begins nursing, but nothing changes," she explained as she demonstrated on her baby (to my amusement/horror). "Did you say 'flick' or 'flip'?" I asked, desperately but unsuccessfully trying not to laugh. "'Flick,'" she answered. "Why? What do you mean by 'flip'?" From that point on I've made it a point to demonstrate the lip flip, instead of just giving verbal instructions.

find it challenging to do on-demand feeding. It does make things a bit unpredictable at first because you can never be 100 percent sure when Baby will want to eat. Scheduling a young breast-fed baby usually backfires, though. You'll just have a hungry (or stuffed), cranky little person on your hands. Or, even worse, your attempts to hold Baby to a schedule may lead to less frequent feedings than she actually requires, and then your milk supply will not develop to be adequate for her appetite.

### Signs that Baby Wants to Nurse

- He's suddenly wide-eyed and alert
- He's making a sucking motion with her mouth
- He's found a finger or fist and is sucking on it
- He tries to latch on to your shoulder when you hold him or latch on to your fingers if you gently caress his cheek

Ideally, Baby shouldn't have to cry or fuss too much to let you know he's hungry. A baby who is crying due to hunger has probably been hungry for fifteen to thirty minutes already. Of course sometimes you'll miss the signs (you may have to take your eyes off her for moments here and there!) and Baby will fuss, but the goal is to watch for the signs that come first, before the cries.

And while we're on the topic of crying . . . feeding on demand doesn't mean that you feed Baby every time she fusses because fussy does not always mean hungry. Over time you will learn to read Baby's cues. A fussy baby may need a diaper change, a change of scenery, or a nap. Or perhaps he is too hot or too cold or uncomfortable for some reason. If it turns out that he does want to nurse, that's OK, too. The point here is not to deny a hungry baby, but to learn how to tell when Baby is indeed hungry so you don't overfeed him or exhaust yourself unnecessarily.

If there are times when you don't think Baby is hungry but he does want to suck, you have a few options. You can put him to the breast for some comfort sucking, you can offer a clean finger for him to suck on, or you can try a pacifier and a cuddle. (It is best to wait to introduce a pacifier until you are sure that breast-feeding is going well for you and for Baby, at least a few weeks after birth.)

There may be days or weeks when you feel like all you're doing is feeding. At first, you'll probably feel this way because feedings can take thirty minutes or more, and after burping and changing you may have only an hour until you have to feed again. As you and Baby learn and practice, feedings probably won't take as long. Baby may also cluster feed in the late part of the day, sometimes to fill up before his longer stretches of sleep at night. Occasionally, Baby may also have hungry days when he wants to feed more often than usual, perhaps due to a growth spurt (typically around three weeks, six weeks, three months, and six months). These frequent-feeding days can be tiring, but they won't last forever. Try to take good care of yourself by eating well and resting whenever possible. If you continue to feed Baby when he is hungry, your body will increase milk production to meet his needs, he'll become satisfied, and he will return to a more manageable feeding routine.

For some Mamas, the seemingly constant demands of feeding and mothering can be overwhelming and even isolating. If you start to feel this way, be sure to talk to other breast-feeding Mamas, especially those who have babies older than yours. Realizing that you're not alone and talking to women who have made it through the challenges of the early days of motherhood will make you feel better.

Here are some ballpark figures to help you understand how often you can reasonably expect to be feeding Baby:

| Baby's Age | Baby Will Probably Eat: | Typical Number of Feedings in 24 Hours |
|---|---|---|
| Birth to 2 months | Every 2 to 3 hours | 8 to 12 |
| 2 to 3 months | Every 2 to 4 hours | 7 to 9 |
| 3 to 6 months | Every 3 to 4 hours | 6 to 8 |
| 6 to 12 months | Every 4 to 6 hours | 4 to 5 |
| 12 months and older | Varies, depending on the child | |

## How Long to Feed

At first, feed Baby from both the left and the right breasts, and alternate which one you start with. Let Baby feed for as long as he wants on the first side. When he stops swallowing or pulls off the breast, you can burp him and then put him back on the other side for as long as he wants. While he's eating, watch how he sucks and swallows. Try to figure out how he acts when he needs to be burped. Over time, probably rather quickly, you will learn how to read his cues, and you will figure out how long he likes to nurse, when to switch sides, and when to take a burping break.

There's no rule for how quickly a baby will finish a feeding. Some babies eat slowly, while others can drain a breast in no time at all. Newborns may take a long time to feed because they aren't very efficient at sucking and swallowing yet, plus they tend to doze off in the middle. After a couple of weeks, however, most babies can get a full feeding in less than thirty minutes—about fifteen minutes on each side. Older babies may be able to get a full feeding in just ten minutes per side. This isn't to say you should cut him off after ten or fifteen minutes, but if he seems to be full and ends the feeding after that amount of time, you can be fairly confident that he has indeed had enough.

Some babies will want to suck for what seems like an eternity. If you feel like your feedings are lasting way too long, observe Baby for clues about what's going on. Is he sucking *and* swallowing for the whole time? If so, maybe he's just a slow eater. At some point he may be done with the milk and stop swallowing but continue sucking for comfort. If you're OK with that, you don't have to do anything about it. Or you can offer a pacifier if you are sure Baby isn't still hungry and you find it doesn't interfere with his latch.

After the first few weeks, some babies may want to nurse only on one side per feeding. As long as Baby is growing well this is fine. Alternate sides so Baby is taking equally from both sides over the course of the day.

## Is Baby Getting Enough?

We know that most babies take anywhere from twenty to thirty ounces of breast milk per day during the first year. Older babies tend to take less, around fifteen to twenty ounces per day, on average. If you're nursing

Baby (as opposed to pumping and serving), it can be disconcerting to never really know how much milk Baby is getting. When he's particularly fussy or you feel that he's not acting "normal," you may wonder if he's hungry. How can you tell? Look for these clues:

1. *The clock.* During the first two months, is he feeding at least eight times in twenty-four hours and sucking (and swallowing) for at least twenty minutes? During Baby's third month, is he feeding at least seven times in twenty-four hours?
2. *The baby.* After Baby pulls off the breast and is burped and changed, is he content? A common term we use for a filled-up baby is "milk drunk." Baby is asleep with milk dripping out of his mouth. Or awake but relaxed and calm, with milk dripping. Or does he seem restless and frantic to continue sucking?
3. *The diapers.* What goes in must come out! If baby has five to eight wet diapers a day, it means she's likely getting enough milk. As for dirty diapers, until around six weeks old, Baby should have three to four dirty diapers a day. After that, anywhere from one to four is considered normal, though it's not necessarily a problem if Baby goes several days without a dirty diaper. Up to seven to ten days can be normal for some babies. Most stools should be yellow with a consistency of gourmet mustard or cottage cheese, with some surrounding liquid.
4. *The growth chart.* Perhaps the best way to make sure Baby is getting enough is to watch his growth. If your pediatrician is concerned, he'll let you know.

| Age | Growth |
|---|---|
| Birth to 1 week | Regain to birth weight by day 10 |
| 1 week to 4 months | 5 to 6 ounces per week |
| 4 to 6 months | 4 to 5 ounces per week |
| 6 to 12 months | 2 to 4 ounces per week |

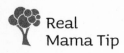
Unfortunately, low milk supply is a common reason Mamas stop breast-feeding earlier than six months or one year. More often than not, however, a low milk supply is not due to anything biological or physical. Problems with low supply are usually due to infrequent and incomplete feedings, not Mama's anatomy. This is good news because it means that the vast majority of women who want to breast-feed are able to make enough milk to do so successfully. A small number of Mamas may struggle to make enough milk even if they're doing everything "right." This could be due to a previous breast surgery, a hormone imbalance, or some unknown problem. If you feel that you fall into this category, a lactation consultant may be able to help you with some strategies for prolonging breast-feeding and maximizing your supply.

## MYTH OR FACT?

*Giving a baby a pacifier or bottle too soon can cause "nipple confusion."*

Fact. Although some newborn babies are unfazed by an artificial nipple, like a pacifier or a bottle, studies do show that introducing them too early can threaten breast-feeding.[20–23] This could be because Baby is in fact "confused" by the different kind of sucking that is required by a pacifier or bottle nipple versus a breast nipple. Or, it could be because the pacifier is used too often as a substitute for the breast and Baby doesn't end up sucking at the breast as much as she should to stimulate milk production. If you decide to give Baby a pacifier early on, make sure you're feeding Baby often enough and not using the pacifier as a way to prolong the time between feeds. To be really safe, wait to introduce a bottle or pacifier until you feel that breast-feeding is well established. This means that it's going well for you and for Baby, and she is latching on correctly, feeding well, and gaining weight. For some Mama-baby pairs this takes only a few weeks, and for most of the others, four to six weeks is enough time.

# Can Baby Get Too Much Milk?

Although it's more common for a Mama to be concerned about having too little milk, sometimes Mamas make too much milk. With oversupply you may have engorged breasts and problems with plugged ducts or mastitis. Baby may be gaining weight fairly quickly, although if it's all from breast milk this is OK. Baby may be fussy at the breast, and may have green and watery stools.

Oversupply usually goes hand in hand with a forceful letdown reflex, when Mama's letdown sends out powerful streams of milk all at once. The forceful flow can cause Baby to gag or choke, pull off the breast right when letdown happens, or to clamp down on the breast as if trying to stop the flow of milk. Baby may be gassy because he swallows too much air when gulping and gagging. If he also has green and watery stools, you may have a foremilk/hindmilk imbalance due to your oversupply. This happens when a large volume of milk is available at each feeding, so Baby becomes full on the foremilk and stops eating before getting enough of the higher-fat hindmilk. The high lactose content of the foremilk, without being balanced by the fat in the hindmilk, can cause gas and green, watery stools.

If you think you have a forceful letdown or oversupply, you can try nursing only on one side per feeding. This may help Baby empty one breast and make it to the high-fat hindmilk. You can also allow Baby to suck for a moment to stimulate your breast and then catch the initial forceful letdown of milk in a burp cloth or towel before putting Baby back on the breast. You can also pump off the first minute or two of letdown milk. To help with the gassiness, burp Baby frequently. Another strategy is to try feeding positions that keep Baby's head higher than his body so gravity isn't working to send milk faster into his mouth. In the cradle hold, instead of sitting up and holding Baby in almost a horizontal position, lean back (support your back with pillows) and let Baby's body rest lower than his head. And hang in there: problems with oversupply tend to go away in time as your body adjusts to Baby's needs and Baby adjusts to your milk flow.

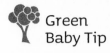

## Green Baby Tip

If Baby takes a pacifier, try the all-natural rubber pacifier from Natursutten (available at many retailers including Giggle, www.giggle.com, and Babies "R" Us, www.babiesrus.com). Other safe BPA-free and phthalate-free options include but are not limited to BornFree's pacifiers (www.newbornfree.com), Gerber's Nuk Classic and Nuk Original (www.gerber.com), and Playtex's Ortho-Pro and Binky pacifiers (www.playtexproducts.com). Check out safeMama.com, a great online resource for parents, for a complete listing of safe pacifiers and teethers.

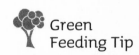

## Green Feeding Tip

Reduce breast-feeding-generated waste by using washable breast pads made of such fabric as cotton, wool, or hemp, instead of disposable ones. (And go one better by choosing pads made with organic fabrics like those by Under the Nile, www.underthenile.com.)

# Vitamins and Minerals for Breast-Fed Babies

Breast milk is designed especially for human babies, and it's meant to be 100 percent nutritionally adequate for babies up to six months old, when solid foods are added to complement the milk. Breast milk contains forms of vitamins and minerals that are very easy for Baby's body to absorb and use. There are only three vitamins or minerals of concern for breast-fed babies who might need a little extra than what they're getting from Mama:

| Vitamin or Mineral | Why It's Needed | How to Provide More |
| --- | --- | --- |
| Vitamin D | Essential for bone health and to help the body make hormones. Exclusively breast-fed babies may need more vitamin D than breast milk alone can provide. | By 2 months, start supplementing with baby vitamin D drops—400 IU per day. Carlson Labs and Sunlight Vitamins make vitamin D-only drops for Baby. |
| Iron | Baby has stored iron from birth and gets sufficient iron in breast milk for the first 6 months. After that, she may need additional iron. | Introduce iron-rich solid foods. Example: HAPPYBELLIES iron-fortified cereals, dried fruits (cooked and pureed), leafy greens, beans, and meats. |
| Fluoride | For healthy teeth. If Baby is exclusively breast-fed after 6 months (no tap water or infant formula), she may need a supplement. | Ask your pediatrician about fluoride drops. Supplementation advice varies according to where you live and how much fluoride is in your water. |

## The Vitamin D Dilemma

If breast milk is supposed to be perfect, why would a breast-fed baby need a vitamin D supplement? Vitamin D is actually a hormone, not a vitamin. It is generated in the skin by exposure to sunlight. Its primary function is to keep calcium levels high in the bloodstream for bone growth. It is also used to make various hormones. In the old days, when babies went outside every day, there was no worry about a deficiency. But now we worry so much about sunlight causing skin cancer that many parents go overboard with sun protection. I chuckle to myself when I see a parent rushing from the grocery store to the car, carefully holding a blanket over the baby so he won't get any "damaging" sun rays.

In my opinion, a baby should get about thirty minutes of unprotected sun exposure every day. This has been shown to be what is needed to generate adequate vitamin D so that a supplement isn't needed. Nature (or God) didn't put very much D into breast milk because he (or she) didn't think we'd become so solarphobic. If your baby doesn't get much sunlight, then supplementing is a good idea. But I prefer the natural way.

# Breast-Feeding as Baby Gets Older

As Baby grows, here are some breast-feeding concerns that may be on your mind:

- *Night feedings and sleep.* All sleep-deprived Mamas eagerly await the night when Baby sleeps through until morning. One way to minimize Baby's need for feeding at night is to feed him enough during the day. Feed on demand, and make sure Baby is getting complete feedings, especially as he starts crawling and playing and is more distractible. At some point, usually when Baby is around six to nine months old, you may sense that at some of Baby's night wakings he needs only comfort, not milk. Instead of instinctually feeding at each waking, try to soothe Baby to sleep in other ways. You may find that you can wean him from night feedings slowly over time this way. It may also help to send your partner to Baby's side for soothing since Baby may demand milk at the sight of you. Of course, there is nothing wrong with simply plugging Baby in at night with each waking, if you don't mind having to do this until Baby is weaned.

- *Teeth and biting.* Sometimes when babies get teeth, they try to bite their nursing Mamas. The first time it happens to you, you'll see that it doesn't tickle! Try to stay calm and gently take Baby off the breast. You can say, "No biting," or you can say nothing if you prefer. After being pulled off a few times Baby should figure it out. Babies can't suck and bite at the same time so you should also watch baby carefully, and when he stops sucking, take him off the breast for a break or to end the feeding. An easy way to get your chomping baby to let go of the breast is to pull his face in close so he can't breathe. He'll have to open his mouth and pull away.

- *Distractibility.* When Baby reaches about four months you may notice that he easily becomes distracted while nursing. The family dog, an older sibling, or a talking parent is suddenly far more interesting than mealtime. At Baby's young age you don't have to worry that he won't get enough or that any shortened feeds may interfere with his growth or your milk supply. Baby's appetite will make sure he gets enough. Help him focus on the task at hand by nursing him in a quiet spot, turning down the lights, and removing all distractions.

Another distracting age is between eight and twelve months,

when Baby becomes mobile. It's far more fun to crawl or walk around and play than nurse. He'll check in with you every so often for a quick nursing snack, but you may find that any serious feeding is reserved for going down for a nap, bedtime, and waking up in the morning. You may experience a decrease in your milk supply, and this is OK. You can let the laws of supply and demand determine how much milk you will continue to produce. Don't take Baby's lack of interest as a sign he wants to wean. Just continue to nurse according to his cues.

## Bottling Your Breast Milk

You may not always be able to be with Baby at feeding time, especially as he gets older and you get back to some of the activities you were involved in before he arrived. Luckily for busy Mamas everywhere, someone invented the breast pump.

Some dads like to take part in feeding Baby, and pumping is a nice way to let Dad share in this duty (especially at night, right?). But don't feel that you *have* to routinely pump to let Dad bottle-feed in order for him to bond better with Baby. If you are exclusively breast-feeding, it's true that you'll have a lot more snuggle time with Baby than anyone else in the household. But there is plenty of time throughout the day for Dad to hold and play with Baby besides feeding time. Dad or others can snuggle, rock Baby, sing to Baby—all great for bonding. Dad can even take off his shirt and hold Baby close for some skin-to-skin contact of his own. If Dad does want to be able to bottle-feed on occasion, wait until Baby is at least one month old and breast-feeding is going well before you introduce a bottle.

Whether you are pumping early on because of nursing challenges, or you need to routinely provide Baby with pumped milk because you also work outside the home, or you want to occasionally leave a bottle with your spouse or a friend to feed Baby so you can have more than two hours of freedom, here are some basic guidelines for pumping, storing, and feeding Baby your milk:

## WHEN SHOULD I PUMP?

There's no blanket rule about when to pump, but here are some suggestions:

| Your Situation | When to Pump |
|---|---|
| You need to begin storing up milk before your return to work or travel | Pick 1 or 2 feedings a day (morning feedings may work best when your supply is high) and pump after Baby finishes. |
| You're going to miss one feeding | Pump in the morning, when your supply is highest. Be sure to nurse right before you leave. |
| Baby isn't eating well because she's sick, teething, or distracted | Pump after Baby feeds, in order to empty your breasts and keep up your supply. |
| You're away from Baby for extended periods of time (e.g., at work) | Pump at least every 4 hours or whenever Baby would be nursing. |

## HOW DO I PUMP?

If pumping after Baby has breast-fed, you can either pump out the rest of the milk on the side Baby didn't finish, or do double-sided pumping. If pumping instead of feeding Baby, double-sided pumping is best. Either way, pump for at least ten to fifteen minutes or until milk flow stops.

## HOW DO I STORE THE MILK?

Most pumps hook up to either storage bags or plastic bottles for catching the expressed milk. To determine where it should go next, decide when you'll likely use the milk:

- *Within ten hours:* Leave the milk on the counter to remain at room temperature (out of any hot sunlight) until Baby drinks the bottle.
- *After ten hours but within eight days:* Store the milk in the fridge. You can pour it into the bottle that you will use for feeding or keep it in the bag or pump bottle for now. If you have more than one bag or bottle in the fridge at a time, label them with the date and time so you can keep track of which you need to use first.
- *More than eight days from now:* Freeze the milk. Freeze in breast milk storage bags or freezer-safe breast milk storage containers. Most that you'll find on the market today are bisphenol A (BPA) free, but check to be sure. Freeze milk in small quantities—one to two ounces for newborns, three- to four-ounce portions for older babies. You want to avoid having to thaw out more than you need at a time. Label frozen milk containers with the date so you can always use the oldest milk first.

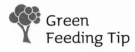

## Green Feeding Tip

For more eco-friendly breast milk storage, freeze milk in small plastic bottles that are free of harmful chemicals, such as bisphenol A (BPA), rather than disposable plastic sandwich bags, which just end up in landfills. When you no longer need the bottles for breast milk storage you can use them to store arts and crafts supplies, herbs, or other small objects. Or find a recycling facility that will take them.

## HOW LONG IS THE MILK GOOD FOR?

For full-term and healthy babies, here are the storage guidelines for expressed milk:

| | |
|---|---|
| Freshly pumped, at room temperature (66–72 degrees) | 10 hours (less if warmer room) |
| Freshly pumped and stored in the refrigerator (don't store in or near door) | 7 days |
| Thawed from frozen, stored in the refrigerator (don't store in or near door) | 24 hours |
| Frozen in a typical freezer (don't store in or near door) | 3–6 months |
| Frozen in a deep freezer | 6–12 months |

Source: La Leche League International, *The Breastfeeding Answer Book.*

# SAFER BOTTLES FOR BABY

By now you've probably heard about the dangers of some types of plastic baby bottles. Clear bottles made of polycarbonate plastic (labeled with a number 7) contain bisphenol A (BPA), an endocrine disrupter that can leach into Baby's milk or formula. The FDA has announced that the current levels of exposure to BPA are safe for our children even though the National Toxicology Program's studies concluded that BPA poses "some concern" over the effects on the brain, on behavior, and on the prostate gland. Critics of the FDA's decision express concern that the FDA's analysis of BPA doesn't include certain types of studies that are more sensitive to certain health concerns. We know BPA leaches into the milk and formula, and we know it's a harmful chemical. Just because the FDA says it's not harmful enough to warrant avoiding doesn't mean it's OK for your baby. We believe using BPA-free bottles is a worthwhile precaution.

Luckily, avoiding BPA in bottles is easy these days. Traditional glass bottles are always an option. If you're concerned about Baby dropping and shattering the glass, the bottles by Babylife (the Wee-go bottles), NurturePure, and Siliskin have nifty silicone sleeves to protect them. If you want to stick with plastic, simply look for bottles labeled BPA-free like the ones from the following companies:

- Adiri Natural Nurser
- Green to Grow—all bottles
- Born Free—all bottles
- Thinkbaby—all bottles
- Dr. Brown's BPA-free line
- Avent's BPA-free line
- Medela—all bottles
- Playtex Original Nurser and Drop-In Liners
- Playtex VentAire Advanced
- Nûby—all bottles

Most bottle manufacturers say that their products are dishwasher safe, but we recommend against regularly exposing any plastics, even BPA-free ones, to the high temperatures of the dishwasher.

## HOW DO I THAW FROZEN MILK?

The best way is to put it into the refrigerator. It will take about twelve hours to thaw. You can also run cool water over the container to thaw more quickly. Don't microwave breast milk because it breaks down some of the beneficial components in the milk. Heating breast milk in a pan on the stove disrupts the milk's proteins and can scald the milk, so skip that method, too. And don't leave it out on the counter to thaw because being at room temperature for too long can encourage the growth of bacteria. Thaw only what you need because you cannot refreeze the milk—if you don't use it in a timely fashion (see table), you have to pour it down the drain (the horror!).

## WHAT TEMPERATURE SHOULD THE MILK BE?

When Baby gets his milk straight from your breast, it comes out pretty warm—your body temp is 98.6 degrees. You don't have to test the milk with a thermometer. Just make sure it's at least slightly warm and can be easily sipped without feeling too hot. At the very least the milk should have the chill taken out. You can heat breast milk bottles using a bottle warmer or by placing the bottle into a bowl of warm water.

## WHY DOES THE MILK LOOK FUNNY?

It's normal for breast milk to separate with a creamy layer at the top. Just swirl the bottle before serving to combine the layers. Don't shake it vigorously because this may actually damage the proteins in the milk.

## HOW MUCH MILK SHOULD I PUT INTO THE BOTTLE FOR FEEDING?

It's impossible to know exactly how much milk Baby will take at a feeding, though we do know that most babies under age one take twenty to thirty ounces a day. Here's how to guess how much to give in a bottle:

| 1. Assume that Baby's intake is the average—25 ounces per day. | 2. Divide 25 ounces by the number of times Baby tends to eat per day. | 3. Round down to the nearest whole or half number. |

You will learn how much Baby likes to take through trial and error. Offer two to four ounces. If Baby is still sucking on the bottle after the milk is gone, he probably needed another one-half to one ounce. If Baby doesn't finish the milk in the bottle, you know you can probably prepare a little less next time. You can serve any unfinished milk at Baby's next feeding, as long as it's only a few hours later. (The same is not true for formula, which needs to be discarded if not finished.)

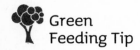

**Green Feeding Tip**

Reduce electricity use by forgoing the bottle warmer. Heat Baby's bottles the old-fashioned way: in a bowl of warm water on the counter.

## BREAST-FEEDING IN ALL SHADES OF GREEN

*The palest green:* Breast-feed. There. You're green!

*A little greener:* Use BPA-free plastics for storage and feeding of expressed breast milk. If you have to supplement with formula, choose a powdered organic iron-fortified formula with added DHA (docosahexaenoic acid) and lactose as the sugar source (see below for a full discussion about formula).

*The deepest shade of green:* Choose glass bottles for feeding Baby expressed milk, and breast-feed Baby until he's at least twelve months old so that he never needs infant formula. Use reusable organic cotton breast pads instead of disposables.

# Weaning

There's no set age when you have to wean Baby from the breast. If you wean before Baby reaches his first birthday, you will need to transition him to infant formula. If you wait until Baby is a year or older, Baby goes straight from breast milk to whole milk. Either way, it's best to wean gradually to give Baby and your body time to adjust to the change. Here are a few tips:

- The most natural way to wean is called the "don't offer, don't refuse" technique. You nurse Baby whenever he asks, but you don't specifically offer to nurse. This doesn't mean you have to drop everything and nurse him every time he demands it. It's OK to be "too busy" if you are in the middle of something. This approach usually extends nursing well beyond twelve months and often until age two years.

- If you really feel ready to wean but Baby isn't slowing down, you can continue the above technique but offer more distractions. You don't need to say no to Baby when he asks, but you can say, "OK, but first Mommy is going to get a drink of water." Or take a walk outside, go get the mail, make yourself a sandwich. Get Baby interested in whatever you are doing. When you are done, immediately move on to something else. Don't sit down. Stay busy. Baby may often forget he asked to nurse. Of course, you will eventually have to settle into a nursing depending on how adamant Baby is. Over a few weeks this approach can limit the nursing to the primary times a baby really needs that comfort: before a nap or bedtime, waking at night, and first thing in the morning.

- If you wean gradually, over a month or two, your breasts should naturally decrease their supply. You may find that you need to pump to relieve your breasts on occasion.

- If Baby is younger than a year and you are thinking of weaning quickly, make sure you try Baby on some formula first before you let your milk supply decrease. If Baby is allergic to several different formulas, you may need to go back to breast-feeding. Use a pump to keep your supply going during this trial period.

- If your breasts get engorged, place cool cabbage leaves in your bra to give you relief (a natural component of cabbage decreases milk production). Engorgement shouldn't last too long. After a couple of days your body will get the point and will slow down the milk supply.
- Don't wean too quickly, or else the retained breast milk may stagnate and become infected (causing mastitis). Cut out one breast-feeding every few days until you are down to only once or twice a day. At that point you can have a "last nursing" ceremony and pump only on occasion when the breasts feel full.

Some babies wean very easily to a cup or bottle, others have a hard time with the separation. Try to be patient and be sure to replace the nursing time with plenty of snuggle time, so Baby doesn't miss out on the closeness you once shared while feeding.

A NOTE FROM DR. BOB

## Cherish These Baby Years

My first child nursed until he was two. The second and third children continued until they were three, but for the entire last year it was really only a once a day at bedtime snuggle routine. My wife and kids were able to cherish this special time without it draining all her energy. I have patients who extend nursing beyond age three or four, and that's OK. There is really no upper limit on the number of years a child can nurse. Well, it would be best if you wean your "baby" before he or she goes on a first date.

# Combination Feeding

We know that not all Mamas will choose to breast-feed exclusively for the first six months and then continue for the next six or more. Many will attempt some kind of combination of breast-feeding, breast milk bottles, and formula bottles. If part-time nursing appeals to you, it's best to wait until breast-feeding is well established before you start to introduce formula. You'll want to make sure you have established a good supply of breast milk before cutting back in any way so that you have enough milk for whatever combination of feeding methods you decide you want to do. If you are supplementing because of milk supply problems from the start, try to keep the supply you do have going for as long as you can.

If weaning before age one, you'll need to replace nursings with formula. Follow the steps we've outlined above for weaning. Gradually eliminate whatever number of feedings you have chosen and replace with formula. Most of the time, a Mama's body will adjust the milk supply to part-time nursing. As long as feedings are complete and regular, she will be able to maintain a supply for as long as she wants to continue to breast-feed. If you're feeding Baby with formula some of the time and at the breast at other times, keep Baby's bottles outfitted with slow-flow nipples so she doesn't start to favor the fast, easy bottle over the slower breast.

# Tips for Overcoming Breastfeeding Challenges

Mamas who breast-feed know that it can be a wonderful experience for Mama and Baby alike, but it isn't always easy. Even though Baby was indeed born to breast-feed, it doesn't mean necessarily that there will be no bumps in the road. Thankfully, there are very few breast-feeding problems that can't be overcome. Here is a list of some challenges new Mamas may face when breast-feeding:

*Nipple pain:* Although breast-feeding isn't *supposed* to hurt, we think it's safe to say that many new Mamas will have some pain in the early weeks, when Baby latches on, for example, or when water hits your nipples in the shower. If Baby is latched on correctly (you can have a lactation consultant check for you to be sure), this pain should subside as your body gets used to feeding over the first few weeks. In the meantime, try the following:

- Avoid washing your nipples with soap since this can dry them out and cause more pain.

A NOTE FROM DR. BOB

## A Lactation Consultant Is Worth Her Weight in . . . Milk!

In my practice I find that at least 25 percent of first-time moms experience latching-on problems or other nursing challenges that warrant a visit with a lactation consultant. Don't take this as a failure. Babies are born knowing how to suck but not necessarily how to latch on correctly. An LC can be a real lifesaver, and money saver. Spending one or two hundred dollars to have an LC help you achieve exclusive and long-term breast-feeding can save you many hundreds of dollars in formula and health-care costs down the road. Many health insurance plans will reimburse you for this. Try to find a consultant who is board certified with the letters IBCLC (International Board Certified Lactation Consultant) after her name. You can also receive free breast-feeding advice over the phone from La Leche League International, or attend a meeting with an LLL group in your area. Visit www.LLLI.org to find a group or advice line in your area.

- Moisturize your nipples with purified hypoallergenic lanolin ointment.
- Express a little milk to rub into your nipples after feeds.
- After feeding, keep your bra open for a while to give your nipples some fresh air.
- If pain continues for several weeks, talk to your doctor or lactation consultant.
- If you have several weeks of pain-free nursing and then feel nipple pain again out of the blue, it could be due to thrush, an overgrowth of yeast. Talk to your doctor for treatment options.

*Other pains: plugged ducts and breast infections.* The most challenging thing about complications during breast-feeding is that you have to continue to mother and feed your baby while you're feeling under the weather or dealing with discomfort. What's best for Baby is also best for Mama in these situations: nursing Baby frequently is usually the best way to speed your healing.

*Plugged ducts.* Sometimes milk builds up in a milk duct in the breast, creating a lump that is tender to the touch. Plugged ducts tend to happen when your breast isn't fully emptied at a feeding or if you go a long stretch without feeding Baby. Underwire bras or tight clothing over the breasts can contribute to the problem, too. Usually, a plugged duct will soften and be alleviated when Baby feeds. If it's stubborn, apply moist heat (like a warm wet washcloth) to the area for fifteen minutes before a feeding. You can also gently massage the area while Baby feeds to try to clear the duct. Be sure to nurse frequently enough, and start each feeding on the side that's affected. Alternating the direction Baby is lying while feeding on the affected breast will also help drain the plugged area (for example, shift between the cradle hold and the football hold). Any breast lump that doesn't go away after a week should be seen by a physician.

*Breast infection (mastitis).* This infection in the breast is caused by bacteria and can happen when germs from Baby's mouth or your own skin enter your breast through a cracked nipple, or when bacteria multiply in milk that's stuck in a plugged duct. Incomplete emptying of the breast at feedings puts you at risk. Mastitis feels like the flu—headache, body aches and pains, chills, and fever. Your breasts may get red and tender, too. If you have these symptoms, call your doctor. You can get antibiotics and feel better within twenty-four hours. Feeding Baby during a breast infection will not make him sick. In fact, frequent feeding is recommended. If nursing is too painful, use a pump to empty the breast instead and feed Baby the expressed milk.

*Nursing in public.* Whether or not it's appropriate for a Mama to nurse her baby in public is often a topic of great debate, but the idea of having to be home for every single feeding for a year is a bit absurd, no? Out of respect for others around you who may not be comfortable, try to be as discreet as you feel is appropriate. You can buy a nursing cover-up or use a basic baby blanket to hide your goods from the guy across the room. One trick that works well is to wear a lightweight cardigan sweater over your other shirt while you're nursing—it helps to cover up the skin that is exposed when you lift your shirt. Fortunately, many states have passed laws that guarantee a mother's right to nurse her baby in any public place.

*Nursing number two (or three or four . . . ).* When your new baby isn't your first baby, you may find that breast-feeding Baby is the easy part—it's taking care of the older sibling(s) that's really a challenge. Fortunately, breast-feeding leaves you with at least one spare hand (two, if you're really adept) for wiping noses, reading books, even getting your toddler dressed. If an older sibling is feeling displaced by the new baby's breast-feeding time, make your feedings into a special time for the older child, too. Have

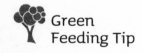

## Green Feeding Tip

If you buy a nursing cover-up, you can choose one made with organic cotton, such as the ones available from the Undercover Baby (www.theunder coverbaby.com) and Bébé au Lait (www.bebeaulait .com).

# Yeast Infection in the Breasts

Any time you take antibiotics, whether during labor (IV antibiotics are commonly given during prolonged labors), to treat mastitis, or for any other illness that comes up, you set yourself up for a vaginal yeast infection. But even more uncomfortable is a yeast infection on the nipples, a very common occurrence when a nursing mom takes antibiotics. The nipples become painful and burn, both while nursing and in between. You may feel shooting pains through the breasts. The yeast from your breasts can also get into Baby's mouth and cause thrush. The best way to prevent this is to take probiotics (ask anyone at a health food store) for about a month during and after the antibiotics. If you do feel burning and pain coming on, apply an over-the-counter antifungal cream (clotrimazole) three times a day after a nursing, and dab a bit of a solution of one ounce white vinegar in eight ounces of water onto each nipple after each nursing. This will help kill the yeast. You can also give Baby an infant probiotic powder available at any health food store. Make a paste with about one-quarter teaspoon of powder with some pumped milk or water, and use your finger to place it into Baby's mouth twice a day to kill any yeast that is likely starting to grow. If you don't improve after several days, speak with your doctor about antifungal medication.

him sit next to you on the couch, read favorite books, or do simple games while you nurse. Depending on the older sibling's age and your family's TV policy, that may be a nice time to let him watch a few minutes of a favorite television show or video.

## A Tip for Taming Sibling Jealousy

Many parents ask me how they can limit the sibling jealousy of a toddler or preschooler when baby number two comes along. One easy way is to avoid interrupting anything you are doing with your older child in order to tend to the baby. Of course, you'll be doing that all day long, but you can do it without your child feeling that the baby is the cause. Whenever your time with your toddler is interrupted by one of Baby's many needs, such as hunger or a dirty diaper, tend to Baby's need right where you are as you continue your interaction with your child. If you are playing a game together, change or nurse Baby right there on the floor as you play. Try to avoid saying, "Wait a few minutes, Johnny, I need to _____ (insert task) *the baby*," or "I can't do that with you right now, I have to _____ *the baby*." Whenever you do say "the baby," make sure it is in a positive light.

# All About Formula

We know there are some circumstances under which breast-feeding is either not possible or not a positive choice for a Mama and baby. There are also plenty of Mamas who combine breast-feeding with formula feeding for a variety of reasons.

Infant formula is second best to breast milk, but of course it's nutritionally adequate and also safe. If you plan to feed Baby with formula, either all the time or as a supplement to breast-feeding, this section is for you. We'll tell you which formulas are best for Baby and show you

## DRESSED TO FEED: NURSING APPAREL

Technically, you don't need any particular piece of clothing to breast-feed Baby. Most Mamas will agree, though, that at least one or two good nursing bras are essential. Your breasts will be inflated, so proper fit and support are important. Toward the end of your pregnancy you can purchase a nursing bra to use right after birth. For the best fit possible, though, wait to purchase the rest of your nursing bras until after your milk comes in at the end of Baby's first week. If possible, go to a shop that either specializes in nursing bras or at least has a very good fitting service. Avoid underwires, as they can cause plugged ducts and discomfort. For green nursing bras, check out Under the Nile (www.underthenile.com) organic cotton nursing bras, and Bravado! Designs (www.bravadodesigns.com) and Motherwear (www.motherwear.com) nursing bras and tanks made from bamboo fibers, a sustainable and green textile material. If you find you need some new clothes to fit your new breast-feeding breasts, here are some tips to keep in mind:

- There are shirts and dresses designed for nursing mothers. They are by no means required, but some Mamas like the ease of nursing in these garments. If you're interested, check out companies like Belabumbum (www.belabumbum.com) and Japanese Weekend (www.japaneseweekend.com).
- Avoid tops that tie at the waist, have belts, or are too tight to pull up.
- Dresses that don't unbutton or otherwise open at the top can be problematic. Keep in mind that you'll have to lift the dress all the way up to feed Baby.
- Patterned shirts are nice because they may hide drops of milk.
- Protect your clothes by wearing breast pads in your bra to catch any leaks.

why organic formula, though certainly green, may not always be the best option.

## SELECTING A FORMULA

The formula section at the store has expanded in recent years. You will find as many as twenty-six different varieties! How do you choose which is best? All infant formulas are similar in their overall nutrient content

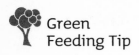
because they're required by the U.S. Food and Drug Administration to contain the same level of protein, fat, carbohydrates, vitamins, and minerals. What differs from brand to brand is the ingredient list.

Most babies, unless your pediatrician advises you otherwise, should get an iron-fortified milk-based formula. Also look for one with added DHA and ARA (arachidonic acid), the omega-3 fatty acid that is found in breast milk and is essential for Baby's brain and eye development.

### Cow's Milk Formulas

The proteins in these formulas—casein and whey—come from cow's milk and have been altered so Baby can digest them (straight cow's milk itself is not recommended until Baby is around a year old because it's not well tolerated). The ratio of casein to whey varies slightly from formula to formula, each trying to mimic most closely the protein profile of breast milk. Standard cow's milk formulas like Earth's Best Organic milk-based formula, Similac Advance, and Enfamil Lipil have mostly casein protein. Other cow's milk formulas are made with a blend of hydrolyzed, or broken-down, proteins that are intended to be better tolerated in babies with sensitive stomachs, for example, Good Start Supreme, Enfamil Gentlease Lipil, or Similac Sensitive. Cow's milk formulas contain milk sugars (lactose) as the carbohydrate source, and each has a slightly different blend of vegetable oils as the fat source. A standard cow's milk protein is a good first formula to try with Baby, as most babies will tolerate it.

### Soy Formulas

These formulas have soy protein instead of casein or whey from cow's milk, so they are an option for vegan families. Rather than lactose (milk sugar) as the carbohydrate source, soy formulas contain sucrose (table sugar) or other sugars.

Although soy formulas are offered as an alternative for babies who don't tolerate cow's milk formulas, we hesitate to recommend them because we know that babies thrive best on milk proteins and milk sugar. Experts don't fully understand the effects of starting babies out on a

## RECENT SCARE: MELAMINE IN INFANT FORMULA

During summer 2008, tens of thousands of Chinese babies were sickened by infant formula contaminated with melamine, an industrial chemical that was being used as a proteinlike filler by unscrupulous formula manufacturers. Months later, after an FDA investigation, traces of melamine were found in a few U.S.-made infant formulas, too, evidently the result of industrial processes, not intentionally added. Fortunately, no U.S. babies became sick from these trace amounts. The level of melamine in the U.S. formulas was a tiny fraction of the levels found in China, and many experts at the FDA consider the levels to be too small to cause any harm.[25] Still, we're not thrilled about babies ingesting *any* melamine so we see this as yet another reason to breast-feed Baby for as long as possible.

diet of soy as their only protein and sugar source. There isn't any scientific proof that soy formula is dangerous to babies, but there isn't good indication that they are helpful, either. They won't help prevent cow's milk allergy, as once thought. Besides, we know that babies who are allergic to milk have a high chance of being sensitive to soy, too. And lactose intolerance is so rare in babies (lactose is the sugar in breast milk, after all) that this is not typically a good reason to switch to soy formulas either. So, the bottom line on soy formulas is that for babies who don't tolerate other formulas, they can be a fine option, but they shouldn't be your first choice. With your doctor's guidance you should try switching to another formula after a month or two of soy.

## Elemental Formulas

These formulas contain proteins that have been fully broken down so that Baby doesn't have to digest them. Enfamil Nutramigen Lipil and Similac Alimentum are two examples. They are considered to be hypoallergenic, so they may be a good option if Baby doesn't tolerate standard cow's milk formulas. Your pediatrician may recommend these formulas if Baby has significant gastroesophageal reflux, eczema, early asthma, or malabsorption problems.

## Organic Formulas Aren't Always Better—Read the Ingredients

Some name-brand organic formulas use corn syrup or brown rice syrup as their sugar instead of lactose, since these syrups are less expensive. This is *not* a wise nutritional move for Baby. Be sure the organic formula you choose uses milk lactose as the sugar source.

### Organic Formulas

These formulas are made with organic ingredients so they are pesticide-free and eco-friendly options. Most of the organic formula brands, such as Earth's Best, Bright Beginnings, and Baby's Only Organic, offer a standard cow's milk formula (made from organic cow's milk that contains no synthetic hormones or antibiotics) and organic soy formula options.

### Formula with Added Probiotics

Adding probiotics to formula is a recent idea, and soon all formulas will likely have them. Today, you'll find them in Good Start Supreme Natural Cultures. These "friendly" bacteria, found naturally in breast milk, help protect Baby against stomach bugs and other infections, and may help protect against food allergies and other allergic disease.

## Bottle-Feeding Basics

All babies have their own appetites and feeding preferences. Just as when you are breast-feeding, with bottle-feeding you have to follow Baby's lead:

- Don't be rigid with a feeding schedule. Instead, carefully observe Baby and respond to his hunger cues.
- Never force Baby to finish a bottle after he's full.
- If Baby is sucking the last drops out of most bottles, this is a clue to start adding another ounce or two.
- Don't expect Baby to drink the same amount of formula at each and every feeding.

If you're formula-feeding your newborn, keep in mind that Baby's stomach is tiny—only about the size of his fist. So start with one to two ounces at a feeding and feed every two to three hours. As he grows, the volume in each bottle will increase (eventually to six to eight ounces per feeding) and feedings will spread out.

Use these guidelines to help you figure out how much to offer Baby at each feeding and then allow Baby to decide when he's had enough. During growth spurts—typically at three weeks, six weeks, three months, and six months—Baby may want to eat even more.

| Baby's Age | Typical Bottle Volume | Typical Bottle Spacing | Typical 24-hour Intake |
|---|---|---|---|
| 0 to 1 month | 1.5 to 3 ounces | Every 2 to 3 hours | Baby's weight (in pounds) x 2.5 ounces = approx. 24-hour intake (example: 10 lb. baby = 25 oz./day) |
| 1 to 2 months | 3 to 4 ounces | Every 3 hours | |
| 3 to 6 months | 4 to 6 ounces | Every 4 hours | |
| 7 to 12 months | 6 to 8 ounces | Every 4 hours | 32 ounces per day (some will want more) |

## SAFE BOTTLE PREPARATION TIPS

Follow these best practices when preparing Baby's formula bottles:

- Always wash your hands well before preparing or feeding a bottle.

# BOTTLED OR TAP?

The question of which type of water to use for reconstituting powdered formula is not an easy one to answer. The quick eco-conscious answer would be to use tap water because bottled water creates about two million tons of plastic landfill waste each year, and plastic bottle production and shipment requires petroleum, a nonrenewable resource. Unfortunately, it's not so simple. A 2005 study by the Environmental Working Group, an independent nonprofit organization, found that tap water in forty-two states contained contaminants including 260 chemicals such as pesticides, industrial toxins, and even pharmaceuticals.[26] These contaminants are concerning for vulnerable consumers like babies, pregnant women, and people with weakened immune systems. So what are we to do? Here's how to sort it all out:

- Find out if your tap water could be contaminated. You can search for your water utility on the EWG's Web site, www.ewg.org/sites/tapwater/. You could also have your tap water or well water tested by a professional. Call the EPA's safe drinking water hotline (1-800-436-4791) to find a testing lab near you or visit www.epa.gov/safewater/labs. You can also purchase home testing kits that can detect some contaminants, such as pesticides, lead, chlorine, bacteria, and nitrates. We recommend Watersafe's All-In-One Drinking Water Test Kit.
- Use a home filtration system (either faucet mounted, pitcher style, or the under-the-sink kind) to remove certain contaminants from your tap water. Look for one that is NSF Standard 53 certified, and then maintain the filter (and change it) as the label directs. A list of all certified filters is found on the NSF Web site, www.nsf.org.
- If Baby gets infant formula exclusively, use fluoride-free water to mix it until she's six months old, and then talk to your pediatrician about whether to continue using fluoride-free water. The concern is that between the fluoride in the formula itself and the fluoridated tap water, Baby could get excessive fluoride, leading to mottling of her teeth (when they eventually come in). If your tap water comes from a fluoridated municipal source, a reverse osmosis water filter will remove the fluoride or you can use bottled distilled or demineralized water instead.
- If you decide to go with bottled water for any reason, make sure you purchase a brand that comes from a clean source. The Natural Resources Defense Council has found that up to 30 percent of all bottled water is just tap water in disguise.[27] The label has to tell you where it's from, but if you can't figure it out, call the bottler directly. Visit bottled water companies' Web sites or call their customer service hotlines to learn about their quality control standards before choosing a brand. Then buy the largest containers possible to minimize the plastic waste.

- Follow preparation and storage instructions on the formula label. Most powdered formula is prepared by adding a level but unpacked scoop of powder for every two ounces of water.
- If formula is at room temperature for more than an hour, discard.
- Prepared formula can stay in the fridge for up to forty-eight hours after mixing.
- If a partial bottle is left at the end of a feeding, discard.
- Store powder formula in a cool dry place like a cool pantry. Use open containers of powder within a month.
- After heating a bottle, always test the temperature before giving to Baby. Heating in the microwave is not recommended because "hot spots" can form and can burn Baby's mouth or throat.
- Never send an older baby to bed with a bottle. This can lead to "bottle rot"—tooth decay caused by milk sugars sitting on Baby's teeth during the night.
- Don't bottle-feed a baby when he's lying down. This can allow formula to drip back into Baby's eustachian tubes (tubes that connect the back of the nose to the inner ears) and could increase his risk of an ear infection.
- Don't leave a baby unattended during any type of feeding. Baby could choke and need assistance.

# Transitioning Away from Formula

By the time Baby turns one year old, his solid food intake will become more nutritionally significant than his liquid feedings. As a result, he doesn't need the high vitamin, mineral, and nutrient levels provided by formula. Instead, cow's milk (or an alternative like goat's milk or soy milk) is recommended, unless Baby is allergic to certain milk proteins. Whole cow's or goat's milk is rich in calcium, vitamin D, and protein, and will provide the fat Baby still needs for his developing brain and

# Don't Got Milk?

Many parents believe their toddler has to start drinking milk in order to be healthy. That is not really true. Milk provides a convenient source of calcium and fat, but there are plenty of other ways for Baby to get those besides milk. Yogurt and cheese are just as good. Dark green veggies have calcium; so do alternative milks like soy, almond, or rice milk. A toddler needs about two servings of something high in calcium every day. It doesn't have to be milk. Toddlers can also get plenty of fat from whole-fat yogurt and cheese, eggs, meat, fish, and nut butters (not peanut until age two years). See page 208 for more foods with calcium and page 210 for other healthy fatty foods.

nervous system. Babies from age one year to two years need at least two cups (sixteen ounces) of milk or the equivalent calcium source each day. We, of course, recommend choosing organic. For more on milk and other beverage choices for Baby, flip to page 217.

It is best to limit regular milk intake to no more than twenty-four ounces each day; sixteen ounces is better. More than that can irritate Baby's intestines, interfere with digestion of certain nutrients, and lower the appetite for foods. Babies need far less milk than they did formula, since foods should now become the main nutrition source.

Most babies will handle the switch from formula to milk very well. If yours doesn't seem to want the new drink, transition him more slowly by mixing half milk, half formula for a few weeks so he can get used to the taste. Gradually go to one-quarter formula, three-quarters milk, and then all the way to a full bottle or cup of milk.

# Choosing a Sippy Cup

Speaking of bottles and cups . . . age one is also a good time to transition away from nipple bottles and over to cups. Continued use of the bottle isn't recommended because the kind of sucking that Baby does with the nipple can hinder his oral and speech development, and may even lead to an increase in cavities. Plus, bottle or pacifier use beyond eighteen months can increase an overbite. Try to switch over to a cup by simply giving Baby his formula or milk in a cup instead of a bottle. Don't worry if he won't take as much as he did from the bottle; he doesn't need very much. Baby may need a little time to get used to the cup, so be patient. If your baby is particularly attached to one or two bottles, like the first bottle of the day or the one that's part of his bedtime routine, get rid of that one last. (Don't forget to brush Baby's teeth before he lies down, though, or he may get cavities.) You may find that once he's used to drinking from a sippy cup, he gladly relinquishes the bottle. If he resists, let him keep the bottle for now and talk to your pediatrician and dentist about when you should push the issue.

There are plastic cups, metal cups, soft spouts, hard spouts, straws—so many to choose from. If you go for a plastic cup, pick one that doesn't contain any concerning ingredients like BPA, and even though it will likely say "dishwasher safe," we recommend hand washing all plastics that touch Baby's foods or drinks. The stainless steel cups, though sometimes more expensive, can be thrown in the dishwasher, so that may make it worth the cost to you. Speech experts recommend straws instead of spouts to encourage better oral development, so consider one of the many straw cups on the market.

Here is a list of just some of the BPA-free plastic or metal sippy cups available in stores. This isn't an exhaustive list, though. More existing brands are going BPA free as time goes on, and new BPA-free products are coming on the market, too. Check your local baby gear stores for even more safe cups.

| Brand/Cup Name | Cup Material | Spout or Straw Material |
|---|---|---|
| Avent Magic Cup | BPA-free plastic | Hard plastic spout |
| Boon Fluid Toddler Cup | BPA-free plastic | Hard plastic spout |
| BornFree Trainer Cup | BPA-free plastic | Soft plastic spout |
| Foogo by Thermos | Stainless steel | Straw or soft spout made from thermoplastic elastomer (TPE) |
| Gerber Graduates Sip & Smile and Fun Grips Cups | BPA-free plastic | Soft spout made from thermoplastic elastomer (TPE) |
| Klean Kanteen Sippy Cup | Stainless steel | Polypropylene (#5 PP) plastic spout |
| Nalgene Grip-n-Gulp | BPA-free plastic | Polypropylene plastic spout |
| Nûby, various models | BPA-free plastic | Soft silicone spout or flip-top silicone straw |
| NurturePure GrowPure Multi-stage Feeder and Sippy Cup | BPA-free plastic | Converts from nipple to soft spout to straw |
| Playtex (all cups except Baby Einstein Sip & Discover line) | BPA-free plastic | Hard plastic spout and silicone straw are available |
| The Safe Sippy | Stainless steel | Polypropylene (#5 PP) plastic lid and soft spout, silicone valve |
| Sigg | Aluminum | Hard plastic spout |
| The First Years Take & Toss line | BPA-free plastic | Hard plastic spout. Marketed as disposable, but please reuse as able. |
| Thinkbaby Trainer Cup | BPA-free plastic | Soft silicone spout |

# Taking It Home . . .

As parents of several breast-fed babies of our own, we know that breast-feeding can be both challenging and personally rewarding. As professionals, we know that breast milk is the perfect first nourishment for Baby. It's also your first opportunity to feed Baby in a green way—it's the most all-natural and low-waste feeding method around. The best practices discussed in this chapter will help you get off to a good start, and will help you establish a sufficient supply and a manageable routine so that you can continue nursing your baby for as long as you and Baby desire. In the next chapter you'll learn how a healthy diet will make your breast milk even more nutrient charged and how a healthy lifestyle will cut Baby's exposures to chemicals in your milk. If you need to supplement with formula eventually, choose powdered formula instead of ready-to-feed to be most eco-friendly, and opt for a formula fortified with iron and omega-3 fats.

# 4

# Still Eating for Two

## What Mama Eats, Baby Eats

Breast-feeding is the most convenient, nutritious, and green way to feed your baby, but you need to do much more than simply plug your baby in every couple of hours. What you eat (or don't eat) affects your body, your breast milk, and therefore your baby. Before Baby, you had only one person's nutrition to worry about—your own. Now everything you eat affects two. Plus, your exposure to toxins in your home and community can put Baby at risk, so now more than ever, a green lifestyle will help protect you and Baby both. In this chapter we will discuss the many choices you will be faced with as a nursing mother, and we will show you the healthy decisions you can make for the next year or two until your baby weans.

Of course, your healthy and green diet won't be just for Baby. The nutrition tips we provide will help you reduce your risk of heart disease, osteoporosis, and even certain cancers. A vitamin- and mineral-rich diet like the one described here also helps your body age more gracefully, helps you achieve a healthy weight, and may even boost your mood—all good reasons to keep up with all of these suggested healthy diet choices long after Baby is weaned.

As you read through this chapter, you may begin to feel over-whelmed with all the dos and don'ts. After all, you have a brand-new baby to take care of. Who has time to worry about healthy eating? And green living, though a worthy goal, may not seem high on your to-do list at the moment. You, like most women, were probably very careful during pregnancy to limit your baby's exposure to artificial substances to insure a healthy nervous system. You ate right, avoided medications, and said no to coffee and alcohol for nine long months. Now you're ready to let loose and party (if you could just find a spare moment!). But because a baby's brain continues to grow and develop over the first few years, it's not the time just yet to give in to some of these temptations. Well, OK—give in a little. Just don't overdo it. We'll let you have some fun, but we'll show you what lifestyle and nutritional commitments are worth the continued effort to help your baby's mind and body thrive to its fullest potential.

If you are unable to breast-feed, most of the information in this chapter will still apply to you as a useful guide to your own postnatal nutrition. And following our suggestions also sets up good lifestyle and nutrition habits for you and your whole family.

## For Nursing Mamas: Eating and Breast-Feeding

You just spent nine months on your best behavior, trying to eat right and be healthy. Well, you're not off the hook just yet. Though the par-ticular food rules may be slightly different now, the idea remains the same: we are what we eat. And when you're feeding Baby your breast milk, she *is* what *you* eat.

We promised you that we would let you have some fun, so before diving into the details of what foods provide which nutrients and what foods you should cross off your grocery list until baby gets older, we want to start with some good news: Yes, you can now eat sushi! Con-gratulations, many of the forbidden-during-pregnancy foods can make their way back to your plate now:

| Foods You Avoided While Pregnant | OK to Eat While Breast-Feeding? |
| --- | --- |
| Sushi | Yes! Enjoy raw and cooked sushi now, but stay away from tuna sushi, as it can be dangerously high in mercury and the World Wildlife Fund considers bluefin tuna to be an endangered species.[1] |
| Soft cheeses and pâté | Yes! The dangerous food bacterium called Listeria may be present in soft cheeses like brie and goat cheese and in pâté, but it won't get into your breast milk to infect your baby. So head to your local farmer's market for a seasonal selection of fresh and delicious cheeses and spreads. |
| Unpasteurized cheeses | Yes! There's always a risk of food poisoning when you eat unpasteurized milk, but food poisoning won't harm your breast milk. |
| Deli meats | Yes! You no longer have to worry about Listeria, a bacterium that can be found in cold deli meats. Steer clear of nitrates and other preservatives by choosing all-natural, organic deli meats. |
| Canned tuna and other fish | No. The mercury in tuna and other fish is still a concern while you're breast-feeding. See page 135 for fish advice. |
| Raw eggs (as in Caesar salad dressing) | Yes! You still run a risk of food poisoning when you eat raw eggs, but it's not going to harm your breastfeeding baby. |
| Alcohol | Yes, but with caution. See page 159. |
| Coffee | Yes, in moderation. The caffeine in one cup of coffee will not cause your baby to be jittery or keep her from sleeping. Green tip: look for coffee that's Fair Trade- or Rainforest Alliance-certified to support environmentally sustainable coffee growing practices. |

## DR. BOB'S RECIPE FOR OPTIMAL BREAST MILK

Your breast milk is really an amazing drink. It contains proteins, fats, vitamins, and minerals—perfectly designed to sustain Baby's impressive rate of weight gain and development. Remarkably, women of all sizes, backgrounds, health profiles, and eating habits make breast milk with almost identical levels of protein, carbohydrates, and total calories. Don't let this fact fool you, though. Your food choices still matter. Many aspects of breast milk's nutritional profile do change depending on Mom's diet. Plus, certain substances in your food and environment can pass through your breast milk into Baby.

You might feel that you're in no state to figure out a whole new "breast-feeding diet." You've got a few other things on your plate right now, to say the least. Well, good news: if you cleaned up your eating habits while you were pregnant, you're probably already eating many of the foods that build better breast milk. On the most basic level, the nutrition advice that we give nursing women isn't really that different from the nutrition advice we'd give any woman. You need sources of vitamins, minerals, and nutrients from all the food groups: fruits, vegetables, whole grains, lean proteins, and healthy fats. You should try to eat foods that are clean and all natural, avoiding foods with pesticides or other toxic chemicals. You don't need junk foods: fried foods, too many sweets, or overly processed foods. And finally, since some of the chemicals you inhale and touch can enter your breast milk, avoiding environmental exposures to certain toxins is important, too.

Here are six steps to making the best, most nutritious breast milk possible:

## 1. Eat Organic

If you haven't made the switch to organic foods yet, now's the time. Many of the chemicals found in conventionally grown foods, like pesticides, make their way into your breast milk. Pesticides aren't exactly the side dish you want to be serving. There are hundreds of pesticides in use, and not all have been thoroughly tested for safety. Plus, as if not knowing their effects isn't scary enough, the knowledge we do have may be even scarier. Many pesticides have been shown to be neurotoxins (substances that kill brain cells) and carcinogens.

Pesticides, like many environmental toxins, accumulate in your body's fatty tissues. Breast milk, with its high fat content, is a prime

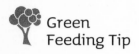

place for them to stay. So is Baby; her body has a higher percentage of body fat than yours. Babies also eat more per pound of body weight than adults, so their exposure in what they eat is relatively greater. Plus, babies lack the enzymes needed to detoxify certain pesticides. All of these factors make their bodies more vulnerable to the effects of pesticide exposure. By choosing organic foods while you're nursing, you significantly reduce Baby's exposure to pesticides and other chemicals (not to mention your positive contribution to the health of the planet).

Please don't allow this information to scare you away from breastfeeding. The multitude of factors that are present in breast milk that can't be duplicated in a laboratory make mother's milk far healthier than formula for any baby. The benefits of breast milk far outweigh any minute amounts of pesticides and other chemicals.

What about buying conventionally grown fruits and vegetables and just being careful to wash them thoroughly? You can't just wash the pesticides off. The only way to really avoid pesticides is to eat organic produce. As for meat and dairy foods, the organic ones will be free from chemicals like antibiotics and growth hormones. Plus, organically raised livestock are fed a chemical-free diet to create cleaner and healthier meat and milk. Throughout the rest of this chapter, whenever we advise you to eat certain fruits and vegetables, meats, and dairy foods, please know that we're recommending you choose organic varieties of these foods.

### 2. Eat the Right Fats

About half of the calories in your breast milk are from fat—that's how Baby gets those delicious sausage-link arms and chubby cheeks. More importantly, fat is the nutrient that fuels her brain development (the brain itself is about 60 percent fat). Your diet does not affect the *amount* of fat in your breast milk. But the *types* of fats in your milk will change depending on the fats that you eat, so give yourself and Baby the right kinds of fats and avoid the "bad" fats.

Of all the good fats, the omega-3 fats are perhaps the most important for you as a nursing Mama. These essential polyunsaturated fats reduce your risk of cardiovascular disease, help prevent certain cancers, and

|  | *Type of Fat* | *Where You'll Find It* | *Why It's Right/Why It's "Bad"* |
|---|---|---|---|
| Preferred Fats | Monounsaturated fats | Olive oil, nuts, avocado, other vegetable oils | These fats don't raise cholesterol levels or clog arteries. |
|  | Polyunsaturated fats, including omega-3 fats | Plant oils like corn, flaxseed, safflower, and peanut oils, and oily fish | These fats are essential because your body can't manufacture them and must get them from your diet. They are also important for Baby's brain development. |
| Fats to Avoid | Saturated fats | Animal sources like full-fat dairy foods and meats. These tend to be solid fats, as a stick of butter, a block of cheese, or marbling in steak. | These fats raise cholesterol levels and clog arteries, increasing the risk of heart disease and stroke. |
|  | Trans fats | In packaged foods like snack foods, bakery items, or anything that contains "hydrogenated" or "partially hydrogenated" oils | These fats, made when unsaturated oils are processed and turn into saturated fats, act like saturated fats in foods and in your body, and may also interfere with Baby's healthy brain function and development. |

may even improve your mood. One particular omega-3 fat, DHA (docosahexaenoic acid) is the major structural component of brain and eye tissue and therefore crucial for Baby's mental and visual development. We American women tend not to eat enough of these fats, and studies show our breast milk is deficient in them compared with women from other parts of the world.[2] To boost the amount of omega-3s in your milk, add these foods to your repertoire:

- cold-water fish, including wild salmon, herring, halibut (see page 212 for details)

- walnuts
- pumpkin seeds
- canola oil
- soybeans and tofu
- kale, collard greens, and brussels sprouts
- flaxseed oil

If you don't get some of these good omega-3 sources on a regular basis, consider a supplement of DHA. The recommended intake for nursing mothers is 300 mg per day. These days, some prenatal vitamin formulations actually include added DHA so ask your doctor to prescribe you one. Or you can find over-the-counter fish oil or algal oil capsule supplements.

## 3. Fortify with Vitamins and Minerals

The dietary recommendations from groups like the Institute of Medicine[3] and the USDA (U.S. Department of Agriculture)[4] advise nursing Mamas to increase their intake of practically every vitamin and mineral, either to ensure an adequate intake for Baby or to preserve mom's own nutritional status. Don't worry, we're not going to list every single vitamin and mineral for you here. For many of them, you'll be fine if you're eating enough food (see above) and eating foods from all the food groups.

Let's just focus here on the vitamins for which your intake will actually affect the level in your breast milk: vitamins A, $B_2$, $B_6$, $B_{12}$, and C. For these, the more you have in your diet, the richer your milk will be. Later in this chapter we'll give you tips for actually getting them on your plate.

*Vitamin D.* Another vitamin that deserves special attention is vitamin D. This vitamin helps build strong bones by aiding the absorption of calcium and phosphorus. It's a unique vitamin because the best source is actually not a food. It's the sun. Vitamin D is formed by your body when ultraviolet rays from the sun hit your skin. If you make sufficient vitamin D, your milk will provide enough for your baby. If you don't, Baby may need a supplement.

| Vitamin | What It Does for Baby | Sources | More Need-to-Know Info |
|---|---|---|---|
| Vitamin A | Antioxidant; supports vision, infection prevention, and cell and tissue growth | Fortified milk and cereal, eggs, and liver | Can be made from beta-carotene, so eat at least one source each day: orange fruits and vegetables like cantaloupe, sweet potato, and carrots, and dark green vegetables like kale and spinach. |
| B vitamins | $B_2$ (aka riboflavin): carbohydrate metabolism and red blood cell production | $B_2$: yogurt, milk, and some enriched bread products | |
| | $B_6$: protein metabolism, immune function, and brain development | $B_6$: spinach, salmon, and bran cereal | |
| | $B_{12}$: nerve function and red blood cell production | $B_{12}$: beef and eggs | Vitamin $B_{12}$ deficiency can lead to problems with Baby's brain development. If you're a vegan nursing Mama, you need a $B_{12}$ supplement. |
| Vitamin C | Antioxidant: protects Baby's cells, collagen production, iron absorption; infection prevention | Citrus fruits, potatoes, tomatoes, strawberries, broccoli, cabbage, bell peppers, and mango | Eat with iron-rich foods to boost the absorption of the iron |

If you're a light-skinned Mama you need at least fifteen minutes of direct sunlight on your unsunscreened face or arms every day to make enough vitamin D. If you are dark skinned, you need more sun time because the melanin in your skin acts as a sunblock, blocking vitamin D production, too. You also need more sun time if you live in a cold place where the sun's rays aren't as direct. It's important to balance your need for vitamin D with the need to protect your skin from

## *Un*cover Your Baby!

For decades doctors have been warning parents to keep their babies out of the sun to help prevent skin cancer. It's almost comical (but sad) to see a parent rushing from the store to the car with a blanket held over the baby, lest the evil sun's damaging rays touch Baby's vulnerable skin. This is a mistake. Babies need some direct sunlight to make vitamin D, a very important hormone that is involved in many body functions, including growth, strong bones, and a healthy immune system. Exactly how much sunlight a child needs isn't known, but the general recommendation is about three hours each week, preferably spread out in fifteen- to thirty-minute increments. And we're not talking early morning or late afternoon sun. Babies need the UV rays during the middle of the day, without sunscreen to block them. Of course, you don't want to let your baby get sunburned. How do you balance it out?

- Don't use sunblock unless you are going out for several hours—to the beach, the park, or other outdoor activity.
- Allow the sun to shine on Baby's unprotected arms, legs, head, and face for those few minutes at a time when you are out and about.
- Purposely take a fifteen- to thirty-minute walk during the warm hours of the day a few times each week with some of Baby's parts exposed. During winter months you'll have to take shorter walks—even five to ten minutes will help and won't let Baby get chilled.

The bottom line on the sun and skin cancer is *not* the actual sun exposure; it is the frequency and severity of *sunburns* that pose a risk. So as long as Baby isn't turning red you know her exposure is OK.

sun damage, though. After your fifteen minutes of vitamin D sunbathing, apply a sunscreen providing at least SPF 15. Dark-skinned women, those in northern states, and anyone whose skin is rarely in direct sunlight should consider a supplement of 400 to 1000 international units (IU) of vitamin D each day.

To boost your vitamin D status, in addition to soaking up the sun, eat foods containing vitamin D including fortified milk, fortified cereals, salmon, oysters, sardines, and egg yolks. Your prenatal vitamin supplement will provide some vitamin D as well.

*Minerals.* In general, your milk's mineral content won't change depending on your food intake. But that doesn't mean you can do without good food sources of these minerals in your diet. They are crucial for your own good health and for preserving your nutritional reserves during lactation:

| Mineral | Benefit to Mama | Best Sources | How Much? | Special Tips |
|---------|-----------------|--------------|-----------|--------------|
| Calcium | Protects bone health | Cow's or goat's milk, calcium-fortified soy milk or juice, yogurt, cheese, sardines (with bones), tofu, blackstrap molasses | 3 servings a day (a serving is 1 cup milk or yogurt, 1½ ounces cheese, 3 ounces sardines, ½ cup tofu, or 2 tablespoons blackstrap molasses) | Dark green vegetables like kale, mustard greens, collards, and broccoli also provide calcium, though in smaller amounts, so eat several cups of these dark green veggies if they are your main source of calcium |
| Zinc | Helps you fend off infection and illness; required for metabolism | Lean beef, lamb, wheat germ, tofu, sunflower or pumpkin seeds, yogurt, cremini mushrooms | You need 12 mg per day (4 ounces of beef contains 6 mg zinc) | Continue taking your prenatal vitamin and mineral supplement to get enough |
| Iron | Helps bring oxygen to your cells and organs | Lean beef, chicken, or pork; fortified breakfast cereals; cooked spinach or Swiss chard; beans; pumpkin seeds; tofu; and dried fruit | Eat 2 or 3 "best sources" each day; you need 9 mg per day (18 mg if your periods have resumed) | Iron from vegetarian sources isn't as absorbable as iron from meat, but eating these with a food that is rich in vitamin C, like an orange, potatoes, tomatoes, or broccoli, will boost your body's absorption of the iron |

You might be wondering if you can just pop a pill to get all these vitamins and minerals into your body. We suppose you could, but it's actually much better to get vitamins and minerals from foods because they are better absorbed and used by your body. If you want to take a supplement as a nutritional insurance plan, it's fine to continue taking your prenatal vitamin and mineral supplement while you're nursing.

## MYTH OR FACT?

*Breast-feeding robs your body of calcium and weakens your bones.*

Myth! During lactation your level of bone calcium does dip slightly, especially if you breast-feed for longer than six months. But as long as you continue to get good sources of calcium in your diet, your bone calcium is restored after you wean, and studies show that you may even end up with stronger bones in the end.[5,6]

### 4. Drink Plenty of Fluids

A nursing Mama needs to stay hydrated with about eight cups (sixty-four ounces) of liquid each day. In general, there's no need to force yourself to drink much more than that. In fact, drinking more than you need won't necessarily increase your milk supply. Any fluids—not just plain water—count toward your eight cups, so having soups, juices, and teas can help you meet your needs. And contrary to popular myth, you don't have to drink milk to make milk.

You do need to drink extra fluids if you notice your urine is very concentrated (it should be pale yellow in color) or you're having issues with constipation—both signs of mild dehydration. You should also drink more fluids if you come down with an illness that causes fever, diarrhea, or vomiting.

Keep a glass of water or diluted juice near the chair where you do most of your nursing and drink it during each feeding. Carry water—in a reusable BPA-free plastic or aluminum container—with you when you go out.

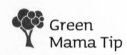

### Green Mama Tip

. . . . . . . . . . . . . . . . . . . . .

REFILL YOUR WATER BOTTLES Be sure to use refillable water containers around the house and on the go instead of opening a single-serve disposable water bottle every time you get thirsty. Refill the containers from your main source of drinking water (tap, filter, or delivered five-gallon bottles). The amount of discarded plastic water bottles that are thrown away each year is staggering, and even recycling them costs money and energy.

## 5. Avoid Sources of Mercury

When you were pregnant, your doctor or midwife probably warned you to avoid certain fish, sources of methylmercury. This toxic element does enter breast milk, so this is one pregnancy food rule that you should continue to follow now that you're breast-feeding.

Mercury is an element that is found naturally in the environment and is also released into the air by factories and industry. It accumulates in streams and oceans in the form of methylmercury, a dangerous toxin. Exposure to mercury in utero may cause problems with brain development leading to lower IQ levels, language and motor problems, and attention deficits.[7] Babies and young children may be developmentally delayed by exposure to too much mercury.

To avoid methylmercury in your diet, don't eat shark, tilefish, swordfish, king mackerel, tuna steaks, canned albacore tuna, and tuna sushi. Don't completely avoid the fruits of the sea, though. Fish is a great source of protein and omega-3 fats. Try to eat up to twelve ounces of safe fish each week. If you want to eat canned tuna, choose light tuna instead of albacore and limit yourself to six ounces per week. The fish listed here are not only low in mercury, but they are also fished in a sustainable way, meaning the fishermen's practices don't contribute to ocean or river pollution, the species isn't in danger of extinction, and they can be fished in a way that doesn't harm the ocean habitat. These fish, therefore, are a great choice for you, Baby, *and* the planet (Monterey Bay Aquarium, www.montereybayaquarium.org).

- anchovies
- arctic char (farmed)
- catfish (U.S.)
- cod (Pacific)
- halibut (Pacific)
- pollock
- rainbow trout (farmed)
- salmon, canned
- salmon, wild
- sardines (Pacific)

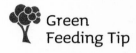 Green Feeding Tip

GO WILD WITH SALMON Salmon is one of the most popular fish on the menu since it doesn't contain mercury. But you have to be careful. Most salmon raised on fish farms in the United States has been found to contain various cancer-causing chemicals, including PCBs that come from factories and pollution in the surrounding area. *Wild* salmon, on the other hand, is caught out in the ocean, away from such pollution. Make sure any salmon you buy or order at a restaurant is wild.

- scallops
- whitefish

## 6. Avoid Environmental Toxic Exposures

Think about how many chemicals you touch, ingest, or inhale each day. Now consider that many of them can actually reach your baby after circulating through your bloodstream and entering your breast milk. Take a "better safe than sorry" stance, minimizing your exposures whenever possible. Here's a list of potentially toxic chemicals that enter breast milk and may be in your home, along with tips for avoiding them.

| Possible Source | Toxins that Enter Breast Milk | Tips for Avoiding Exposure |
|---|---|---|
| Tap water | Lead, bacteria, industrial chemicals | Test your water with a home testing kit. Temporarily switch to bottled water, if need be, or install an under-the-counter reverse osmosis water filter, or use a pitcher-type activated carbon filter instead. These remove lead, chlorine, and many other contaminants. |
| Plastics in the kitchen | Phthalates, BPA—can leach into foods, beverages | Don't microwave in plastic—use microwave-safe ceramics or glass instead.<br><br>Don't cover hot foods with plastic wrap—use a plate or a plain, bleach-free paper towel instead. |
| Beauty supplies | Phthalates, parabens | Avoid synthetic perfumes—choose products scented with plant-derived oils instead.<br><br>Avoid products with parabens (these are listed on the ingredients label).<br><br>Choose mineral makeup, which typically has fewer chemical preservatives and additives.<br><br>For a list of safe beauty products, see the Environmental Working Group's Cosmetic Safety Database (www.cosmeticdatabase.com). |

| | | |
|---|---|---|
| Nail and hair treatments | Solvents, plasticizers, or even formaldehyde | Skip the mani, pedi, and perm until you stop nursing.<br><br>Bring your own phthalate-free nail polish to the salon.<br><br>Opt for highlights instead of a full head of dye. |
| Secondhand smoke | Nicotine | Don't smoke, and ask people not to smoke in your home. |
| Air fresheners and candles made from paraffin wax | Volatile organic compounds (VOCs) | For household odors, open windows to air out rooms.<br><br>Use a paste of baking soda and water to clean the smelly household objects.<br><br>Place an open box of baking soda in the bathroom and fridge to absorb odors.<br><br>Choose candles made from soy or beeswax instead of paraffin wax (which is made from petroleum—a nonrenewable resource). |
| Cleaning supplies | VOCs, chlorine compounds, phosphates | Choose eco-friendly cleaning products or use natural cleaning alternatives—See chapters 9 and 10 for ideas.<br><br>When cleaning, open windows to ventilate the room. |
| Paint and paint removers | Lead, VOCs | If possible, skip the painting projects while nursing.<br><br>Call professionals for removing paint from before 1978.<br><br>When anyone is painting, properly ventilate rooms to dissipate fumes. |
| Mattresses, furniture, electronic equipment | Bromine-based flame retardants, such as PBDEs | Look for PBDE-free mattresses, electronics, furniture, carpet pads, and baby gear (the Environmental Working Group provides a handy list of these products at www.ewg.org/pbdefree).<br><br>Reupholster or replace any furniture with exposed foam cushions. |

## A GREEN BEAUTY ROUTINE FOR THE NURSING MAMA

*The palest green:* While you're nursing, avoid anything unnecessary, like wearing perfume and having salon nail or hair treatments.

*A little greener:* Switch your hand soap, body cleanser, and body lotions—the products you use most often and which cover more body area—to paraben-free and phthalate-free products. Parabens will show up on the label. Phthalates may be disguised as "fragrance," so choose products scented only with plant-based oils.

*The deepest shade of green:* Read ingredients for all your beauty products and choose only all-natural and organic ingredients.

All-natural and organic beauty products are easier than ever to find. Here are some brands that are widely available: Nature's Gate (www.natures-gate.com), Avalon Organics (www.avalonorganics.com), JASON (www.jason-natural.com), Aubrey Organics (www.aubreyorganics.com), Burt's Bees (www.burtsbees.com), and Kiss My Face (www.kissmyface.com).

## Putting It All Together—"What (Exactly) Should I Eat?"

If you're like us, your eyes start to glaze over when you read nutrition advice that tells you to eat $x$ number of servings of this food group each day, $x$ number of servings from another group, and so on. We've found that most women, especially Mamas with young children, don't have the time or energy to count everything and keep track like that. Rather, they just want advice about what meals to make and snacks to buy so

# Perfume Is Nice, But . . .

Some new moms love to get all dressed up, put on makeup, and apply the favorite perfume that they used to enjoy wearing before they became pregnant. Well, I hate to be the bearer of bad news, but you should probably keep the perfume hidden away for a while longer. The strong odor, while very nice for us men, isn't good for babies to inhale day after day. Some makeup and body lotions also have a nice but strong odor. For baby's first year of life, it's best if you keep these items to a minimum (such as date night with your spouse or partner).

# Breast Is Best!

Reading about all the chemicals that *could* be in your breast milk may prompt any new mom to think that maybe formula would be safer. Nothing could be further from the truth. There are chemicals in formula as well, especially nonorganic formulas. What's so distinct about breast milk is the multitude of growth- and immune-building factors, brain-building ingredients, cancer-fighting properties, natural anti-inflammatories, and other substances that can't be duplicated in a factory. Plus, every few years we discover something new in breast milk that we didn't know about before. There are ingredients with benefits that we can't even imagine. We hope that you take our warnings here about chemicals the right way. Clean up *your* life and diet to optimize your breast milk for your baby. Don't take the easy way out and turn to formula.

# MEDICINES AND HERBALS FOR NURSING MAMAS

Most medications do find their way into breast milk, and some may even affect Baby's developing body or your milk supply. Although there are plenty of over-the-counter and prescription medications that are approved for use by nursing women, we recommend extreme caution when taking medications or herbs, especially when Baby is very young. Of course sometimes medications can't be avoided, for example, if you get a bacterial infection, or if you need to treat a serious chronic health concern like high blood pressure. Discuss your options with your doctor and she'll help you find a safe approach. If another health care provider has recommended a treatment (over-the-counter, prescription, or herbal), you should still call your pediatrician's office to verify it's OK for nursing.

In some cases, you may be able to avoid medications by treating your symptoms with simple home remedies. Here are some breast-feeding-friendly ideas:

| Symptom | Home Remedy |
|---|---|
| Nasal and sinus congestion | Use a cool mist vaporizer while you sleep. Regularly use a nasal saline spray or sinus-cleansing neti pot. Inhale steam in the shower or from a bowl of steamy water (be careful not to burn yourself). |
| Cold symptoms | Eat warm chicken soup—it's not just an old wives' tale! |
| Cough | Swallow a spoonful of honey. |
| Tension headache | Dab peppermint oil on your temples. |
| Sore muscles | Use an old-fashioned hot-water bottle. |

they can be on their way. If you're sitting there, nodding your head, you're in luck. Here are some practical tips for you—food lists and meal and snack ideas.

## A Healthy Mama's Weekly Grocery List

First, a grocery list to keep you on track. Fill your cart with some of these foods (and then eat them!) and you will be on your way. When it's time to make a meal, you'll have the best ingredients available to you. You'll notice this list leaves out junk foods and treats (except dark chocolate). This doesn't mean you can never have a slice of pie or a cookie. This isn't some kind of torture diet! It's just that these foods aren't important to include on a daily or weekly basis, so they didn't make this shopping list.

| Food or Drink | Vitamin A | B Vitamins | Vitamin C | Calcium | Iron | Zinc | Omega-3s | Protein |
|---|---|---|---|---|---|---|---|---|
| **Fruits** | | | | | | | | |
| Apple, pear, plum | | | ✓ | | | | | |
| Avocado | | ✓ | ✓ | | | | | |
| Banana | | ✓ | ✓ | | | | | |
| Berries: blueberries, strawberries, raspberries, blackberries | | | ✓ | | | | | |
| Cantaloupe | ✓ | | ✓ | | | | | |
| Citrus fruits: orange, grapefruit, tangerine | | | ✓ | | | | | |
| Dried fruit: raisins, prunes, apricots | ✓ | | | | ✓ | | | |
| Mango | ✓ | | ✓ | | | | | |

| Food or Drink | Vitamin A | B Vitamins | Vitamin C | Calcium | Iron | Zinc | Omega-3s | Protein |
|---|---|---|---|---|---|---|---|---|
| Peach | ● | | ● | | | | | |
| Pineapple | | | ● | | | | | |
| **Vegetables** | | | | | | | | |
| Bell pepper | ● | ● | ● | | | | | |
| Broccoli | ● | ● | ● | | | | | |
| Brussels sprouts | ● | ● | ● | | | | | |
| Carrots | ● | | ● | | | | | |
| Cauliflower | | ● | ● | | | | | |
| Collard greens, turnip greens, Swiss chard | ● | | ● | ● | ● | | | |
| Corn | | ● | ● | | | | | |
| Garlic | | ● | ● | | | | | |
| Kale | ● | ● | ● | ● | ● | | | |
| Lettuce greens | ● | ● | ● | | ● | | | |
| Mushrooms | | ● | | | | ● | | |
| Onion | | ● | ● | | | | | |
| Potatoes, sweet | ● | ● | ● | | | | | |
| Potatoes, white | | ● | ● | | | | | |
| Spinach | ● | ● | ● | ● | ● | ● | | |
| Summer squash and zucchini | ● | | ● | | | | | |

| Food or Drink | Vitamin A | B Vitamins | Vitamin C | Calcium | Iron | Zinc | Omega-3s | Protein |
|---|---|---|---|---|---|---|---|---|
| Tofu | | | | ● | | ● | ● | ● |
| Tomatoes | ● | ● | ● | | | | | |
| Winter squash | ● | ● | ● | | | | ● | |
| **At the Meat/Poultry/Fish Counter** | | | | | | | | |
| Beef (choose lean cuts) | | ● | | | ● | ● | | ● |
| Chicken | | ● | | | ● | | | ● |
| Fish (choose from the safe fish list above) | | ● | | | | | ● | ● |
| Pork (choose lean cuts) | | ● | | | ● | ● | | ● |
| Turkey | | ● | | | ● | | | ● |
| **Canned and packaged foods** | | | | | | | | |
| Almonds | | ● | | | | | | ● |
| Beans | | ● | | | ● | | | ● |
| Bread (whole grain, all-natural) | | ● | | | ● | | | |
| Breakfast cereal (whole grain, low in sugar) | | ● | | | ● | ● | | |
| Canned vegetable soup (low-sodium) | ● | ● | ● | | ● | | | |

| Food or Drink | Vitamin A | B Vitamins | Vitamin C | Calcium | Iron | Zinc | Omega-3s | Protein |
|---|---|---|---|---|---|---|---|---|
| Canola oil | | | | | | | 🥄 | |
| Chocolate, dark | | 🥄 | | | | 🥄 | | |
| Flaxseed oil | | | | | | | 🥄 | |
| Granola and granola bars | | 🥄 | | | 🥄 | 🥄 | | 🥄 |
| Hummus | | 🥄 | | | 🥄 | | | 🥄 |
| Lentils | | 🥄 | | | 🥄 | | | 🥄 |
| Oatmeal | | 🥄 | | | 🥄 | | | 🥄 |
| Pasta | | 🥄 | | | | | | |
| Peanut butter | | 🥄 | | | | | | 🥄 |
| Pumpkin seeds | | | | | | 🥄 | 🥄 | |
| Quinoa | | | | | 🥄 | | | 🥄 |
| Salmon, canned | | | | | | | 🥄 | 🥄 |
| Sunflower seeds | | 🥄 | | | | 🥄 | | |
| Walnuts | | | | | | | 🥄 | 🥄 |
| Wheat germ | | 🥄 | | | 🥄 | 🥄 | | |
| From the Dairy Case | | | | | | | | |
| Cheese (low-fat varieties) | | | | 🥄 | | | | 🥄 |
| Eggs | | 🥄 | | | | | | 🥄 |
| Fruit juices | | | 🥄 | | | | | |

| Food or Drink | Vitamin A | B Vitamins | Vitamin C | Calcium | Iron | Zinc | Omega-3s | Protein |
|---|---|---|---|---|---|---|---|---|
| Goat's milk, low fat | ✓ | ✓ | | ✓ | | | | ✓ |
| Milk, nonfat | ✓ | ✓ | | ✓ | | | | ✓ |
| Soy milk | ✓ | ✓ | | ✓ | | | | ✓ |
| Yogurt | | ✓ | | ✓ | | ✓ | | ✓ |
| From the Freezer | | | | | | | | |
| Burritos and pocket sandwiches | | ✓ | | | ✓ | | | ✓ |
| Frozen berries | | | ✓ | | | | | |
| Frozen pastas | | ✓ | | | | | | |
| Frozen vegetables (e.g., broccoli, spinach, green beans, squash, peppers, corn) | ✓ | ✓ | ✓ | | | | | |
| Veggie-topped frozen pizza | ✓ | ✓ | ✓ | | | | | |
| Waffles, whole grain | | ✓ | | | ✓ | | | |

## EAT ENOUGH AND EAT RIGHT

It takes calories to make calories. But how many do you need? The standard nutrition advice is for lactating women to eat an extra five hundred calories each day. This is probably a good idea during the first

# BREAST-FEEDING NUTRITION BY THE NUMBERS

If you're the kind of person who craves numbers, this next chart is for you. It shows how many servings of each food group you need, and it gives you serving sizes. To be sure you are getting adequate vitamins, minerals, and nutrients, you need to eat this minimum number of servings of each food group daily:

| Food Group | Recommended Daily Intake | What a Serving Equals |
|---|---|---|
| Breads, cereals, pasta, and grains | 6 servings | 1 ounce slice of bread, 1 ounce dry cereal, ½ cup cooked cereal, ½ cup cooked rice or other grain, ½ cup cooked pasta, 3 to 4 crackers, 3 tablespoons wheat germ, 1 small tortilla, ½ bagel |
| Fruit group | 2 servings | 1 apple, orange, or other whole piece of fruit; ½ cup cut fruit or berries; ¼ cup dried fruit; 6 ounces 100 percent fruit juice; ½ grapefruit |
| Vegetable group | 3 servings | ½ cup chopped raw vegetables, 1 cup raw leafy greens, ½ cup cooked vegetables |
| Protein foods such as beef, chicken, beans, tofu, and eggs | 3 servings | 2 to 3 ounces of meat or fish, 2 eggs, ½ cup tofu, ½ cup ground meat, ½ chicken breast, 1 medium pork or lamb chop, 4 tablespoons peanut butter, ⅔ cup nuts, 1 cup cooked lentils or beans |
| Milk, yogurt, and cheese group | 2 to 3 servings | 1 cup milk, 1 cup yogurt, 1 to 2 ounces cheese, 1 cup cottage cheese |

few weeks of nursing, when your body is ramping up for breast milk production and healing from childbirth. Sufficient calories will help you get off to a good start. Beyond that, though, the research doesn't entirely support the idea that every single nursing woman needs to eat extra calories in order to make enough milk.

Rather than counting calories, our advice is to let your body be your guide. Did you gain a little extra padding in your behind and thighs during pregnancy? That was your body's way of storing up some energy to be used later for breast milk production. In general, if you have some weight to lose, from pregnancy or otherwise, you probably don't need to eat extra calories because your body can tap into these energy stores.

You probably do need extra calories if you're very lean or underweight, or if you feel like you're starving all the time. Your body may not have enough energy in reserve that a new mom needs. You may also need extra calories during Baby's growth spurts, when she feeds more frequently and nursing is more physically demanding.

After you've been breast-feeding for six months or so, reevaluate whether you might need additional calories. By that time, if you've lost all your baby weight, your body may not have enough stored energy left. If so, increase your food intake by adding one or two healthy snacks (totaling three hundred to five hundred calories per day) to support continued breastfeeding.

## HEALTHY MAMA MENUS

So, you have the list of foods to include in your diet, the list of ones to avoid, you're eating organically, you know which foods to buy at the store . . . what's next? Well, you have to eat! Here's how to put it all together. Over the next few pages you'll find some of our favorite meal and menu ideas to help you translate the nutrition info you just read into actual food on your plate.

### "Pile-On" Meals

Certain kinds of meals are perfect for piling on the vitamins, minerals, and nutrients. Consider the basic bowl of spaghetti and marinara

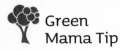

### Green Mama Tip

MSG SOUP  Most canned
and dried soup mixes have
MSG (monosodium gluta-
mate) to enhance the flavor.
MSG is very bad news for
a growing brain.[8] Many studies have shown how MSG
disrupts the normal levels
and functions of chemicals
and hormones in our brain.
Some brand-name soup
makers are starting to take
MSG out, and hopefully,
all makers will follow suit.
Be sure to read the label of
every soup you buy.

sauce. It's an easy and comforting meal. But it also gives you an opportunity to raise the nutritional quotient of your dinner by adding lots of
vegetables and a protein source like chicken, tofu, or even shellfish to
the sauce. It doesn't take much more time, but you get much more out
of it. Here are some more ideas to help you pile on the good stuff:

- *Salads:* Pick your favorite salad greens (vary your lettuces and/
  or use spinach), and then add some of the following foods to
  up the nutritional value: tomatoes, red and green bell peppers,
  raw or blanched broccoli, kidney beans, canned salmon, tofu,
  chicken, steak, hard-boiled egg, low-fat shredded cheese,
  walnuts, dried cranberries or raisins, sunflower or pumpkin
  seeds, and a canola oil vinaigrette.
- *Sandwiches:* Start with a 100 percent whole grain bread or pita
  and choose your favorite healthy fillings—all-natural sliced
  turkey breast, low-fat cheeses, roasted or raw vegetables, and
  healthy spreads like guacamole or hummus.
- *Soups:* A bowl of soup can be a simple way to get lots of
  vegetables at a single meal. If you're starting from scratch,
  chop up whatever vegetables you have and throw them into
  the broth. Add beans and whole grain pasta, and you have
  yourself a filling bowl! You can also find canned soups made
  from organic ingredients and packed with vegetables,
  lentils, and/or beans (opt for the low-sodium varieties if
  possible).
- *Oatmeal:* Instead of just a plain bowl of oatmeal, consider these
  ways to pack in the nutrition: Make it with milk instead of
  water, add a tablespoon of wheat germ and/or ground flaxseed,
  top it with fresh or frozen berries, or add dried fruit.
- *Yogurt:* Make a smoothie of yogurt, low-fat milk or soy milk,
  and fresh or frozen chopped fruits. For a nutrient-loaded
  parfait layer yogurt, add whole grain granola and dried or fresh
  fruits. Up the value of either yogurt treat with a generous sprin-
  kling of wheat germ or ground flaxseed on top.

A NOTE FROM DR. BOB

# Breakfast Smoothies Instead of Coffee

Many of us need that caffeine boost in the morning. New moms are no exception. I have found a good-tasting and effective substitute that really gets me up and running for a morning in the office. When you read the ingredients, you may say to yourself, "Good tasting? Are you serious?" Well, admittedly, it may be an acquired taste. But I think they are great! Here's what goes into my own personal smoothie each morning:

- 1½ cups milk (any kind)
- ¾ cup plain yogurt
- 2 tablespoons peanut butter
- Frozen blueberries, strawberries, mango—about 1½ cups total, to taste
- Half banana
- Honey (if you need sweetener)
- Two scoops of smoothie protein/vitamin/mineral powder from a health food store—check for all-natural ingredients
- 1 tablespoon ground flaxseed meal
- 1 tablespoon oat bran

(Hint: save time by mixing about 3 parts of the protein powder to 1 part each of flax and oat bran and store in a larger airtight container. It's less to have to scoop each morning.)

Sound yummy? You can change it up, add things, and take things away according to your own taste. But the key here is protein, omega-3 fats, fiber, and antioxidants. I can (almost) guarantee you won't need to stop by Starbucks (as often) if you make this part of your breakfast.

## More Meal Ideas

*Breakfast:* A well-rounded breakfast consists of a high-fiber grain product, a source of protein, and a fruit. Breakfast is also a great place to squeeze in some calcium in the form of dairy or fortified soy milk or juice. Here are some ideas for you:

- Bran muffin with cottage cheese and sliced peaches
- Whole wheat bagel with low-fat or tofu cream cheese and ½ grapefruit
- Oatmeal made with milk or soy milk (instead of water), and topped with dried fruit, ground flaxseed, and a touch of honey or brown sugar
- Egg sandwich on whole grain bread made with one or two scrambled eggs, a slice of low-fat cheese, served with fruit salad
- Buckwheat pancakes topped with blueberries and maple syrup, a wedge of cantaloupe, and a glass of milk or soy milk
- Yogurt parfait made with nonfat or low-fat plain yogurt, a touch of honey, with a low-sugar granola and fresh berries
- Unsweetened multigrain cereal with milk
- Whole grain toast with peanut butter (or other nut butter) and sliced bananas, fruited yogurt

*Lunch and dinner:* For these meals try to include a healthy starch, some vegetables, healthy fats, and some protein. Try also to let go of the idea that dinner needs to be so formal—a good sandwich and a bowl of soup is a fine dinner! Heck, scrambled eggs, toast, and fruit are great. Try also to make ahead and freeze easy dishes like lasagna or baked ziti, meatloaf, and soups so you have something fast to grab in a pinch. Here are some more relatively quick and easy ideas:

- Grilled chicken breast with a baked sweet potato and steamed green beans
- A quesadilla made with whatever leftover meat or tofu you have in the fridge, shredded low-fat cheese, and whatever veggies you have on hand. Top with guacamole and salsa.
- Tofu and vegetable stir-fry with brown rice
- Baked fish with roasted potatoes and asparagus

- Turkey burger on a whole wheat bun with lettuce, sliced tomato, and avocado. Serve with sweet potato oven fries and coleslaw.
- Grilled salmon with whole wheat couscous and sautéed zucchini and summer squash
- Vegetable lasagna with a side salad of greens, chopped raw vegetables, and vinaigrette dressing
- Baked potato topped with broccoli and shredded cheese

## ABOUT CONVENIENCE FOODS

OK, we know what you're thinking: "Are you kidding me? I'm spending about twelve hours a day feeding my baby right now and you think I'm cooking dinner?!" No, we know that some days (many days!) it will be virtually impossible to actually cook dinner and get it on the table. Luckily, there are lots of convenience foods that are actually good for you. These days, grocery stores are filled with all-natural and even organic options. Instead of resorting to fast food or ordering yet another pizza, try some of these überquick and easy options:

- Frozen burritos and pocket sandwiches
- Frozen pastas like ravioli and tortellini
- Canned chili and soups (look for low-sodium varieties and no MSG)
- Frozen burger patties (choose organic beef or turkey) or chicken breasts (choose antibiotic-free or organic chicken)
- Frozen fish fillets or precooked shrimp. (See page 212 for a list of sustainable fish choices)
- Frozen stir-fry vegetables to add to quickly cooked chicken, steak, or tofu
- Frozen veggie-topped pizzas

Look for some of these all-natural brands in the freezer case: Amy's Kitchen (www.amys.com), Health is Wealth (www.healthiswealthfoods .com), Kashi (www.kashi.com), Cascadian Farms (www.cascadian

A NOTE FROM DR. BOB

## Where You Shop May Be Just As Important As What You Buy

It used to be that only "weird" people shopped at those strange healthy grocery stores like Trader Joe's, Whole Foods, and Mother's Market. I thought *my* mom was strange for shopping there when I was a kid. Now there's one in every neighborhood because consumers are sick and tired of having to read every label to make sure any convenient and packaged food they buy doesn't have hidden chemicals or surprise ingredients like MSG, high-fructose corn syrup, hydrogenated oil, food coloring, artificial sugars, or preservatives. Shop at a healthy store and you'll be hard pressed to find such "bad" words on the label. Conventional grocery stores, on the other hand, still carry a lot of that junk. They *are* getting better and carrying more organic and natural choices, but you still have to be careful.

farms.com), Seeds of Change (www.seedsofchange.com), and Applegate Farms (www.applegatefarms.com).

### HEALTHY SNACKING

Always have some good snacks around to grab between meals. Don't buy empty junk foods with little nutritional value. You can find better options than a candy bar or a bag of potato chips. Most moms like to keep a stash of healthy foods that require only one hand for eating. You can grab these to eat while you're nursing, pushing your stroller, or simply holding your baby.

- Granola bars
- Trail mix or dried fruit and nuts
- Homemade or store-bought yogurt drinks
- Fresh fruit like apples, bananas, grapes, berries, cut melon, orange slices
- Sandwiches—every few days, make a couple of sandwiches, cut them into quarters, and put in the fridge for easy grab-and-go eating
- Low-fat organic cheese slices or cubes
- Carrot sticks or baby carrots
- Dry cereal for snacking
- Guacamole with dippers like baked tortilla chips and sliced veggies

## TWO SAMPLE MENUS FOR THE NEW MAMA

### 1. For the "It's Three O'clock and I Haven't Eaten Breakfast Yet" Mama

Don't become so occupied by the day-to-day tasks of raising a baby that you forget to eat. A strategy that we think works well for busy moms is to put together small, frequent meals throughout the day—almost like having many large snacks. Here's a sample day:

7 a.m.—Plain or fruited yogurt topped with granola and berries

10 a.m.—Multigrain toast with peanut butter and a glass of orange juice

1 p.m.—Grilled cheese sandwich on multigrain bread

4 p.m.—Low-sodium minestrone soup with pretzels

7 p.m.—Mixed green salad topped with grilled chicken, sunflower seeds, cherry tomatoes, and carrots with canola oil and vinegar

9 p.m.—A cookie with a glass of soy or nonfat milk and a sliced apple

## 2. For the "I Never Miss a Meal" Mama

If you're more of a three square meals type of gal, here's a sample day for you. There are some healthy snacks thrown in between the main meals to keep your energy up and to provide more of the nutrients that you need:

Breakfast—oatmeal made with nonfat or soy milk with dried apricots

Midmorning snack—carrot sticks with hummus

Lunch—all-natural sliced turkey breast on 100 percent whole grain bread with mustard, lettuce, and tomato; a side salad with mixed greens, sunflower seeds, cherry tomatoes, and an olive oil-based dressing; pretzels, an orange

Afternoon snack—yogurt parfait made from nonfat plain yogurt, honey, granola, and fresh berries

Dinner—tofu or chicken and frozen stir-fry vegetables, stir-fried in canola oil and served with teriyaki sauce and rice

Dessert—a small square of dark chocolate (it's actually good for you!)

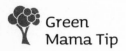
### Green Mama Tip

Gather friends together for an all-organic potluck dinner party. Potluck dinners are a great way to entertain without spending too much money or time. Challenge even your nongreen friends to use all-natural and organic ingredients, and be sure to swap recipes to add some new healthy meals to your own repertoire.

# Mama Nutrition FAQs

*Are there foods or herbs that help with low milk supply?*

Certain foods and herbs, called galactagogues, stimulate milk production and can be used safely by nursing Mamas. Two simple ones to try are oatmeal and dark leafy green vegetables. Have a bowl of oatmeal each morning or an oatmeal cookie for a snack. Use whole oats instead of the instant varieties to get the benefit of the active ingredient beta-glucan. Include plenty of dark leafy green vegetables in your diet, too. If you're so inclined, try a shot of wheat grass each day for a plentiful milk supply.

Herbs such as fenugreek, blessed thistle, fennel, anise, hops, and alfalfa are available in capsule, tincture, and tea form for stimulating milk production. You can find these herbal remedies in natural food stores or pharmacies, but if you suspect that you're having milk supply issues (either too little milk or too much) talk to a lactation consultant and take other appropriate measures to correct the problem before attempting to treat yourself with herbs. For example, make sure Baby is nursing often enough and has a good latch, and that you're eating and drinking enough.

Be aware that some herbs, such as sage, peppermint essential oil, and parsley, can actually hinder milk production. These may be found in medicinal grade teas or other products for health concerns unrelated to lactation (e.g., in cold or digestion remedies). It's best to avoid these until you are no longer nursing.

For more information about herbs and lactation, refer to *The Nursing Mother's Herbal* (Fairview Press, 2003), an excellent reference by Sheila Humphrey, BSc, RN, IBCLC.

*I know Baby isn't supposed to have honey until she's a year old. Can I eat honey while I'm nursing?*
Yes. Honey is not allowed for babies under age one because botulism spores in honey could potentially sicken young babies. These toxic spores do not enter breast milk, so enjoy this sweetener any time.

*If I have an alcoholic drink, will it affect Baby?*
Most pregnant moms don't mind missing out on that glass of nice wine with dinner or a celebratory cocktail at a special event. Once Baby arrives, you can again enjoy an alcoholic drink now and then. Caution and moderation is warranted, though, since alcohol does enter breast milk, and the effects of exposure to alcohol aren't fully understood.

When you have a drink, the alcohol travels in your bloodstream and will show up in your milk within about thirty to sixty minutes. It will be present in your milk until the alcohol has worked its way out of your system about two to three hours later. Avoid feeding baby during those two to three hours. Since large amounts of alcohol may cause drowsiness and weakness in Baby and may inhibit your milk letdown, if you overindulge and get drunk, it's best to "pump and dump" (express your milk and discard it) until you feel sober again. Good rule of thumb: if you are too tipsy to drive a car, you are too tipsy to feed your baby.[9]

If you want to have one drink, have it right after you feed your baby so that it's out of your system by the time she needs to eat again. One drink equals one twelve-ounce beer, an ounce of hard liquor like vodka or gin, or four ounces of wine.

Speaking of beer, you may have heard that it can increase your milk supply. This may be true, but it's not the alcohol in the beer that helps you, it's the barley hops. So if you want to see if beer will increase your supply, try a nonalcoholic brew instead.

*Are there foods I should avoid if my breast-fed baby is fussy?*

Interestingly, research doesn't support the notion that specific foods in Mama's diet give Baby a gassy tummy. To that some Mamas say, "research smeesearch!" Veteran moms may tell you how their baby became a gassy sleepless mess when they ate a particular food. Some babies may respond to at least one or two foods in Mama's diet, however, most babies couldn't care less what Mama eats. What this boils down to is that you should never avoid a food as a precautionary measure just because you have heard it gives babies gas.

While it's tempting to blame your own diet when Baby is very gassy or fussy, first rule out some other causes. Make sure Baby is feeding properly—that she has a good latch on the breast or, if she takes a bottle, that you are holding it at a 30- to 45-degree angle, and that the baby's mouth is making a good seal with the bottle's nipple. Make sure you are successful in getting a good burp out of Baby with each feed. Also consider if you're pushing her to take a pacifier too often in the day and night. Sucking on a pacifier often introduces air into a baby's digestive tract and can cause gas.

Next, observe her symptoms. If your baby is not only fussy but also has a skin or diaper rash, diarrhea, vomiting, persistent nasal congestion, or green mucous stools, she may be showing signs of a food allergy. You'll need to identify the offending food and eliminate it from your diet. If your baby is extremely fussy with symptoms of colic (crying for several hours a day, several days a week, usually in the evening) she may benefit from you avoiding the common food allergens listed below and taking a probiotic supplement.

Still suspect that it's something in your diet? If it is a food that's causing the problem, it's more likely to be one of the following:

- "Gassy" vegetables like cabbage, broccoli, onions, and peppers
- Caffeine from coffee, tea, soft drinks
- Chocolate
- Citrus fruits or tomatoes
- Highly allergenic foods like cow's milk, peanuts, tree nuts, corn, soy, eggs, fish, or shellfish

To track down the culprit, keep a diary of what you eat and Baby's symptoms. A food that you eat will show up in your milk within four to six hours, on average. If there's a food that seems to precede all of Baby's fussy outbursts, try eliminating it for two to three weeks to see if Baby is less gassy or fussy. It might take a week to see the effects of eliminating the offending food.

If you eliminate a food and you find that baby's gas or fussiness clears up, avoid that food until Baby is older. Then reintroduce it and see what happens. Many babies outgrow sensitivities by the time they are about four to six months old.

If you do decide to stop eating a particular food or food group, be sure to replace that food with others that provide the same nutrients. If you eliminate cow's milk, for example, be sure to find other sources of calcium, vitamin D, and protein. If you need to cut out multiple food groups, it might be a good idea to talk to a dietitian about how to maintain an adequate diet despite all your restrictions.

*Do I need to avoid spicy or heavily seasoned foods if I'm nursing?*
Your breast milk takes on some of the flavors from the foods that you eat, giving Baby a little preview of meals to come. Most babies tolerate these flavors with no problems, so there's no reason to avoid certain

seasonings. This early exposure to flavors actually helps set the stage for the development of Baby's future food preferences. Some flavors, like garlic and vanilla, seem to be especially appealing to babies.

As we said before, though, all babies are different, so pay attention to yours. If you notice, for example, that after a big helping of your favorite spicy chili your baby seems uncomfortable or doesn't feed as well as usual, maybe lay off the Tabasco for a while.

*Can my diet protect my breast-fed baby against food allergies?*
Breast-feeding itself may be the best protector against food allergies—babies who are breast-fed exclusively for at least four months seem less likely to develop them.

If any of Baby's close relatives (a parent or sibling) has an allergic disease like asthma, eczema, or food allergies, your baby is considered at risk for developing a food allergy. Some studies suggest that avoiding common allergens—peanuts, tree nuts, cow's milk, fish, shellfish, wheat, and soy—while breast-feeding may protect your baby by delaying her exposure to these foods.[10] Even though the evidence isn't strong enough for groups like the American Academy of Pediatrics to make a blanket recommendation to avoid certain foods, it is prudent to avoid or at least limit the most allergenic foods if you have a strong family history of food allergies.

Another proactive step to help prevent allergies is to take a probiotic supplement while you're nursing. Probiotics are "friendly" bacteria that protect the immune system. Some research shows that when Mama takes a probiotic supplement her breast milk is higher in certain immune factors that help reduce eczema and allergic disease. Look for probiotic supplements in the gastrointestinal health section of your local drugstore.

*Can I go on a diet and lose weight while I'm breast-feeding? How can I eat to lose this baby weight?*
Now that you're holding Baby in your arms instead of your midsection, getting back to your prepregnancy weight (or at least getting back into your old jeans) is surely on your mind. And it should be—studies show

that if you gained a little too much weight during pregnancy and don't lose it within six months of Baby's birth, chances are you're going to hold onto that weight for at least another decade.[11] This could mean starting your next pregnancy at an unhealthy weight and opening yourself up to all kinds of risks.

Though it's a hotly debated topic, most evidence does suggest that breast-feeding helps women lose their pregnancy weight. For many women, the weight just comes off on its own. Others may find losing it more of a struggle. Whether you're breast-feeding or not, the basics of weight loss still apply: don't eat more than you need, and don't just sit on the couch.

Let us repeat: Don't eat more than you need. Eat plenty of fruits and vegetables, lean proteins, whole grains, and healthy fats. But limit or avoid the stuff you just don't need: desserts (you may *feel* that you need that chocolate cake, but really, you don't), unhealthy snacks, foods full of saturated or trans fats, and alcohol. Don't starve yourself. Cutting too far back on your food intake will just backfire—too few calories could affect your breast milk supply, your energy levels and mood, and may lead to cravings and overeating. It can also lead to loss of muscle tissue instead of loss of body fat.

If you want to lose weight and you're nursing, wait until Baby is about four to six weeks old and your breast-feeding is well established. Then aim to lose one pound a week. This rate of weight loss doesn't appear to affect milk production at all. Losing more weight or overly restricting your diet can have negative effects on baby's weight gain and even her temperament (she could get grumpy from a sudden drop in milk production).

*Do artificial sweeteners get into my breast milk?*
Many artificial sweeteners, like aspartame and sucralose, do enter your breast milk. We find it shocking that these sweeteners are generally regarded as safe to consume while breast-feeding. Evidently, research has not proven them to be hazardous for a nursing infant. Despite that, we're not confident that we know all there is to know about these chemicals, so feeding them to Baby just doesn't sit well with us. We recom-

# Might As Well Just Eat Sugar!

I am not a fan of artificial sweeteners. There hasn't been nearly enough research to show they are safe for babies. In fact, some research shows they may be harmful. I advise any parent (or older child) to just go ahead and drink regular soda, chew regular gum, and eat regular *anything* instead of the sugar-free equivalents. Of course, it's best to limit these things anyway. Beware of the "No Added Sugar" label. This usually means an artificial sweetener was added instead.

mend that you avoid these and any artificial chemical food ingredients while you are nursing.

*I'm exhausted! Can I eat anything to increase my energy levels?*
Having a new baby is exciting and fun, but relaxing it's not. Undoubtedly, you've learned how brutal sleep deprivation can be. While no food can undo a sleepless night or replace a power nap, the way you eat can help you beat fatigue and feel a little more alert. Here's how:

- *Get some protein:* The protein in foods can increase your brain's levels of dopamine and norepinephrine, neurotransmitters that help you be alert. Try to include a good source of protein with every meal and snack. Protein comes from foods such as eggs, yogurt, milk, cheese, nuts, meat, poultry, fish, tofu, and other soy foods.
- *Skip the sugar high:* The simple sugars in sweet foods like candy and soda will provide you with a quick burst of energy, but this burst may be followed by a drop in energy and a craving for

more sweets. If you're craving something sweet, go for nature's candy: fresh and dried fruits.

- *Eat breakfast:* Yes, it's the most important meal of the day. Eating a healthy breakfast will help you be alert throughout the morning, minimize cravings, and may even help you manage your weight. The best breakfasts include some high-fiber carbohydrates and some protein. Here are a few examples: an egg on whole grain toast, a high-fiber breakfast cereal with soy or skim milk, or a low-fat yogurt with granola.

- *Stay hydrated:* You need the fluids for breast milk production and you need it for energy. Aim for at least six to eight cups of fluid a day.

- *Go easy on the java:* Though after a sleepless night you may feel like downing the whole pot of coffee, we don't recommend it. One mug of coffee will help perk up your morning, but if you drink more than that, your body might actually experience some minor withdrawal symptoms later in the day. And it could irritate your nursing baby, too. If you do choose to have caffeinated drinks, enjoy only one or two servings (a serving is eight ounces of coffee, not a super grande mega twenty-ouncer), and finish them before 3 p.m. or your nighttime sleep may be affected, too.

- *Mineralize:* If you are deficient in iron or magnesium you might feel low in energy. Your prenatal vitamin has iron—keep taking it. To get iron from foods, enjoy some lean organic ground beef once or twice a week, and choose other sources like fortified cereals, beans, dried fruit, dark leafy greens, and egg yolks. Magnesium is found in nuts; soybeans and tofu; spinach; whole grains like shredded wheat, wheat bran, and oatmeal; and yogurt.

# Taking It Home . . .

Even after your baby arrives, your nutritional obligations to her continue. (But yes, you can finally eat sushi!) Eat a balanced, clean diet full of all-natural foods from all the food groups. Here's a reminder of our ultimate recipe for nutritious breast milk:

- Eat organic
- Eat healthy unsaturated and omega-3 fats
- Get plenty of B vitamins, vitamins A and C, and other vitamins and minerals
- Stay hydrated
- Avoid high-mercury fish
- Avoid environmental toxic exposures

Getting all the necessary nutrients onto your table might feel like a challenge, but some simple throw-together meals and snacks will have you on your way. You can also eat in a way that helps you get back to your prepregnancy weight. Spending a little extra time and effort on this now will pay off by giving you a positive attitude and more energy to spend on yourself and your new baby.

# 5

# Your Hungry Baby

Starting the Solid Food Adventure

Most aspects of parenting are fairly intuitive, and parents can usually get by with simply trusting their instincts. But when it comes to a baby's nutrition, many moms and dads have numerous questions and concerns. When should you begin solids? What are the best foods for a baby? What foods can cause allergies? How much and how often should you feed? What if your baby refuses to eat? How can you know if your baby is too thin or too plump? Do vigorous eaters grow up healthier than picky ones? What are the best ways to help a baby learn to be a good eater?

The first six months of a baby's nutrition are easy. Just breast-feed eight to ten times a day or more often if Baby asks, or give Baby whatever amount of formula seems to satisfy her. Baby's weight gain at her checkups will be the proof in the pudding (hopefully, not literally—no pudding for babies!). But when you get the green light to begin solid foods at six months, you now have many choices to make. Fruits or veggies first? Make your own baby food or buy it at the store? Jarred or frozen? Organic or conventional?

Throughout this chapter you will learn the answers to all these questions and more. We will focus on the best foods to feed your baby and how to prepare or buy them. You will learn creative ways to get your baby interested in food and how to lower Baby's risk of food allergies. But even the best advice can go unheeded by a baby who has a mind of her own.

What is a parent to do when you've done everything right and prepared the best food for your baby, but when you sit down for that first feeding all you get is tight lips and a turned head? And as you try and try again, your baby continues to give you clear indications that she is not interested. Should you panic? Is your baby going to wither away? A baby must begin solid foods at six months in order to thrive, right? Wrong.

The truth is, breast milk is complete nutrition for the entire first year of life. Formula also provides all the calories a baby needs for about a year. A baby could actually not eat any solids at all until she is one year old and be just fine. Food in the first year is mainly for fun, to get baby interested in the concept of eating, and to prepare baby's taste buds and palate for later on when he is weaned and must rely on foods for growth and nutrition.

Here's a general rule when it comes to understanding babies: if at least 25 percent of babies do it, it must be normal and nothing to worry about. And this is certainly true when it comes to picky eaters. Many babies are picky and may refuse solids for months, and as a pediatrician and a nutritionist we have watched thousands of such babies grow and thrive just as well as those who do eat. So we have learned not to worry about the overall health of these babies. We know they will be fine in the long run.

But we can't seem to get moms to stop worrying about their picky eaters. There's just something about Mamas that must see food go into their baby's mouth. More power to you! Because you were physically connected to your baby for nine months, and you were Baby's only source of nutrition in the womb and for the first six months of breast-feeding, it's only natural that you are so concerned that your baby eats well. Dads (like Dr. Bob) just don't seem to worry as much. You are right to pay attention to your baby's nutrition. Healthy eating is important;

just don't lose sleep over it if your baby isn't jumping right into solids. In the next chapter we will share with you creative approaches to solving your picky eater problems.

On the other hand, many babies love food and just can't get enough. For these little ones it's even more important that what goes into your baby is healthy, since there will be so much of it. These first three years are a critical time for brain growth and development. What goes into a baby's mouth (and therefore into her brain) must be pure and natural. Organic eating is a must. Pesticides are poisonous to brain cells. Hormones can harm a baby's metabolism. These and other chemicals can affect a baby's immune system. We'll show you how to feed Baby a pure and natural diet without driving yourself (too) crazy.

There is another important reason that babies should eat only natural whole foods. It's a concept we call shaping young tastes. What a baby eats in the early years actually programs the taste buds to crave those flavors and textures. So a baby or toddler who eats only real fruits and veggies, whole grain foods, healthy meats, poultry, and fish, and other healthy foods will actually crave those foods throughout childhood. Such foods will just feel right to their palate as they grow. A baby who eats mostly processed foods, bland jarred baby foods, and crunchy snack carbs like crackers will have taste buds that will mainly accept such foods as they get older and shun the natural taste of whole foods. Sure, even healthy eaters will learn to love sweet foods and treats, but they'll always enjoy everything that's healthy as well.

The bottom line on feeding your baby is that food should be fun for both of you. If it isn't, back off. The goal for feeding in the first year is to help your baby learn to want to eat eventually, not to have a perfect and plentiful eater right away. This chapter will show you how to reach that goal, naturally!

## Raising a Happy Green Eater from Day One

As Baby starts her solid food adventure you certainly want the solids that you feed Baby to provide her with healthy nutrients that will contribute to her growth and development. But perhaps even more important is for Baby to learn *how* to eat and that eating is a positive experience. She needs to master certain eating skills like swallowing, chewing, and feeding herself. She also needs to learn how to navigate the social and sensual aspects of eating. Through her early eating experiences she will join others at a common table, assess smells and flavors of foods, and hopefully, learn some table manners. The best ways to teach her all of these skills is to feed her with the rest of the family, to feed her a variety of healthy and flavorful foods so she gets used to the mechanics of eating different textures and the experience of a wide spectrum of flavors, and, as soon as possible, to start feeding her the same types of foods that are being eaten by those around her at the table.

Later in the chapter we'll discuss how Baby's early eating experi-

A NOTE FROM DR. BOB

## Holding Off the Hungry Four- and Five-Month-Old

The official policy of the American Academy of Pediatrics is to wait until Baby is at least six months old before you feed him anything besides breast milk or formula. However, some babies are eager to get started earlier. In years past the usual advice was to start foods (like rice cereal) at four months, so many parents (and grandparents) still believe that's OK. If your baby wants food now but you really want to wait, you can trick Baby into thinking he's joining in the family meal by letting him play with a cup and spoon at mealtime. Let him sip some water out of a sippy cup. Give him something to gnaw on that he can't really eat (like a peeled carrot stick). This may hold him off for a few weeks until you are ready to start.

ences will help shape her food preferences for years to come. What better time than now to introduce fresh, all-natural, and organic healthy foods to Baby? Whether she *eats* her greens or not, green she will be!

# Ready, Set, Eat!

While some babies may not show interest until later in the first year, most are good and ready at six months. At this age, babies will benefit from exposure to more flavors, textures, and eating skills, and most babies are physically and developmentally ready to handle solid foods. This means Baby:

- can hold her head up straight when sitting
- can sit with support (i.e., in a high chair)
- no longer has the tongue thrust reflex (pushes everything out of the mouth)
- has the head control to turn her head toward or away from food
- appears interested in food when other people are eating, for example, she reaches for food on your plate or mimics chewing motions

Your baby may hit these milestones before the six-month mark, but there are many reasons to wait until this age before starting solid foods:

- Introducing solids too soon may actually sabotage breast-feeding because as Baby eats more and more food, she may be less interested in nursing and consequently your supply may suffer.
- Waiting until six months may help to prevent food allergies, especially if your family has a strong history of allergies. By this age Baby's intestinal tract is mature enough to handle new and foreign substances without prompting an allergic reaction.

- On a less serious note, one more reason to wait is because you don't need something else on your to-do list! You should try to just enjoy the relative ease of your baby's early months when all she needs is a breast or a bottle.

Despite these reasons to wait, don't be surprised if your pediatrician OKs solids once Baby hits four months old. If you have a really big baby who gulps down her breast milk or formula and then looks for more, it may seem that she needs food in order to be satisfied. Or maybe you ask your doctor if you can start food so Baby will sleep through the night. Sounds like a great plan, but unfortunately, it's not likely to work. Young babies don't usually wake up because they're hungry—they wake up because their little brains and bodies just can't stay asleep for very long stretches. Of course, when they *do* wake up they realize they're starving.

Even though it might be tempting to start solids early, our advice is to wait it out. Six months will be here before you know it.

## HOW-TOS FOR FIRST TIMERS

### Baby's First Food

You've probably heard that you should start Baby on rice cereal. Rice cereal is a very common first food because it has the right texture, is easy to digest, and it's very unlikely that your baby will have an allergic reaction to it. Other single-grain, wheat-free cereals, like oatmeal and barley cereals, are also good choices for these reasons. Infant preparations of these cereals will be supplemented with iron—a nice bonus since Baby does need some extra iron at this stage.

Starting with rice cereal is common, but in truth this is more a feeding custom than a feeding law. Although we think infant iron-fortified cereals play an important role in the diets of six- to twelve-month-old babies, you don't have to start with this as Baby's very first food if you don't want to. If you prefer, you can choose one of these foods, which are mild, unlikely to be allergenic, and are appealing to a baby's taste buds:

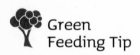 Green Feeding Tip

Choose organic foods for Baby's first eating experiences—they will be free of pesticide residues and may even taste better.

## KEY NUTRIENTS IN FIRST FOODS

| Food | Key Vitamins and Minerals | Comment |
|---|---|---|
| Fortified infant cereals | Iron | Our organic HAPPYBELLIES cereals also provide important probiotics—healthy bacteria to keep Baby's gut healthy and to prevent allergies and eczema |
| Orange and dark green fruits and vegetables | Vitamin A | Examples: carrots, squash, sweet potatoes |
| Other fruits and vegetables | Vitamin C | Examples: apples, pears, potatoes |

- bananas
- peaches
- pears
- applesauce
- avocados
- sweet potatoes
- winter squash
- carrots

### Equipment

For the first few feedings, you don't need many supplies. Use a spoon made especially for babies or a tiny sugar spoon that fits easily in Baby's tiny mouth. You can even use your clean finger instead of a spoon, if you prefer. Though your older relatives may have used a baby bottle to feed their babies infant cereal, this is no longer recommended as it can be a choking hazard. The most important equipment for these experiments: a bib.

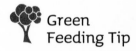

## Green Feeding Tip

Stainless steel cocktail spoons are a nice alternative to plastic spoons, which may contain polyvinyl chloride (PVC) or phthalates, chemicals that can leach into Baby's foods. Bamboo spoons are great, too. Bambu (www.bambuhome .com) makes a set of small bamboo utensils especially for Baby. If you do opt for plastic, look for ones labeled "PVC free."

# Veggies First? Does It Matter?

No. In my opinion it doesn't matter whether Baby tries fruits, veggies, or cereal first. Many people believe that if you start a baby on fruits, she'll get used to sweet foods and won't take veggies later. This theory has never been researched. No one has taken a group of a thousand babies, started different groups of babies on various foods, and monitored which group become the better eaters later on. I believe it's more important that a baby's first experiences are with organic unprocessed whole fruits or veggies. No bland jarred baby food for beginners. Fruits and veggies may even be better than cereal since they have much more flavor and more interesting flavor. If you are worried about fruits first, sure—go ahead with a veggie. But follow it up with a fruit a few days later. Don't agonize over your decision about which food comes first. Soon enough, Baby will be eating all the foods on this list and the order in which they were introduced won't matter.

## Timing

For Baby's first few tastes of solids, choose a time when Baby is alert, happy, and not too hungry. Consider your own needs, too, and don't pick a time when you're rushing to be somewhere else. If you're concerned that Baby's sensitive tummy will have a hard time with food (if she's had stomach issues in the past), you may want to give new foods during the first half of the day so that if something doesn't agree with her, she'll likely work through the symptoms before she goes to sleep that night. It would be unfortunate (mostly for you!) to have a food reaction ruin a good night's rest.

Look at Baby's first solid foods as snacks in between her meals of breast milk or formula. For instance, if Baby nurses or takes a bottle every three or four hours, you could pick a time about one to two hours after a feeding to try solids. If you wait too long and Baby is too hungry, she may get frustrated with the food. Too soon and Baby may not care to eat any food. After the solids, Baby will let you know when she is hungry again for her milk. It may be a little later than if she hadn't eaten food, but eating solids will rarely prompt a baby to skip a nursing or bottle-feeding entirely.

Experiment to find the routine that works best for you and Baby. The only rule at this stage: don't replace Baby's liquid meals with solids. Breast milk or formula will be Baby's main source of nutrition until she's a year old. In fact, if your breast-fed Baby seems to develop a preference for solids over breast milk, it's recommended that you nurse her throughout most of the day and then feed her solids only at the end of the day, when you probably are making less milk anyway.

First Food Texture

Up to this point, Baby has been swallowing only liquids, so make Baby's first-ever solid feeding almost liquid in consistency—it should pour off the spoon. Never give solid foods in a bottle, no matter the consistency. As Baby gets used to swallowing food, prepare her foods to be thicker (more like the consistency of a porridge) by adding less liquid.

- *Cereal:* Prepare iron-fortified infant cereal by mixing a small amount of cereal with one or two teaspoonfuls of expressed breast milk or infant formula. This will give it the right texture and a pleasing familiar flavor.
- *Fruit or vegetable:* Use a single-ingredient thin puree. You'll need to cook the vegetable, then blend it with breast milk or formula to get the right consistency. Many first fruits don't need cooking. See page 173 for a full discussion about making baby food.

## Technique

Offer Baby the spoon or your clean finger with a tiny amount of the food on the tip. Let her open her mouth to accept the food instead of forcing it between her lips. Be enthusiastic and say things like "Mmmm!" and "Yummy!" as you feed her. Don't overwhelm Baby, though. If you hover over the high chair and put too much pressure on Baby to love the food, your efforts could backfire and she'll reject your overly eager attempts. So, be encouraging but remain low-key. This advice will become even more important as Baby gets older and becomes a toddler.

Baby should happily accept the food and show eagerness for more. The expression on a baby's face when she tastes a new food, thinks about the taste, then decides she likes it and wants more, is priceless. You shouldn't have to keep coaxing Baby to get in that next bite, or ten. If all she wants is that one bite, it's better to stop and try again at the

### A NOTE FROM DR. BOB

## Beware of Constipation

Many of the typical starting foods (bananas, rice cereal, and applesauce) can be constipating for some babies. If you notice your little one getting a little backed up, stop these foods and incorporate some pureed prunes or peaches into Baby's daily diet. Once things start moving again you can ease these foods back in and see what Baby can tolerate. My first child needed a daily dose of prunes, peaches, or diluted prune juice for the first two years of life once we started solids. You can also feed Baby some frozen baby foods with probiotics (or buy an infant probiotic powder to add to foods). These are great for helping things move along.

next meal. Pushing Baby into more will create a negative experience and make feeding her more difficult next time.

## How Much and How Often

For the first few days, offer about a tablespoon of food once a day. Don't be surprised if Baby takes less, though. If she seems to want more, you can go get another teaspoon or two. Once she is easily accepting food (this could be after one meal for some babies or after several weeks for others) you can give her more food and add more meals. The ultimate goal in all of this is for Baby to eventually join the family at the table for three meals a day. It's OK if it takes the next few months to get to this goal.

As Baby gets used to eating and progresses through a list of new foods, her intake will increase. Let her tell you how much she wants. Watching for her cues will help make feeding times a nice experience for both of you.

### "Feeding Time at the Zoo" Cues

- waving arms and legs excitedly when food is offered
- smiling during the feeding
- cooing happily when fed
- opening the mouth for the spoon
- moving toward the spoon

### "Do Not Feed the Animals" Cues

- falling asleep
- getting fussy
- spitting out the food
- pushing away the spoon
- closing the mouth
- turning the head when the spoon approaches

Remember that nutritionally, food is just the icing on the proverbial cake. Breast milk or formula will still provide the bulk of Baby's nutrients at this age. The best clue to whether Baby is getting the right amount of calories from her combined diet of breast milk or formula and food is her growth. If she is following a reasonable growth curve as charted by your pediatrician at regular checkups, and her doctor is not concerned about too little or too much weight gain, chances are her intake is on target. Although we can't predict how each baby will eat, we know it's helpful to have some basic parameters as a guide, so here you go:

| Age | How Many Meals per Day * | How Many Different Foods per Meal * | Typical Serving Size * |
|---|---|---|---|
| 6 to 8 months | 1, 2, or 3 meals, depending on Baby's level of interest and mood | 2 foods (e.g., cereal and fruit or fruit and vegetable) | Up to ½ cup of each food |
| 9 to 12 months | 3 meals | 2 or 3 foods (e.g., a protein, vegetable, and starch) | Fruits, veggies, or starch: ¼ cup<br><br>Meat, chicken, beans, or tofu: ⅛ to ¼ cup<br><br>Yogurt: ¼ to ⅓ cup |

* Important: These are ballpark figures of what you may reasonably expect, not recommendations for how much Baby needs to be taking.

What if Baby Won't Eat?

Even if the calendar points to Baby being ready to start solids and she's exhibiting the signs listed above, it doesn't mean she's going to go after the solids with unbridled passion. Some babies enthusiastically take to eating, but others need more time. Many parents are quite shocked when Baby absolutely refuses to open her mouth for the first full week of attempts at feeding her.

If your baby is like most and absolutely refuses to take any food the first time, don't force the issue. It could be that she's not ready or needs to get used to the idea. Try again the next day or give her a week before another attempt. Her refusal could also mean that she simply doesn't

## Don't Worry About Exact Amounts of Food

During Baby's first year of life you really don't need to worry about the quantity of food she eats. Baby's appetite will ensure she's eating enough. If she doesn't eat much food one day, she'll ask to nurse more often or fuss for an extra bottle. This may vary from day to day, or a baby might be extra picky with foods for a few weeks and then chow down the next month to make up for it. Say, a baby doesn't eat enough whole grains for a few days. Or she doesn't care so much for dark green veggies. Who cares? Hopefully, not you. You have so many other things to worry about that the day-to-day minutiae of a baby's diet aren't worth worrying over. We present this information to you for education, not as a required menu. The ultimate proof that Baby is eating enough is her growth measurements at each checkup.

like the food you've selected for her. Try switching foods (for example, from rice cereal to oatmeal or peaches). Then, once Baby is settled and accepting solids without problems, you can try the original food again. Never give up on a particular food altogether because Baby rejects it the first time. She may need ten to fifteen encounters with a food before she decides she likes it.

If after several weeks of attempts at solid feeding you feel that there has been no progress and you are concerned, talk to your pediatrician. Most of the time, there's nothing to worry about. You'll probably be advised to just keep trying, and over time Baby will decide she wants to try the food. Occasionally, a baby's reluctance to eat could be a sign that

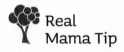

Real Mama Tip

"I found it easier to get him to try a new food that he was hesitant about by giving it to him and to my friend's baby (who is about the same age) when they were together. I guess peer pressure works—in a positive way—even in infancy!"

—Pam, San Diego, California

she's having difficulty figuring out how to swallow or is uncomfortable from an undiagnosed digestive issue like gastric reflux. If your doctor suspects a problem, she may refer you to a gastrointestinal or feeding specialist for an evaluation. Don't worry. Most feeding concerns are easy to address, and Baby will be eating in no time.

# Moving Ahead: New Flavors and Textures

From six to eight months, Baby's menu will consist of cereals, fruits, and vegetables. After Baby takes her very first food once a day for a few days in a row, try another food from the list. Introduce just one new food at a time so you can easily figure out if something new causes a reaction. You can add a new food to foods she's already eaten, if you want. So, for example, if she's had rice cereal for a few days already and you want to try pears next, you can mix the pears with her cereal. You don't have to give the pears by themselves.

Most six-month-old babies will do best on pureed textures, but soon Baby's feeding and eating skills will progress to being able to "chew" more lumpy or chunky solid foods. Some babies master purees very quickly and will be excited to have lumpy mashed foods. Others will have a harder time figuring out how to swallow these thicker textures and may even appear to gag on certain foods. If that's the case, stay with purees until both you and Baby are comfortable enough to move on.

Usually, by seven or eight months of age babies are used to taking pureed foods and are ready to try more variety of textures. If you are buying commercial baby foods, you can advance to "stage 2" foods at this time—HAPPYBABY calls these foods "smooth combos." If you're making your own foods, simply blend the foods with less liquid to make them a little thicker, and leave some soft lumps. Giving Baby more texture will help her development of mouth skills like moving food around the mouth, chewing motions, and swallowing safely.

Next, at around eight or nine months of age, Baby will probably be ready to progress to even more chewing and mashing with her gums. Try "stage 3" foods now—HAPPYBABY's are called "sorta chunky." You can also add protein foods to her menu at this time. These include pureed or finely ground meats and poultry, mashed beans, mashed tofu, plain whole milk yogurt, mashed egg yolk (wait until one year to offer the white), and mild cheeses.

This table provides ideas for new foods for every age.

| 6 months old: Start with pureed, strained foods. Offer 1 to 2 tablespoons (equivalent to 1/2 to 1 cubes of frozen baby food) | | | |
|---|---|---|---|
| *Cereal/Grains to Introduce* | *Fruits to Introduce* | *Vegetables to Introduce* | *Proteins to Introduce* |
| Brown Rice cereal | Peaches | Peas | None |
| Barley cereal | Pears | Green Beans | |
| Oatmeal | Apples | Winter Squash | |
| Rice (pureed) | Banana | Sweet Potatoes | |
| | Apricots | Carrots | |
| | Avocado | Summer Squash | |
| | Plums/Prunes | | |
| **7–9 months old:** Add coarsely mashed or finely chopped foods | | | |
| *Cereal/Grains to Introduce* | *Fruits to Introduce* | *Vegetables to Introduce* | *Proteins to Introduce* |
| Mixed Grain | Mango | Spinach | Yogurt* (plain, whole fat) |
| Wheat Cereal* | Pineapple | Broccoli | |
| Other cooked grains (quinoa, barley) | Papaya | Cauliflower | Egg yolk, hard-boiled and mashed |
| | | Cucumber | |
| May be ready for dry "O" type cereal, bits of soft breads* | | | Pureed or finely ground chicken, turkey, beef, lamb, or pork |
| | | | Beans, mashed |
| | | | Lentils, mashed |

| 9–12 months old: Add more finger foods | | | |
|---|---|---|---|
| *Cereal/Grains to Introduce* | *Fruits to Introduce* | *Vegetables to Introduce* | *Proteins to Introduce* |
| Finger foods including teething crackers or biscuits, dry "O" type cereal, soft cooked pasta (preferably whole grain)* | Finger foods, including small pieces of soft fruit like banana, ripe pear, cooked apple (skins removed) and cooked peach (skins removed) | Finger foods, including small pieces of soft cooked vegetables, skins removed | Cottage cheese* <br><br> Soft, mild cheeses* (pasteurized) <br><br> Tofu*, mild fish like wild salmon or cod* |

*These foods may cause allergic reactions. See page 167 for more information.

Here's an example of a seven-month-old baby's menu:

| *Time of Day* | *Food or Beverage* |
|---|---|
| Wake-up | Breast milk or formula |
| Breakfast | 2 tablespoons (some babies may take up to ¼ cup) iron-fortified cereal, such as HAPPYBELLIES Organic Brown Rice Cereal, and 2 tablespoons* pureed fruit, such as HAPPYBABY Wiser Apple |
| Midmorning | Breast milk or formula |
| Lunch | 2 tablespoons pureed vegetable, such as HAPPYBABY Yes Peas, and 2 tablespoons pureed fruit |
| Midafternoon | Breast milk or formula |
| Dinner | 2 tablespoons iron-fortified cereal and 2 tablespoons pureed vegetable |
| Before bed | Breast milk or formula |
| All night long, perhaps! | Breast milk or formula |

*One cube of HAPPYBABY or homemade frozen baby food is 2 tablespoons, or about 1 ounce.

# Too Many Rules?

We provide you with feeding charts for various ages as a guideline. But you will notice some variations between our information and the feeding charts you may find in other books or online. Who is right? How do we know exactly what is right to feed a baby at various ages? The truth is that no one really knows for sure. These feeding charts are based mainly on common sense and what doctors have observed over the years. The main reason we provide such lists is to make sure a baby doesn't eat foods that might be highly allergenic before a baby is ready. So, we are going to sum up the main rules you *really* need to know when it comes to feeding what foods at what age. Everything else on our feeding chart is fairly flexible.

- Don't give any cow's milk products (yogurt, cheese, or butter) or corn before eight months.
- Don't give any straight cow's milk, egg whites, honey, or nut butters before age one year.
- Don't give any shellfish or peanut products before age two years.
- Don't give chokable foods (see list, page 169).

That's it! Those are really the only rules you have to make sure not to break when it comes to feeding your baby. Any other accidental or purposeful deviations from our food chart are probably harmless in the long run. So, be free!

Here's an example of a ten-month-old baby's menu:

| Time of Day | Food or Beverage |
|---|---|
| Wake-up | Breast milk or formula |
| Breakfast | ¼ cup iron-fortified cereal and ¼ cup mashed or chopped fruit |
| Midmorning | Breast milk or formula |
| Lunch | ⅓ cup plain whole milk yogurt with ¼ cup mashed or chopped fruit, handful of O-shaped dry cereal |
| Midafternoon | Breast milk or formula |
| Dinner | 3 ounces (¼ to ½ cup) of a mixed dinner, such as HAPPYBABY Chick Chick* (or 2 tablespoons minced chicken with 2 tablespoons mashed or chopped vegetable and 2 tablespoons rice or other starch) |
| Before bed | Breast milk or formula |

* 3 cubes of HAPPYBABY or homemade frozen baby food is 3 ounces.

# Next Step: Finger Foods

Around eight or nine months of age, when Baby can sit up without help, is good at eating varied textures from a spoon, and has the pincer grasp figured out (she can pick up small objects between her forefinger and thumb), she may be ready for finger foods.

Finger foods are simply any soft food that Baby can pick up with her fingers and feed to herself. Cut them into bite-size pieces (the size of a pea) and give them to her along with her other foods at mealtime. Try some of these:

- Soft cooked or canned apple, pear, peach, apricot
- Tofu cubes (no need to cook first)

- Banana
- Avocado
- Cooked sweet or white potato
- Overcooked (i.e., soft) carrots or parsnips
- Freezer waffles (choose an egg-free variety until Baby is one year old)
- Soft cooked pasta
- O-shaped no-sugar dry cereal
- Spinach or potato pancakes (eggless)
- Rice (starchy short-grain rice works well because it sticks together)
- Mild cheese
- Fish cakes made with minced low-mercury fish (a salmon cake, for example)

When Baby starts feeding herself, things will get messy. Throw something like an old towel or a shower curtain under her high chair and let her go at it. Allow baby to use her hands, even on foods that aren't usually consumed that way (a handful of yogurt really hits the spot, or the face!).

If you're really brave, you can encourage her to try a spoon as well. Many babies want to use the spoon themselves but are not able to actually get the food from bowl to mouth. If mealtimes are all mess but no sustenance and you find Baby is getting frustrated, try offering spoonfuls of food in between her self-fed bites. Just be sure to read her cues and avoid stuffing her with food after she's no longer hungry.

Some babies start to reject mashed and pureed foods once they move on to table foods and that's OK. In fact, that's the goal: to help Baby move from baby foods to table foods. You may need to shift to meals of mostly finger foods with spoon-fed foods as a side dish.

Stuck with a freezer or pantry full of baby food and a baby who seems to not want it so much anymore? You can use those leftover purees in creative ways. Here are some ideas:

# Get Messy

Letting Baby feed herself, and get messy in the process, is good for development. Not only does self-feeding exercise the fine motor pincer grasp and hand-to-mouth coordination, it also helps Baby become accustomed to the variety of messy and sticky sensations on the hands and face. I was shocked to read in one baby book the advice to teach a baby how to raise her hands during meal-time to allow only a parent to do the feeding. This was intended to teach Baby cleanliness, neatness, and obedience. Can you imag-ine? Babies aren't supposed to be neat and clean. And obedience? What's that to a nine-month-old? Of course, when the food starts flying across the room it's time to get down.

- Veggie puree can be a sauce to serve over noodles
- Older children or adults in the home can use fruit purees as a dip for French toast sticks or pancakes
- Mix fruit puree into plain yogurt or hot oatmeal
- Mix ground beef, turkey, or chicken with vegetable purees for moist burger patties
- Use fruit puree instead of oil in homemade muffins or cookies

## MYTH OR FACT?

*Babies without teeth can still eat finger foods.*

Fact! If she doesn't have any teeth, Baby will be able to "chew" soft foods with her gums. In fact, the teeth that babies tend to get first, the ones in the front, don't do much chewing anyway, so even babies with front teeth are mashing their food with their gums. That's why Baby's foods should always be soft and in tiny bite-size pieces to reduce her risk of choking, regardless of how many teeth she has.

## A Beverage for Baby

Babies typically stay well hydrated with adequate breast milk or formula. Extra fluids are required only when one of the following is true: Baby has had significant fluid losses from sweating or an intestinal illness with vomiting or diarrhea, or Baby is constipated since starting solid foods.

Even though Baby doesn't necessarily *need* extra fluids, at around seven or eight months of age it's time to introduce water as a mealtime beverage to help her develop a taste for it and to give her something to wash down her food with. It's also a good time to introduce a cup—a sippy cup or an open cup. You can give Baby expressed breast milk or formula in a cup if you want to. For a full discussion of safe sippy cups, turn to page 103.

As we discussed back in chapter 3, although tap water has been generally considered safe for babies, in recent years we've heard alarming reports about contaminants in our water supply—by-products from the chlorination process, industrial chemicals, agricultural chemicals, even pharmaceuticals.[1] What's a green Mama to do? Baby will be exposed to less water (tap or bottled) if she's breast-fed, so this is yet another reason to stick with nursing until age one year or beyond. You can also use a faucet-mounted or pitcher-style water filter to remove some contaminants, like lead, copper, cadmium, and mercury. Buying bottled water isn't exactly an inexpensive or eco-friendly option, but you have to weigh the pros and cons here. If you buy bottled water for baby, buy the largest containers possible to minimize plastic waste and recycle these containers whenever possible. If you've switched to bottled water for your breast-fed Baby, she may need a fluoride supplement for her growing teeth. Ask her pediatrician about this.

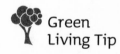 Green Living Tip

Do your part to reduce tap water contamination. Use fewer household chemicals, support organic farming, and dispose of any chemicals or potentially toxic household waste carefully. Most communities have special trash pickup days for these hazardous items. And don't flush old medications down the toilet or pour them in the sink. Ask a pharmacist or your local department of public works how to dispose of these safely.

## ABOUT FRUIT JUICE

Fruit juice is not nutritionally necessary for Baby. It's a good source of vitamin C, but it also has a lot of fruit sugar, which can cause hyper behavior, contribute to cavities, and cause a baby to develop a sweet tooth. For babies and young toddlers, it's better to foster a preference for plain water than for a sweet beverage like juice. If you do choose to serve juice:

- Wait until baby is at least six months old and then give Baby 100 percent juice only (apple juice is a good choice).
- Heavily dilute juice with water to make it less concentrated and sweet.
- Avoid all juice drinks and other beverages with added sugar or sweeteners.
- Offer juice in a cup (not a bottle) and serve with a snack rather than a meal so it doesn't interfere with the appetite.
- Limit Baby to no more than four ounces, or one-half cup, of juice per day.
- Look for juice blends that contain vegetable juices, like those from First Juice (www.firstjuice.com), as these are often low in sugar.

### Why is my baby turning orange?

After a couple of months of eating orange fruits and vegetables like squash, apricots, peaches, and sweet potatoes, Baby's skin may actually take on an orange hue. You may notice this skin tone, like that of some adorable science fiction creature, only in photographs. If this happens, don't panic. The color is due to all the beta-carotene in these foods and will go away as Baby's diet becomes more varied. Rest assured that it's not dangerous. You can cut back on the orange and push the green, if you want to.

# Spotting Food Allergies

As you introduce new foods to Baby, observe how she reacts to each food, looking out for allergies or intolerances. Since reactions don't always appear immediately following a first exposure, feed her a new food for two to four days before starting another new food. Spreading out the new foods this way will help you determine the culprit if a reaction does occur.

Signs of a food allergy include:

- a new skin rash
- diaper rash—redness around the anus
- swelling of the face or tongue
- a stuffy or runny nose lasting more than two weeks
- rattling in the chest or wheezing
- mucous diarrhea
- vomiting

Some babies may also experience a food intolerance that isn't an actual allergy. Symptoms could include:

- fussiness or night waking
- upset stomach, gas pains, vomiting
- runny or mucous stools, diarrhea

Occasional changes in the color and texture of Baby's stools aren't usually cause for concern, although if *most* of Baby's stools become more runny or mucous for more than several days, this may indicate a sensitivity.

Luckily, the vast majority of children (96 percent)[2] will not develop a single food allergy. If Baby does develop a food allergy, there's a good chance it will be to one of these eight foods, responsible for more than 90 percent of food allergies in children:

- cow's milk products
- wheat
- soy
- egg white
- peanuts
- tree nuts (e.g., almonds, cashews, and walnuts)
- shellfish
- fish

We generally recommend waiting until age one year to start many of these foods in order to help avoid an allergy to them. Some forms of these can be started around nine months, such as cheese, yogurt, baby cereals, teething biscuits, breads, egg yolk, mild fish like wild salmon or cod, and tofu.

If Baby has a strong family history of allergies—one parent or a sibling with food allergies—you should delay all forms of these potentially allergenic foods until Baby is at least one year old. Waiting until two years is even better.

Other foods that may not be tolerated well by young babies or that may cause allergic reactions include chocolate, citrus fruits, strawberries or other berries, and tomatoes. If you prefer to be extra cautious, you may want to wait until at least Baby's first birthday to offer these foods.

If you think Baby is allergic to a food, eliminate it from her diet to see if the symptoms also disappear. Ask your pediatrician about any new symptoms or if you suspect a food allergy. If you suspect food allergies, a blood or skin test can be done to determine which foods are the culprits. If Baby ever has a severe reaction to a food and she is having trouble breathing, call 911.

Can food allergies be prevented or avoided? We don't know for sure. Based on the current research, it seems that the best ways to reduce Baby's risk of developing a food allergy are to give her only breast milk until four to six months old, wait until six months to introduce solids, and then follow the most conservative guidelines about when to introduce common allergens.

## Fixing Food Allergies

Figuring out food allergies doesn't have to be complicated. Here's what I do in my office. First, I take the baby off all forms of cow's milk (yogurt, cheese) since this is the most often the cause, and I also advise my patients to change to a hypoallergenic formula if they are not nursing. If the allergies don't improve within two weeks, I take the baby off wheat (and continue going cow's milk-free). If problems continue, Mom and Baby stop all eight foods: wheat, cow's milk, egg white, shellfish, fish, soy, peanuts, and tree nuts. This may be tough on Mom's diet, but it's easy for a young baby since she can rely on breast milk or formula. If the allergies continue, *then* I do blood allergy testing or send the baby to an allergist for skin testing.

# Foods to Skip (For Now)

### CHOKABLE FOODS

Foods that can cause choking are hard foods that require too much chewing for young babies and small round foods that can lodge in the throat. Avoid most of these choking hazards until age four years or older:

*Hard foods:* Nuts, seeds, popcorn, raw carrots (or any hard vegetable), whole grapes, hard fruit (like apples), whole hot dogs or sausage links, hard candy, or large chunks of meat or other tough foods.

*Soft but sticky foods:* Chewing gum, marshmallows, and jelly candies can also get lodged in the throat and should be avoided.

## NO HONEY UNTIL AGE ONE YEAR

Honey may contain spores of *Clostridium botulinum*, the organism that causes botulism. The immune systems of older children and adults systems can handle a small amount of these spores, but babies younger than one year are susceptible to a life-threatening reaction to the toxins they produce. These spores are even heat resistant and may survive in baked goods. So, no honey for your honey until she's at least twelve months old!

# Choices: Jarred, Frozen, and Homemade Baby Foods

When Baby begins solid foods you have some choices to make. Will you feed her jarred food? Homemade? Frozen? Organic? Conventional?

These days there are lots of options at the market. Truly, we think that the gold standard is to make your own baby food from organic, fresh, all-natural ingredients. In fact, HAPPYBABY offers baby-food-making classes around the country to help moms (and dads) get started. But we live in the real world, too, and know that some parents won't be able to make their own, even if they recognize the benefits. So, that's where we come in with our line of organic fresh-frozen baby meals. Before we jump into baby foods, let's first discuss jarred baby food.

## JARRED BABY FOODS

The most abundant option on the shelves of your local store is likely to be jarred baby food. While jars may be a convenient and inexpensive option, there are reasons we encourage moms and dads to "think outside the jar." Jarred foods are prepared using very high heat, and this heat processing actually destroys certain vitamins in the food. This is not to say that jarred foods are not nutritionally adequate per se, but they are not as rich in certain nutrients as more freshly prepared foods like homemade foods and home-style fresh-frozen foods.

Personally, we aren't thrilled that the color, texture, and taste of jarred foods bear little resemblance to the fresh ingredients. Picture feeding a baby jarred bananas for a few months. Then when you give her a real banana one day, she may think, "Hey, this is not a banana!"

That said, even parents who make their own food or buy home-style frozen baby foods may need to reach for a jar now and then. If you use jarred foods, choose organic options and avoid any varieties with added sugars, like baby custards. Baby certainly doesn't need dessert—she's sweet enough already.

When feeding Baby jarred foods, always spoon her portion into a separate bowl before serving. Refrigerate the open jar and throw it away after two to three days. Remember that Baby's saliva contains bacteria, and you don't want this touching the portion of the food that you plan to save for another feeding. If you feed directly from the jar you will need to discard any unused portion.

Jarred foods can be served at room temperature, chilled, or warmed—it's simply a matter of Baby's preference. Our advice is to try to get Baby used to eating her food straight from the pantry or refrigerator, rather than heated. It's definitely easier to feed her on the go if you don't need to find a way to heat her food. If you do heat the jarred food, you can spoon it into a small saucepan or microwave-safe dish. When using a microwave be very careful to stir the food well and test the temperature before serving, as hot spots can develop and can burn Baby's mouth and throat.

## FROZEN BABY FOODS

This category of baby foods is relatively new to the market, and our brand, HAPPYBABY, was one of the first. Shazi Visram and Jessica Rolph started the line for the moms they knew who wanted to give their babies the best possible foods but felt they had only two choices: open a jar or spend time they didn't have toiling away in their kitchens to make it homemade. Since there's enough guilt and stress that goes along with motherhood already, they decided to make our line of products a high-quality equivalent to homemade.

Why did we choose to do frozen foods? Freezing preserves the com-

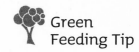

## Green Feeding Tip

*Reduce, reuse, or recycle those jars.* In one year, American families throw out more than two million tons of glass food containers, including baby food jars.[2] You can cut that number by:

- making your own baby food
- recycling empty jars (only 15 percent of the glass food containers thrown out in 2006 were recycled.[3] We can do better than that!)
- finding new uses for empty jars, such as holding sewing or craft supplies and storing office supplies

ponents in fruits and vegetables that provide their vibrant and nutritious color. Heat processing, as in the jarring process, can destroy some of these components. When you do a comparison of frozen baby foods to jarred foods, you will see that the color of a batch of frozen pureed peas, for example, does not even resemble that of a jarred variety. The frozen ones are a bright appealing green (like the color of fresh peas); jarred peas are a dull gray-green.

What you can't see in your visual comparison, however, is that freezing preserves the nutrients and flavor, too. Other methods of processing and preserving can break vitamins down as a result of postharvest handling and exposure to heat, light, and other elements. Freezing may halt this breakdown. Frozen fruits and vegetables may even be more nutritious than fresh. In one study, when comparing frozen green beans with fresh, researchers found that the frozen green beans had more than twice the vitamin C as green beans that had been displayed in the store and then stored in the fridge before eating.[4]

As for taste, if you do a taste test of flash-frozen baby food products like HAPPYBABY's baby meals and compare them to jarred foods, you will notice a much fresher flavor—one that is closer to the taste of the real thing. In fact, we consider our meals to be home-style—as fresh as homemade but without the work. We created them as an alternative for moms who want to make their own food but who may not have the time to make it all. Check out your grocery store's freezer case for frozen options for Baby.

To serve frozen baby foods you'll need to thaw the food first, following the instructions on the package. Then serve Baby's food at room temperature or slightly warmed, depending on your preference. HAPPYBABY's frozen cubes can be prepared several different ways:

· Microwaving: Place frozen cube(s) in a ceramic or glass microwave-safe dish. Heat for twenty to thirty seconds, and then stir well to distribute the heat and eliminate any hot spots that can occur in the food. Then test the temperature carefully with your lip before serving to Baby.
· Warming on the stove top: Simply throw the frozen cubes into

a small saucepan and heat on low, or use a double boiler. Once thawed, stir to distribute the heat and always test the temperature before serving to Baby.

· The food doesn't actually have to be warm, just thawed to a comfortable temperature. This will vary depending on whether you are giving Baby some fruit for a snack or a chicken meal for dinner.

· In the refrigerator: Place the frozen food into a sealed container and leave in the refrigerator overnight. Once thawed, serve within one day.

· In a sealed container, on the go: Pop out Baby's portion of frozen cubes into a sealable container and bring with you either in a cooler bag or just tossed in the stroller. Once the food is thawed, serve immediately.

## MAKING YOUR OWN

Making your own baby food may seem like a lot of work, but trust us, it's far less work than it may seem, especially as Baby gets past the puree stage and into lumpier textures and finger foods. It's not really cooking as you might think of it. For example, let's say you want to feed Baby sweet potatoes. Here's the recipe: take a sweet potato, bake it in the oven or microwave, scoop out the orange flesh, and mash it with a fork until it's the right consistency. Voilà! You've made your own baby food. Not exactly the kind of thing that requires culinary school. Many of the homemade foods you give Baby can simply be items that you are already preparing for yourself that you just have to mash up a little when you sit down to eat together.

Some parents choose to make their own baby food because they want the nutritional benefit of homemade fresh foods. Others feel that the more processed jarred options are not as tasty or appealing and don't provide the kind of eating experience they wish to give their families. Making your own food may also reduce your household's waste—fewer food packages coming in and out.

If you make some or all of your baby's food at home, there can indeed be a nutritional benefit. First, you pick all the ingredients yourself, so you can choose the freshest and healthiest foods that are available. You also control exactly which foods and flavors you give your child. Further, homemade food is not heated to the degree to which jarred foods are, and this translates to fewer nutrient losses in processing. While it is work, some parents find that setting time aside once a month to prepare meals in bulk and then freeze them for later use is a helpful way to handle it.

As for flavor and appearance, there is no doubt that homemade foods taste better than jarred foods. As we said earlier in the chapter, sustenance is just one thing you want to provide your baby in this stage. Providing her with flavors and a food experience that resembles real food is one of the best ways to assimilate her to the family table.

During the first several months, while Baby is eating pureed and slightly chunky foods, you will need some basic equipment and supplies to make her food:

- Something to steam fruits and vegetables—either a steamer basket or electric steamer is best. In a pinch, a small saucepan will work, too.
- A food processor, food mill, or blender. You don't have to use one especially for baby food, but if you're in the market for one, we like Kidco's BabySteps food mill or BabySteps electric food mill, both made with BPA-free plastic (www.kidco .com).
- BPA-free and phthalate-free ice cube trays with plastic covers (OXO Good Grips, www.goodgrips.com, makes one) or other plastic trays made especially for freezing baby food, such as Fresh Baby's So Easy food trays (www.freshbaby.com) or Kidco's BabySteps freezer trays.
- Freezer-safe storage containers made of BPA-free plastic with tight-fitting lids (or freezer-safe zip-top bags, if you must).
- Freezer-safe plastic wrap (if your plastic tray doesn't come with a cover).

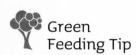 Green Feeding Tip

Many plastic blenders and food processor bowls are made of hard clear polycarbonate plastic and contain BPA. If you're in the market for a small appliance for making baby food, choose a BPA-free one. Vita-Mix's 5200 model is a BPA-free blender (www .vitamix.com), the Beaba Babycook food processor is BPA free (available at www .williams-sonoma.com), as are all Kidco brand baby-food-making products (www .kidco.com). If you already own a food processor made of polycarbonate plastic, take steps to reduce Baby's exposures to BPA: never pour hot food into the plastic bowl or blender, and hand wash the plastic parts rather than putting them in the dishwasher. Another option is to use a handheld immersion blender to blend Baby's foods in a stainless steel or ceramic bowl instead of a plastic one.

Once Baby is a bit older and eating more finger foods and mashed foods, you will need only a stove or microwave and a fork and a knife.

## Step 1: Ingredients

When Baby is new to solid foods, you'll be creating single-ingredient purees. Then, once you establish her tolerance to different fruits and vegetables, you can start to combine foods to make tasty mixtures.

Popular homemade single-ingredient purees:

| | |
|---|---|
| Applesauce | Pears |
| Avocados | Peas |
| Bananas | Potatoes |
| Carrots | Sweet potatoes |
| Green beans | Winter squash |
| Peaches | |

Choose organic produce whenever possible. A complete discussion about organic foods starts back on page 30. For optimal freshness and food safety, it's best to use fruits and vegetables within one to two days of purchase, and always check the expiration dates on all packages of meat, poultry, and fish. If fresh varieties of Baby's favorite foods aren't available, you can use frozen organic instead.

## Step 2: Prepping

Before you begin, wash your hands well with an organic and all-natural soap, like a vegetable-oil-based castile soap, and prepare a clean workspace in your kitchen. Then wash the produce well, and if needed, peel thick skins and remove any pits. If you have a strainer or food mill, you can leave the skin on during cooking because it will be strained out later in the preparation. If you are cooking poultry, meat, or fish, you can wait to remove the skin and bones until after cooking.

# NITRATES IN HOMEMADE BABY FOOD

Parents are sometimes warned to avoid using certain ingredients in homemade baby food due to concerns about the amount of nitrates in the food. Nitrates are chemical compounds that are found in the soil and water, and tend to be highest in root vegetables like beets, turnips, and carrots, as well as in spinach and collard greens. Once in the body of a young infant, nitrates get converted into a substance that can rob the cells of oxygen, leading to a potentially fatal type of anemia called blue baby syndrome. All commercial baby food companies, including HAPPYBABY, screen for nitrates in their batches of food and discard any food with dangerous levels. Still, all baby food has at least some level of them.

Although blue baby syndrome is certainly a scary prospect, the good news is that most experts, including the American Academy of Pediatrics, agree that nitrates from foods do not pose a significant threat for babies older than six months old. By this age babies have enough hydrochloric acid in their tummies to neutralize the nitrates and get rid of them through a metabolic pathway, drastically reducing the risk of blue baby syndrome.[5] If you're concerned about nitrates, be sure to choose organic produce because although nitrates occur naturally in soil in small amounts, a significant source of nitrates is the chemical fertilizer used in growing conventional foods.

## Step 3: Cooking

For babies up to eight months old, most fruits and vegetables need to be cooked before pureeing or mashing. Cooking helps to soften the flesh and the fibrous parts of fruits and veggies, making them easier to digest. The exceptions are the naturally soft papaya, banana, and avocado. Canned fruits, like pears and peaches, are already cooked, so you don't need to cook them further. Chicken, turkey, beef, lamb, pork, and fish also need to be cooked before you serve them to Baby, of course. Tofu, on the other hand, does not.

When you're cooking a food for Baby, cut it into small (¾ inch) pieces to help it cook faster. If you plan to puree the food, you need to cook it to a very soft texture, even slightly mushy. If you're just going to be mashing or chopping the food (when Baby has moved past purees), cook until tender, but be sure to stop before the food becomes mush. You can use any of these methods to cook Baby's foods:

- Steam them in an electric steamer or use a steamer basket in a saucepan on the stovetop. See the chart below for approximate steaming time for some common baby foods.
- If you don't have an electric steamer or steamer basket, steam the food(s) in a saucepan on the stove. Put an inch or so of water in the bottom of the pan, add your cut-up ingredients, bring to a boil, and then reduce heat and simmer with the pan tightly covered until the food is done.
- Bake or roast the food in the oven. For basic baking, preheat the oven to 350 degrees and cook the food in a lightly greased (with olive oil, canola oil, or butter) covered baking dish. To roast, preheat the oven to 425 degrees and cook in a single layer on a baking sheet. Most foods will roast better when tossed in a little olive oil or canola oil.

Try not to boil fruits and vegetables because they'll lose vitamins and minerals. In fact, whenever you use a wet cooking method like steaming or simmering, reserve any cooking liquid that remains in the pot—this liquid will contain some vitamins that are lost in cooking, and you can use this when blending the food into a puree. Here are some approximate steaming times for common baby foods:

| Food | Approximate Steaming Time | Comments |
| --- | --- | --- |
| Apple | 10–12 minutes | No need to peel before cooking. Skin will come off easily. |
| Apricot | 2–4 minutes | No need to peel before cooking. Skin will come off easily. |
| Beef (ground) | 4–5 minutes | Cover with liquid to cook; always check carefully for doneness. |
| Broccoli | 10–15 minutes | |

| Food | Approximate Steaming Time | Comments |
| --- | --- | --- |
| Carrots | 15–20 minutes | |
| Cauliflower | 10–15 minutes | |
| Chicken or turkey breast (boneless) | 8 minutes | Dark meat or boned poultry is fine for Baby, too. Cooking times may vary. Always check carefully for doneness. |
| Dried fruit (prunes, dried apricots) | 5–10 minutes | |
| Fish | 15–20 minutes | Cover with liquid to cook. Fish is done when it's opaque and flakes easily. |
| Green beans | 15 minutes | Use fresh or frozen. |
| Peach | 2–4 minutes | No need to peel before cooking. Skin will come off easily. |
| Peas | 10–15 minutes | Use fresh or frozen. |
| Potato | 10–12 minutes | Or cook in the microwave. Pierce several times with a fork, cook on high 4–6 minutes. |
| Root vegetables—turnips, rutabaga, parsnip | 15 minutes | |
| Spinach | 3–4 minutes | |
| Squash, summer | 10–12 minutes | |
| Squash, winter | 12–15 minutes | |
| Sweet potato | 12–15 minutes | |

If your family cooks with herbs and spices, like garlic, sage, coriander, cumin, and cilantro, feel free to add these to Baby's foods as well. This will help Baby get used to the flavors of your family's meals. See the recipe for Baby Ganoush on page 183 as an example of how to incorporate spices. You can also add chopped onion to the pot when you're steaming a food and blend it in to add flavor. Avoid salt, though. Baby's young kidneys are not equipped to process added sodium, and you don't want to foster a preference for salty foods.

Once Baby is about eight months old, she can handle some raw fruits.

Ripe peaches, pears, and apricots, for example will be soft enough to mash up without cooking. Just remove the skin before serving. Other things, like broccoli and bell peppers, though technically can be eaten raw, should probably be cooked until Baby has a full set of teeth and can effectively chew them up—closer to age two.

### Step 4: Pureeing, Mashing, or Chopping

Once the food is cooked (or otherwise soft enough to serve) you need to get it to the right consistency for Baby. Depending on your baby's age and stage this could be a soupy puree, a thicker puree, or even a coarse mash (see page 158 for tips on texture).

For purees, use a blender, a food processor, a food mill, or a ricer to blend the food into a smooth or slightly lumpy texture. You don't have to buy a special baby food maker to make baby food. Your standard blender should work fine. Depending on the food's consistency, you may need to add liquid as you're pureeing to get it right. Use the cooking liquid that you reserved from steaming or use expressed breast milk or infant formula.

For coarser textures like a chunky mash, you can use a blender if you wish, or you can just use a fork. For finger foods, just cut the cooked or prepped food into tiny bite-size pieces (about the size of a pea) with a fork and knife.

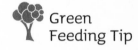

**Green Feeding Tip**

Use a hand-cranked food mill for small batches of pureed baby food to reduce your electricity use.

### Step 5: Serving and Storing

Once a food is cooked and at the right texture, you can feed it to Baby or store the food for future use. Don't worry if the food is still warm—there is no need to cool it down before storing in the refrigerator or freezer. If you plan to serve the food within the next one to three days, it can go into the refrigerator in a sealed container. If you will be storing the food for a longer period of time, you will need to freeze it.

To freeze, pour the pureed or mashed food into a freezer tray, cover, and place in the freezer. If your tray doesn't have a cover, use freezer-safe plastic wrap instead. Once the cubes are frozen, transfer them to freezer-safe bags or containers for storage; cover tightly to reduce loss of nutrients to light and air and to minimize flavor transfer from other

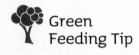
foods in the freezer. Label the batch with the list of ingredients and the date, and use within three to six months.

When it's time to serve your tasty creations you must thaw the cubes. If you have time, you can thaw them in the refrigerator overnight in a covered container. Or, you can gently heat the cubes to thaw them. On the stove top, place the cubes in the top saucepan of a double boiler while the water boils in the bottom. If you don't have a double boiler, make one. Set a heatproof glass bowl or small saucepan into a pot of boiling water. The stove-top method will take about ten to fifteen minutes. If you wish to use the microwave, you can do so safely if you take certain precautions. First, never microwave in plastic, and use only microwave-safe glass or ceramic. Heat slowly, testing the temperature every ten to fifteen seconds to avoid scorching the food. Beware of hot spots that can develop in microwave heating. Always stir well and test the temperature before giving to Baby.

## Flavor Fusion for Babies

Don't be afraid to mix and match flavors for Baby (once you're sure she tolerates the separate ingredients). One way to do this is to prepare single-ingredient purees and mix those together before serving. Or, if Baby has a favorite, mix larger quantities of pureed and mashed fruits and veggies and store them that way. There are so many delicious combinations to try— use your imagination! All fruits and vegetables listed here are cooked unless otherwise indicated.

### SIX MONTHS

A Is for Avocado
    Avocado (uncooked) and apple

Autumn Harvest
    Apple and squash

# QUICK GUIDE TO SAFE AND
# GREEN KITCHEN STORAGE

In order to make meals ahead for Baby or safely store leftovers you'll need some reusable containers with tight-fitting lids. Here's a guide to choosing the best materials for food storage for Baby (and the rest of the family, too!):

*Glass.* A very safe food storage material, glass is also recyclable, so it's particularly eco-friendly. We like the covered glass containers for refrigerator, freezer, and pantry storage from Pyrex (www.pyrex.com) and Anchor Hocking (www.anchorhocking.com).

*Ceramic.* Choose covered ceramic containers made especially for food storage and reheating, such as the dishwasher- and microwave-safe containers from Corning Ware (www.corningware.com).

*Plastic.* Since they are petroleum based and often not recyclable, plastics are not the top choice for the eco-conscious Mama. However, they are lightweight and practical, and an informed Mama can make safe plastic choices by avoiding the hard clear polycarbonate plastic, labeled with the recycling code 7 or the initials PC, because it may contain bisphenol A (BPA), a chemical that disrupts hormone function. Instead, choose any of the following:

- polyethylene terephthalate, labeled with recycling code 1, PET, or PETE
- high-density polyethylene, recycling code 2 or HDPE
- low-density polyethylene, recycling code 4 or LDPE
- polypropylene, recycling code 5 or PP

Many of the reusable plastic containers from Glad (www.glad.com), Ziploc (www.ziploc.com), Rubbermaid (www.rubbermaid.com), and Tupperware (www.tupperware.com) are made with polypropylene and are considered to be safe. Check for the recycling codes 1, 2, 4, or 5 when making your selections. You'll also find several options at the Container Store (www.containerstore.com).

Spring Garden
>   Peas and carrots

Little Jack Horner
>   Plums, apricots, and winter squash

## SEVEN TO NINE MONTHS

Green Mango
>   Spinach, pear, and mango (uncooked)

Baby's First Burrito
>   Black beans and banana (uncooked)

Bananas and Cream
>   Banana (uncooked) and yogurt (at nine months)

### GRRREAT GREENS

Makes about eight ½-cup portions or 32 1-ounce cubes that you
can freeze for up to 6 months in a sealed container in the freezer.

This is a delicious and nutritious way to get baby to eat greens because the
sweetness of the mango and pear balance the bitterness of the spinach. It's
good for babies 7 months and up.

3 medium pears, peeled, cored, and chopped

1 large ripe mango, peeled, pitted, and chopped

3 cups spinach, hard stems discarded and leaves chopped

1. Using an electric steamer or steamer basket in a pan on the stovetop, steam pear for four minutes, or until pear is tender. Transfer fruit and any remaining steaming liquid into a bowl to cool while you do the next step.

2. Steam spinach for 3 minutes, until wilted and bright green. Transfer into a bowl and gently press out any excess water.
3. Puree the cooked pear, mango, and cooked spinach in a food processor or blender. Add liquid from the pears if needed. Puree until you have a smooth mixture.
4. Store as described in this chapter.

## BABY GANOUSH

Makes about 1.5 cups; Typical serving for 9–12 month old will be ¼ cup.

This mild version of the Middle Eastern eggplant spread Baba Ganoush is a way to introduce Baby to new flavors. Serve alone or mixed with plain yogurt and bite-sized pita bread pieces.

1 large eggplant                   1 Tablespoon olive oil
3 cloves garlic                     ½ tsp cumin

1. Preheat the oven to 425 degrees F.
2. Wash the eggplant well and cut off the two ends. Remove the peel from each garlic clove.
3. Slice the eggplant down the middle lengthwise. Place skin-down on a baking sheet or in a baking dish. Place the garlic cloves next to the eggplant.
4. Pour the olive oil into a small dish. Use a basting brush to brush the oil on the flesh of the eggplant, and on the surface of each garlic clove. (If you don't have a brush, pour the oil on top of the vegetables and use your fingers to spread.)
5. Place the pan in the oven on the middle rack and roast for 35 minutes. After about 20 minutes, check the garlic cloves—they are done when soft and golden brown. When the eggplant is done, remove from the oven.
6. Let the garlic and eggplant cool in the pan or on a plate for 10 minutes.

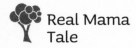
Then, flip the eggplant over so the skin side is up. Using a fork or a knife, gently loosen the skin and peel off in strips until all skin is removed. Alternatively, use a spoon to scoop the flesh out of the skin. (Discard or compost the skin.)

7. Cut the eggplant flesh into 6 to 8 large pieces. Cut the garlic cloves in half. Place two or three pieces of food at a time into the blender or food processor. Blend on low speed for several moments and turn off. Add two or three more pieces of food and blend again. If the food is getting stuck and not combining you may need to stir it with a spoon before blending each time. Continue until all the eggplant and garlic has been added and the mixture is the right consistency for your baby. If it is too thick, add 1 to 2 tablespoons of water to smooth the mixture and thin it out.

8. When the right consistency, transfer into a bowl with a tight-fitting lid to be used in the next 2 to 3 days or pour into baby food or ice cube trays for freezing, as described on page 171.

## SHAPING BABY'S TASTES

Don't become so distracted by the logistical details and the mechanics of feeding Baby that you miss the bigger picture. Infancy is a key time in the development of her future food preferences—and your first opportunity to encourage Baby to enjoy the foods that will help her become a healthy eater.

Some likes and dislikes are influenced by genes and anatomy. For example, researchers have found a specific gene that heightens the experience of bitter flavors. Presumably, babies who have this gene may not easily accept foods like spinach or kale. We also know that the concentration of taste buds on our tongues can affect how we experience flavors. One in four people are "supertasters" with a very high concentration of taste buds on their tongues. These people taste things really vividly, so they tend to have less preference for bitter vegetables, coffee, and other foods with strong flavors, like hot peppers and olives. On the other side of the spectrum are people with fewer taste buds. These "nontasters" may accept many foods but just have a general lack of zeal for eating. (The rest of us are simply tasters—we ex-

## BETTER BABY FOOD IN ALL SHADES OF GREEN

You don't have to immediately become a homemade baby food guru. Take it in stages (the way Baby is!). Here's how:

*The palest green:* Rely less on jarred foods and opt for organic frozen varieties or fresh foods instead. When you do need to use jarred food, choose organic varieties without additives like sugar.

*A little greener:* Prepare some simple baby foods in your kitchen, and then use frozen or fresh commercial baby foods to supplement. Offer a quickly mashed banana or a soft-cooked, then mashed pear, for example. Choose organic fruits and vegetables whenever possible.

*The deepest shade of green:* Make all of baby's food at home using the freshest organic produce you can find. Prepare meals in advance and freeze them, or just puree or mash up the family's dinner (unsalted, of course) and serve it to Baby right then and there.

perience a broad spectrum of flavors, none of them too strong or too weak.)[6]

The chapter would end here if only our genes and our bodies determined which foods we like. But that's not the whole story. We also can learn to like and dislike foods. Exposure to foods is one of the most powerful factors in the development of food preferences. This means that as parents we actually get a chance to shape Baby's food preferences.

Your baby's exposure to foods actually began long before she took her first bite of solids. When she was in the womb, around eight weeks after conception, her taste buds appeared. Later, during the second trimester, she used those taste buds as she started swallowing and inhaling amniotic fluid and tasting the hints of the flavors from the foods you ate that day. By the time she was born she could already distinguish between sweet and bitter flavors (not surprisingly, most babies prefer sweet). Baby's flavor lessons continued with every sip of your breast milk, which took on the flavor of some of the foods in your diet.

The more times a baby or child is exposed to a flavor or food, the more likely she is to accept it. Experts suspect that this is why breast-fed babies, with their early exposure to a variety of flavors in breast milk, are less likely to be picky eaters. Infant formula, on the other hand, tastes the same every single day. Consider this: children in India eat curries and Asian babies accept ginger. Ask many American moms if their young toddlers eat such "exotic" fare and the answer is likely to be no. Do Indian and Asian children have more sophisticated palates? Not at all. They were simply introduced to these flavors from a very early age—from before they were even born—and are now used to them.

### Dr. Bob's Tips for Growing a Healthy Eater

1. Make a concerted effort to introduce a variety of healthy, fresh, natural, and good-tasting foods from day one. Choose organic whole foods for Baby's meals.
2. Keep Baby away from junky processed foods as long as possible, preferably past her second or third birthday.
3. Introduce Baby to the flavors that are in your family's typical meals so that she begins to develop a taste for those same foods. For example, if you eat foods that are seasoned with garlic, let Baby experience that flavor, too, in mild doses.
4. Babies may need to be exposed to a food ten to fifteen times before accepting it. So if Baby rejects carrots the first time, don't give up. Try again every few days over the next few weeks. You may be surprised one day when she decides to give them a try.
5. Don't push it if Baby isn't a fan of solids at six months. Eat in front of her as a family and she'll get the picture soon.

The foundations for Baby's food preferences are being laid right now, in infancy. If you wait until she's two or three, it may be too late. Plus, now is the time when you have the most influence and control

# LOOKING AHEAD TO AGE ONE AND BEYOND

When Baby turns one, breast milk and/or formula may begin to play a smaller (but still important) role in overall nutrition. Parents often wonder how to best balance foods and milk and make sure Baby is getting enough. The table below shows the recommended minimum intake for twelve-month-old babies. When babies first start solids, they will probably eat less than this. However, as the months go on and your baby approaches her first birthday, she should be working toward this level of food intake. If your pediatrician is concerned about her growth or if her food intake seems far below these recommendations at age one, you may want to talk to a dietitian to see if Baby needs more calories or might benefit from a multivitamin.

| Nutrient | Best Food Sources | Recommended Minimum Intake After Age 1 | Comments |
| --- | --- | --- | --- |
| Protein | Lean beef, poultry, pork, eggs,* milk and milk products,* fish,* beans and lentils, nut butters* | About 3 to 4 tablespoons (2 ounces) per day by age 1 | No shellfish or peanut products until age 2 |
| Carbohydrates | Bread and bread products;* cereals;* grains, including rice, oats, barley, and quinoa | About ½ to 1 cup per day by age 1 | Aim for whole grain foods whenever possible |
| Fat | Whole milk dairy products, including milk, yogurt, butter, cheese;* avocado; olive oil; canola oil | Include several food sources per day. Do not restrict fat intake. | Essential for brain development. Babies need more fat than adults do. |
| Vitamin A | Sweet potatoes, carrots, spinach, winter squash, apricots | At least ¼ cup (about 2 ounces) per day by age 1 | In general, vitamin A food sources are dark green, yellow, or orange. |

| Nutrient | Best Food Sources | Recommended Minimum Intake After Age 1 | Comments |
|---|---|---|---|
| Vitamin C | Broccoli, cauliflower, citrus fruits,* 100 percent fruit juice, mango, potatoes | At least ¼ cup (about 2 ounces) per day by age 1 | |
| Vitamin D | Breast milk and formula, fortified dairy products,* eggs* | Formula-fed babies don't need additional vitamin D. If breast-feeding, ask your pediatrician about whether Baby needs a supplement of this vitamin. | Sun exposure helps Baby produce this hormone |
| Other vitamins and minerals (e.g. potassium, B vitamins) | Apples and applesauce, green beans, bananas, peas | ¼ cup (about 2 ounces) or more per day by age 1 | |
| Iron | Breast milk and fortified formula, fortified infant cereal, meat and poultry, beans and lentils, spinach, egg yolk | At least 1 serving (4 tablespoons) of iron-fortified infant cereal per day plus 1 other iron source. | Vitamin C helps the body absorb iron so serve sources of C with iron-rich foods. |
| Calcium | Breast milk and formula, milk and milk products,* dark green leafy vegetables, tofu | Will need 2 servings per day starting at age 1. One serving is 1 cup milk or yogurt. (1 cup tofu = ½ serving of calcium.) | Each breast-feeding session is probably ½ of a serving of calcium. Active nursers don't need other calcium sources yet. |

*These foods may cause allergic reactions. See page 167 for more information.

over what she eats and which foods she will like. When Baby becomes a toddler or preschooler, her food choices will start to be influenced by a whole host of other factors. At two, she may start to refuse to eat certain foods just to assert her independence, not because she doesn't like them. And three-year-olds will be influenced by their peers' food choices and may be persuaded that certain foods are "yucky." So feed your baby healthy foods now, and start down the road to good health together from day one!

## Taking It Home . . .

You're embarking on a great solid food feeding adventure! It might seem like a daunting task—figuring out what and how and when to feed your little one. It doesn't have to be overwhelming, though. Here are the basics:

- Start when Baby is ready—ideally around age six months.
- Choose from the list of appropriate first foods, and just work your way down the list, offering each food for a few days before adding another to the menu.
- Alter the texture of Baby's foods to suit her stage of development, starting with purees and progressing through lumpy purees, mashes, and chopped foods.
- Give Baby the opportunity to touch and smell and taste her foods with her hands. It might make a mess, but that's how she is going to learn.
- Be on the lookout for allergies or intolerances. If something doesn't agree with Baby, avoid it for now.
- Try making your own baby foods. It's easier than you think.
- When you can't make your own foods, try home-style frozen baby foods to expose Baby to organic, minimally processed, flavorful foods.
- Introducing all-natural, fresh-tasting, wholesome foods from day one to help Baby develop preferences for healthy foods.

# 6

# What's on the Menu?

## Growing Healthy Babies from Healthy Foods

During the first few months of Baby's starting solids, healthy eating is fairly automatic. It's mostly fruits, veggies, and cereals. Now that Baby is one and turning into a toddler, her choices expand, and so do your responsibilities. Convenient snack foods, treats at parties, the junk foods your best friend lets her baby eat—these all become temptations you will be faced with. Not temptations because your baby will want them (she doesn't even know about them yet)—the temptation is yours! Do you just let your toddler eat whatever is easy to buy, simple to prepare, and conveniently packaged to take on the go, or do you stick with whole foods that you prepare and serve fresh? Do you let your child get stuck on sweetened and processed foods that are yummy and filling because you know she'll eat them, or do you stay consistent with natural foods that she might not be as eager to chow down? Do you just buy whatever is cheap and popular for kids, or do you take the time to read labels to avoid artificial ingredients and to limit fat and sugar? And does it really even matter?

Yes it does! And we know that you know it does! That's why you are reading this book. We won't lie, though—providing healthy food does take more effort. Throwing a can of fish-shaped crackers into the diaper bag is so much easier than packing some fresh fruit. You *know* your toddler will eat a plateful of mac and cheese, so why bother serving her some of the fresh salmon you plan to make for dinner?

The reason that some parents choose convenience over quality can be summed up in one word—quantity. Parents want their toddler to eat lots of food. They think that how much a child eats is more important than what they eat. And the sweeter, fattier, and more processed the foods, the more a child will eat. It's quantity that determines how well a child will grow, right? Wrong. Eating lots of processed food may put more fat and weight on a child, but is the child actually growing *better*? No.

We would like you to believe us when we tell you that the most important aspect of eating for this next year is the *quality* of the food—the types of carbs, protein, and fat, as well as the vitamins and minerals, in the foods you feed your baby. Quantity is a secondary concern. And it's not just what's in the food that matters, it's also what is *not* in the foods you choose: chemicals, artificial additives, sweeteners, and colors. That's just as important.

Here's a little tip you should know about toddlers—many kids go through a slimming stage between one and two. Fat babies often slow down and gain very little weight. Slimmer babies may become even more so. Parents naturally want to fatten their kids up. If you have a toddler who eats anything and everything, you may be able to keep him looking big and chunky (in a healthy way) by letting him eat large quantities of healthy foods. But the reality is that most toddlers are somewhat picky. They won't eat much at a time. Therefore, they slim down. We view this as a simple fact of nature. Trying to fatten a kid up on unhealthy foods doesn't benefit him in the long run. In fact, it may set up preferences for processed and fatty foods for years to come that can cause harm in the long run.

So, we ask you to set aside expectations of how much your toddler may eat, and to trust us when we say your child will be fine. Let's focus on how to shape your toddler's tastes for healthy food and set up good eating habits that will last a lifetime. We'll show you what foods should be on your toddler's weekly menu, what foods provide the best nutrition, which foods to limit or avoid altogether, what types of beverages are best for Baby, and how to navigate confusing food labels so you can make sure your baby is getting the best. We will offer suggested quantities to shoot for as a goal but not a requirement.

Feeding Baby all-natural and healthy foods when she's a toddler will set her up for a lifetime of healthy eating habits. It may even minimize your future dinner table struggles because Baby will view whole foods—as opposed to processed ones—as the norm. She'll begin to expect nothing less than unadulterated healthy ingredients. And all the while you'll be helping to sustain her planet. What could be better?

## Three Essentials for Green and Healthy Eating

By the time Baby reaches her first birthday you will be moving her away from baby foods and offering mostly table foods—foods that you are eating but have modified slightly to be appropriate for her development (e.g., cut into small enough pieces, cooked enough, etc.). Food will now become the main source of nutrition in her diet. An entire world of choices opens up for Baby, with very few limitations. You no longer need to offer Baby formula, and if you are breast-feeding, your milk can continue to be an excellent source of nutrition for Baby as long as you want it to be. Our baby and toddler feeding philosophy can be simply expressed as three feeding essentials:

- Essential 1: Choose organic foods.
- Essential 2: Provide Baby with foods from eight key food groups to meet her nutritional needs.
- Essential 3: Choose all-natural and whole foods while limiting processed foods with artificial ingredients.

## Feeding Essential 1: Choose Organic

In chapter 1 we explained all about organic foods and why they are better for Baby and better for the environment. Just to recap, here are our five reasons to choose organic:

1. Organic farming is green farming. It generates far less waste, doesn't send chemicals into surrounding lands and waterways, is humane to animals, and is better for the planet.
2. Organic foods cut Baby's exposure to pesticides, which are known to kill brain cells and cause cancer in laboratory studies.
3. Organic foods don't contain hormones and don't contribute to antibiotic resistance.
4. Organic foods often contain more vitamins, minerals, and nutrients than conventionally grown foods.
5. Organic foods taste better!

It's simple enough in theory: Just buy organic foods whenever you can. In practice, there are other considerations for many families. One is availability. Although organic foods are way more widely available than they ever have been in the past, some communities still don't have great access to organic foods.

Another is cost. Any discussion with parents about organic foods always turns to money. It's true that organic foods are often more expensive than conventional foods. It could be because organic farming methods are more labor-intensive. It could also be because organic farms produce lower yields than conventional farms, so they need to

Labels give clues to how organic a packaged food is:

| If the Label Says . . . | What It Means |
| --- | --- |
| 100 percent organic | Every ingredient in the food meets the definition of organic. |
| USDA Organic | At least 95 percent of the food's ingredients are organic. |
| Made with organic | At least 70 percent of the ingredients are organic, and the label will tell you which ones. |

charge more to make the same profit. We encourage you to look at the money you spend on organic food, particularly for your baby, as an investment into his long-term health.

## OUR BANG-FOR-YOUR-BUCK ORGANIC SHOPPING LIST

The good news is that nobody would expect you to switch to a 100 percent organic existence in one fell swoop. You don't have to throw out your pantry and start over. (In fact, that would be pretty wasteful!) You can slowly transition over to organic foods. And it may make more sense for your family to switch to organic versions of a select group of foods that give you the most bang for your buck—nutritionally and financially speaking. We would advise you to start with these foods:

1. *High-pesticide fruits and veggies.* Certain conventional fruits and vegetables tend to be more contaminated with pesticides than others. Keep this "dirty dozen" list near your grocery shopping list on the fridge. When you put one of these foods on the shopping list, write an "O" after it so you remember to choose organic.

| Apples | Grapes (especially imported) | Kale |
|---|---|---|
| Bell peppers | Nectarines | Strawberries |
| Celery | Peaches | Spinach |
| Cherries | Pears | Lettuce |

(Source: Environmental Working Group)

2. *Milk and other dairy products.* A recent study found that 30 percent of nonorganic milk samples contained pesticide residues.[1] Nonorganic milk may also have traces of the antibiotics and hormones used to treat the cows. Since it's likely that milk and dairy products will be a staple in your child's diet for the next

few years, choosing organic will significantly decrease her exposure to these chemicals. Also, during these early years when you're a particularly big milk consumer (my household goes through at least a gallon a week), you'll be doing your part for the planet by supporting dairy farms that produce less waste, treat animals humanely, and don't contribute to the problems of antibiotic resistance.

3. *Beef and chicken.* Although the FDA says they are safe for human consumption, we don't like the idea of feeding Baby foods made with synthetic hormones and antibiotics. The price of organic meat may dissuade you from picking it up, but consider the fact that only one or two ounces of meat provides Baby's protein for the whole day.

4. *Any food that Baby eats in large amounts.* Maybe your baby goes through several pints of strawberries each week during the summer. Or maybe she dips everything in ketchup. If there are foods that Baby eats every day or several times a day, mitigate any risks by making the switch to organic. (Bonus: organic ketchup not only is pesticide free, but it's also higher in antioxidants than conventional ketchup.[2] Plus, it doesn't contain high-fructose corn syrup like the conventional variety.)

We certainly encourage you to buy organic foods whenever you can, even if they aren't on the list above. But if you are going for the phase-in approach to buying organic foods, you can let yourself off the hook for the following list of fruits and veggies that tend to have the lowest amount of pesticide residues:

*Safest nonorganic produce:*

| Asparagus | Cauliflower | Onion |
|---|---|---|
| Avocado | Corn | Papaya |
| Cabbage | Kiwi | Peas |
| Watermelon | Mango | Pineapple |

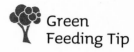

**Green Feeding Tip**

In the produce section the little stickers on the fruits and vegetables will help you determine if something is organic or not. Organic produce has a 9 in front of the 4-digit PLU code that identifies it. For example, a conventional tree-ripened peach is 4044, and an organic one is 94044.

## GO ORGANIC OR STAY LOCAL?

Today, many people are trying to eat locally—choosing foods that are grown close to their hometown so they can support their local farming communities and minimize the amount of resources it takes to get their food from farm to table. But let's say you live near a farmer's market and some of the offerings there aren't labeled organic. Is it better to go over to the grocery store to buy organic food that has been shipped across the country or flown in from South America? The answer isn't a clear yes or no—it depends on how the local farm operates. Before you decide, talk to the farmers directly at the market or look up the local producers online. Many small producers use sustainable farming methods and minimal chemical pesticides in their farms, but they don't seek the official organic certification from the USDA. If this is the case, go for the local food. If not, turn to the "dirty dozen" list above and choose organic versions of those foods, and buy the local conventional versions of the others to support the local farmers and minimize the environmental impact of your meal.

# Feeding Essential 2: Feed Baby the "Great Eight"

Here is a list of the eight key food groups for babies and toddlers. Try not to look at it as a daily checklist, though. Instead, aim for Baby's diet to include these foods over the course of several days or a week. For each food group, we'll explain why it's on the list, how much your baby needs, and tips for getting it on the table (and, more important, into Baby's mouth). There are lots of tips here for you, so don't get overwhelmed; you don't need to commit this stuff to memory. Just earmark these pages so you can refer to this section when you need it most—for example, when you run out of fruit ideas or if Baby decides she's not eating meat anymore.

## 1. NATURE'S CANDY: FRUIT

This is an easy one to start with because fruits are pretty darned tasty and usually accepted by young children. That is, if they are offered. We

## Bedtime Snack

It's inevitable. You get your child ready for bed, and she says, "I'm hungry!" One rule we set up in our house is that the children are allowed to eat only fruit for a before-bedtime snack. There's nothing more enjoyable than seeing your child munch on an apple or banana while you read a bedtime story. We always save the toothbrushing for after stories.

were surprised to learn that a huge study of three thousand infants and toddlers found that more than 25 percent had not had a single bite of fruit in the prior twenty-four hours![3] Most kids will gobble up fruit as if it's candy (unless there's actual candy around to distract them).

*Why?* Fruits add vitamins and fiber to Baby's diet. They are sources of vitamins A and C, B vitamins, and potassium. They are also sources of phytochemicals—plant chemicals including carotenoids, flavonoids, and isoflavones, which are antioxidants that protect against cancers, heart disease, and other conditions. Although these chronic diseases are probably not at the top of your worry list for your baby at this young age, remember that now is when she will get into the habit of eating healthy foods and lay the foundation for a healthy future.

*How much?* One serving of fruit for a one- to two-year-old is about two tablespoons to one-quarter cup. By age two it's recommended that Baby eat a full cup of fruit each day. To get there you'll need to serve her fruit a few times a day. Get in the habit of serving at least one fruit with breakfast and one with each snack.

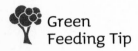

- Older toddlers love to dip their food. Give Baby strips of French toast, pancakes, or waffles, and provide a fruit puree (home-made or store-bought like HAPPYBABY's Wiser Apple or Paradise Puree) as the dip.
- Mix fruit purees into Baby's oatmeal or other hot cereal. Use in muffin and cookie recipes, too. (See Recipes on page 257.)
- Add frozen blueberries to hot oatmeal—the berries cool off the oatmeal and the oatmeal thaws the berries!
- If fresh fruit isn't available or in season, canned or frozen varieties can be nutritious substitutes. You may even be able to find organic ones. These fruits have been frozen or canned at the peak of ripeness and preserved in that delicious state until you take them out in your home. If you're going for a can, be sure to choose fruit that is canned in water or its own juice instead of heavy sugary syrups.
- Add fruit to a yogurt smoothie for a yummy (and calcium-filled) snack. Kids love mango, berries, or bananas in their smoothies. (See Recipes.)
- And don't forget: it's easy to get into an apple/orange/banana/ pear rut. Don't overlook berries of all types and tropical fruits, such as mango, papaya, kiwi, and pineapple.

## 2. EDIBLE HEALTH: VEGETABLES

Studies consistently show that people who eat more vegetables have lower rates of disease. Vegetables could really be three separate items on our list because Baby will get specific benefits from three different types: orange or yellow vegetables, green vegetables, and other vegetables.

*Why?*

- Oranges and yellows: These brightly hued beauties, such as orange bell peppers, sweet potatoes, and carrots, provide beta-carotene, an antioxidant that the body can convert into vitamin A.

# KEY VITAMINS FOR BABY

## Vitamins C and A

Among the fruits and vegetables you give Baby each day, make sure there is at least one excellent source of vitamin C and one excellent source of vitamin A. Her daily vitamin C needs (15 milligrams per day) will be met with any of the following: ¼ cup diced cantaloupe, 3 medium strawberries, ¼ orange, 2 tablespoons papaya, 2 tablespoons of broccoli, or ½ cup mashed potatoes plus ¼ cup tomato. Other good sources include kiwi, papaya, grapefruit, raspberries, and tangerine. Fruit and vegetable sources of beta-carotene will provide Baby her vitamin A for the day. Her minimum vitamin A needs are met with any of the following: 1 tablespoon cooked carrots, 2 tablespoons sweet potatoes, ¼ cup butternut squash, 1 tablespoon cooked spinach, 1 tablespoon cooked kale, ¼ cup cantaloupe, or ½ cup chopped apricot.

Beta-carotene and vitamin A strengthen the immune system and are essential for healthy vision.

- Greens: The benefits of green veggies make a pretty impressive list. The leafy greens, like lettuce, spinach, Swiss chard, mustard greens, and kale, are highly protective against cardiovascular disease. Other green vegetables, like broccoli and bok choy, have anticancer properties. The pigments that give green veggies their color, lutein and zeaxanthin, protect the eyes from dangerous free radicals and prevent vision problems. The carotenoids in these vegetables have antioxidant effects and prevent the growth of breast, skin, lung, and stomach cancer cells in laboratory tests. Green vegetables' folate may decrease pancreatic cancer risk, and their fiber may help prevent colorectal cancer. We could go on and on.
- Other vegetables: Tomatoes, onions, garlic, mushrooms, cauliflower—their phytochemicals prevent disease, and their fiber is good for digestion and regularity.

# Heart Disease? In Children?

Everyone thinks that it's only us adults who have to pay attention to diet and exercise regularly to prevent heart disease. Well, cardiovascular disease begins in toddlerhood. Autopsy studies done on young children have shown fatty deposits will begin to build up in kids' arteries as young as age three.[4] By twelve years of age, many kids will already have some hardening of the arteries (enough fat has built up to interfere with the arteries' ability to dilate and bend). Ensuring a diet rich in fruits and vegetables helps to keep these fatty deposits flushed out.

*How much?* Try to work up to about a cup of vegetables per day by age two. A serving size is about ¼ to ½ cup, so that means offering veggies several times a day.

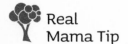

## Real Mama Tip

"We always served the kids pizza with veggies on top, but around age three my son realized it doesn't automatically come that way and started asking for 'just sauce, cheese, and crust, please, Mommy.' Oh well, it was good while it lasted!"

—*Colleen, New York, New York*

### Veggie Tips

- Vegetables aren't just for lunch and dinner. Add chopped spinach or squash to your omelets at breakfast. Serve baby carrots or sliced bell peppers as snacks with some healthy dip like guacamole or hummus. You may be surprised to learn your child will snack happily on broccoli florets. If raw carrots, peppers, and broccoli are too hard for your toothless baby to munch on, lightly steam them first and then chill in the fridge until snack time. (Steamed and then chilled baby carrots make a great on-the-go veggie snack.)
- Noodles can be a great vehicle for vegetables, and we've yet to meet a toddler who doesn't like them. Buy frozen ravioli filled

with spinach or mushrooms. Order steamed vegetable dumplings at your favorite Asian restaurant. Try potato and onion pierogi.

· Use homemade or HAPPYBABY pureed vegetables as dips for pita bread, carrot sticks, or crackers. Add purees to spaghetti sauce or soups to boost the vitamin content.

· When making ground meat dishes like burger patties or meatballs, add shredded carrots and spinach to the mix. Not only will this increase the nutrient content of the dish, but the moisture from the veggies actually makes for a juicier finished product.

· If you serve your toddler foods like pizza, quesadillas, or macaroni and cheese, always give them to her with veggies added. Tiny broccoli florets work well in mac and cheese. Chopped spinach is great in quesadillas. Thin-sliced zucchini is good on pizza.

· Condiments and sauces like spaghetti sauce, salsa and guacamole all count toward Baby's one cup of vegetables each day.

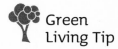

## Green Living Tip

. . . . . . . . . . . . . . . . . . . . .

Composting is a great way to make good use of scraps of vegetables that Baby picks at but doesn't finish. For a composting how-to guide, visit www.compostguide.com.

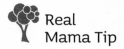

## Real Mama Tip

. . . . . . . . . . . . . . . . . . . . .

"I buy lots of green beans, berries, and other goodies at the farmers' markets when they are in season, and then I freeze them to use throughout the winter."

—Lindsay, Portland, Oregon

A NOTE FROM DR. BOB

## It's All in the Presentation

When it comes to feeding toddlers, you have to become a marketing expert. Find creative ways to present food to your kids. As a child I remember loving "egg canoes"—hard-boiled eggs sliced into quarters. My kids loved to pretend they were giants munching on broccoli trees. But my favorite marketing pitch was the "green candies" my first child would down by the handful—peas! He couldn't get enough of them. We still tease him to this day (he's sixteen) about how he fell for it.

## 3. ENERGY POWERHOUSES: GRAINS

The low-carb craze may have demonized foods like pasta, bread, cereal, and crackers, however, they are nutritionally important, especially for toddlers and children. But you have to make sure you are giving your child *whole grains*. Whole grains like whole wheat, buckwheat, rye, brown rice, amaranth, or whole oats have not been stripped of any of their components—the bran, the endosperm, or the germ. If a food is made from a whole grain it will say "whole" right in the ingredient list. But some labels can fool you. A product may say "made with whole grains," "whole grains added," or "enriched." This doesn't mean that all the grains in the food are whole grains. The manufacturer has just added enough to meet the labeling requirements. Foods that are "enriched" have had part of the grain removed, and then some vitamins and minerals were added back.

*Why?* Grain foods are complex carbohydrates that give Baby energy for growth and for activity. Whole grain foods contain fiber, vitamins like niacin and other B vitamins, vitamin E, selenium, and minerals like zinc and iron. These foods help to prevent cardiovascular disease, type 2 diabetes, and possibly even childhood asthma.

*How much?* A serving of grains or breads is typically about a quarter to a third of an adult serving size, though many toddlers eat much more than this. Baby's total intake for the day should be at least two to three ounces of grains. An ounce is a slice of bread or one-half cup cereal or cooked starch like pasta or rice.

### Grain Tips

- Give your toddler a grain food with every meal. Cereal, toast, waffles, or pancakes at breakfast. Bread, pasta, rice, or cooked grains like bulgur or barley at lunch and dinner.
- Serve grain foods for snack. You'd be hard pressed to find a toddler who will refuse a cracker, pretzel, muffin, or rice cake. Just be sure to check the labels on these foods to avoid trans fats from partially hydrogenated oils.
- Breakfast cereal is highly fortified with vitamins and miner-

als and can really boost Baby's iron intake. It makes a good breakfast or snack, either dry or with milk. Choose a low-sugar variety—the label should say it has fewer than 5 grams of sugar per serving.

- Frozen waffles and pancakes are good to keep on hand. Try the whole or multigrain varieties. Gluten-free options are also available.

- If you make cookies, muffins, or quick breads (for instance, banana bread) at home, substitute whole wheat flour for half the flour. You can also add homemade or HAPPYBABY fruit puree as a substitute for half the oil or butter. See Recipes.

- Make silver-dollar-size pancakes. Instead of offering maple syrup, serve plain or with fruit purees for dipping. Look for all-natural pancake mixes in the baking section of your grocery store or make homemade. See our oatmeal pancake recipe on page 258.

- Experiment with grains like quinoa, barley, bulgur, and buckwheat. Instructions for cooking will come right on the box or

A NOTE FROM DR. BOB

## Grains as Mother Nature Intended

Nature knows what our bodies need. If we alter a food too much, we lose out on many benefits. Nowhere is this more true than with grains. Whole grains are perfectly designed with complex carbs, protein, and fiber. Combined this way, the carbs are a natural and long-lasting energy source. Without protein and fiber, the carbs are basically just sugar. So make sure that the majority of your child's breads, cereals, crackers, and pasta are as whole as they can be!

bag. Typically, all you have to do is boil some water or broth and cook the grain until done.

· Stretch beyond basic wheat, rice, and oat breakfast cereals. Try multigrain varieties or flakes made from amaranth, a super nutritious grain that is rich in lysine, an essential amino acid.

· Give spelt breads, pastas, crackers, and pretzels a try. This ancient grain is related to wheat but is higher in many vitamins and minerals.

· Serve Baby brown rice, whole wheat pasta, and whole grain breads from a young age so she doesn't balk when you try to give them to her later.

## 4. MUSCLE BUILDERS: PROTEIN FOODS

Protein is the main component of Baby's muscles, including rather important muscles like her heart and other organs. Protein foods—meat, fish, dairy foods, beans, and soy foods—should be a part of every meal and, ideally, snacks, too. They are more effective at satisfying hunger than carbohydrate foods alone, so add some beans to your pasta dishes and chicken to your noodle soups.

*Why?* Baby needs protein for her growth, and foods that provide protein also offer many other vitamins and minerals that contribute to good health. Animal sources of protein provide vitamin $B_{12}$, zinc, iron, vitamin $B_6$, and niacin. Vegetable sources like beans and tofu provide B vitamins, iron, magnesium, and other minerals.

*How much?* If your toddler is a picky eater you may be pleased to learn that he requires only 15 grams of protein to meet his minimum needs. That means that he gets enough protein by drinking just two 8-ounce cups of milk. Or by drinking one 8-ounce cup of milk and having an ounce of chicken or turkey. To get the benefit of all the vitamins and minerals that are protein's partners, aim for Baby to get 2 ounces of meat or the equivalent in vegetable protein sources most days. One ounce of chicken or fish or beef is about 2 tablespoons, and it's equivalent to ½ cup beans, an egg, or ⅓ cup (3 ounces) of tofu.

## Protein Tips

- Vegetable sources of protein like beans, tofu, and quinoa aren't just for vegetarians. On the contrary, these healthy foods should be staples in all kids' diets. There's an easy tofu stir-fry recipe on page 267.

- Young children don't seem to mind the taste or texture of uncooked tofu, making it one of the easiest foods to give a toddler, hands down. Just drain off the water, cut into small cubes (or mash for young babies), and serve. Tofu cubes with brown rice and cooked vegetables (frozen or fresh) and an all-natural teriyaki sauce is a great go-to meal for busy weeknights.

- Although tofu and soybeans are good for Baby, avoid processed soy foods that are made from texturized soy protein or soy protein isolate instead of whole soybeans. Some experts have raised concern over the potential health effects of this highly processed soy protein, especially for developing babies and pregnant women. That means skip the meat substitutes like soy cheese, soy burgers, soy crumbles, and soy deli meats. Instead, choose soy products made from whole soybeans, like the blocks of tofu you find in the produce section of the supermarket. Organic Nasoya brand tofu (www.nasoya.com) is widely available and it's a good choice.

- Eggs are an inexpensive and quick protein. Try hard-boiled or scrambled eggs, or egg salad. Quiche is a simple dish to make (or buy), and most kids like the mild cheesy taste. After age one, serve both the egg white and the yolk; before age one, serve just the yolk—half the egg's 6 grams of protein and many of the egg's other nutrients are found in the yolk.

- Ground or shredded meats have an easy-to-chew texture that many toddlers enjoy. Try burger patties, meatballs, meatloaf, or simply sautéed ground meat. When selecting ground beef, 85 to 95 percent lean ground sirloin or ground round is a fine choice. (When cooking for the whole family, opt for the leanest ground beef available, since Baby's the only one who can afford to eat a high-fat diet.) If you're grinding your own meat, choose

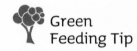

## Green Feeding Tip

. . . . . . . . . . . . . . . . . . . .

When buying meat, poultry, eggs, and dairy, support sustainable producers. Sustainable livestock-raising practices are humane to the animals, fair for the farm workers, and do less damage on the environment. Sustainable producers avoid the use of synthetic hormones, unnecessary antibiotics, and animal by-products that may contain these chemicals, making it a healthier choice for Baby, too. Visit www .sustainabletable.org for guidance on how to identify sustainable farms.

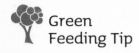

## Green Feeding Tip

Be sure to include vegetarian protein sources like tofu and beans in Baby's diet. Compared with animal proteins, vegetarian ones tend to be contaminated with fewer environmental toxins, such as persistent organic pollutants. Plus, eating less meat is great for the environment: it takes a hundred times more water to grow a pound of beef than to grow a pound of vegetable protein and far more fossil fuels, too.

A NOTE FROM DR. BOB

## Don't Bother Counting Grams of Protein

Many moms in my office tell me they don't think their toddler is getting enough protein. Well, protein should be the least of your worries because kids don't need to eat very much to meet their daily requirement. A toddler needs only about 15 grams each day. As long as you are presenting a healthy variety of protein sources, the quantity takes care of itself.

cuts of beef that have light marbling (the fat that makes little white lines throughout the meat), such as top sirloin or eye of round. See the Recipes section for a healthy burger recipe.

· And don't forget beans! Beans are another simple, inexpensive, and easy source of protein. Don't worry about beans' gassy reputation—Baby may not mind. Use mashed beans as a filling for a quesadilla, give whole black beans right on Baby's tray as finger foods, and serve hummus or other bean dips for snacks.

## 5. BONE BUILDERS: CALCIUM AND VITAMIN D SOURCES

Calcium and vitamin D are the nutritional dynamic duo for Baby's bones. Osteoporosis, the thinning and weakening of the bones, is considered a disease of the elderly, but really it has its roots in childhood and adolescence, when the bones develop most of their strength. Getting Baby started now with a diet rich in calcium and vitamin D will not only build her strong bones and teeth now, but it will help her develop a preference for the good sources of this pair to keep her bones strong for years to come.

*Why?* In addition to its important role in the health of Baby's growing bones and teeth, calcium helps her muscles function and may play a role in preventing childhood obesity and cancer. Vitamin D, once thought only to help build bone, may also help prevent many different conditions including cancer, diabetes, multiple sclerosis, and arthritis.

*How much?* Your one- to two-year-old needs 500 mg of calcium each day and 400 IU of vitamin D. Dairy foods are the best food sources:

- Each cup of cow's milk provides 300 mg of calcium and 100 IU of vitamin D. Goat's milk provides even more calcium—325 mg per cup (along with 30 IU of vitamin D).
- Half a cup of yogurt provides about 190 mg of calcium.
- An ounce of cheese has 150 to 300 mg calcium, depending on the type.

Vegetable sources of calcium shouldn't be overlooked either. Spinach and other dark greens provide about 80 mg of calcium in every ¼ cup. A half-cup of tofu provides 100 mg calcium. Soy milk, an alternative for children who don't tolerate cow's milk, is usually fortified to provide as much calcium as cow's milk.

The best source of vitamin D is sunlight. If you live in a warm climate that allows your family to get some healthy sun exposure year round, you probably don't need to worry about dietary sources of vitamin D. If you routinely use sunscreen (which blocks the ultraviolet rays that the body needs to produce the vitamin), or live in parts of the country that are too cold for shorts and T-shirts part of the year, you will need some vitamin D in your diet. Fish and eggs are among the only natural (nonfortified) food sources of vitamin D. Each ounce of salmon provides 100 IU of vitamin D, half Baby's needs for the day. One egg yolk offers 25 IU. Fortified foods like milk and cereal will provide the bulk of Baby's vitamin D. If Baby isn't exposed to direct sunlight each day and eats few vitamin D-fortified foods, it may be a good idea to give her a supplement. See page 216 for details.

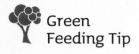
## Calcium and Vitamin D Tips

- Yogurt smoothies are a delicious way to give your family a calcium-rich snack. See Recipes.
- Offer cheese either with meals or as a snack. This can be cheese sticks, spreadable cheeses, sliced cheese, or cottage cheese. Make sandwiches, quesadillas, homemade pita or mini-bagel pizzas (and don't forget to shred in some hidden veggies wherever you can!).
- An intolerance to lactose, the natural sugar in cow's milk, is a challenge for some children and adults (an estimated 75 percent of the world's population has trouble digesting lactose).[5] But lactose intolerance is very uncommon in babies under age two years. When children react to cow's milk, it's usually due to an allergy to the protein, not the lactose. So even if you don't tolerate lactose, don't assume your baby won't. If it does cause her tummy troubles, buy lactose-free whole milk or soy milk instead.
- Dark green leafy vegetables like spinach, kale, and collards are fairly good sources. Since they are not the most toddler-friendly veggies (they're a little bitter), you may want to sneak them into your toddler's diet by shredding or pureeing them and then hiding them in foods like spaghetti sauce or burger patties.

### MYTH OR FACT?

*Babies and toddlers must have dairy foods as part of a healthy diet.*

Myth. Although dairy foods are indeed packed with good nutrition for growing bodies—fat, protein, calcium, vitamins A and D—it is possible to create a healthy dairy-free diet for your child, if need be (e.g., if she's allergic to cow's milk). The main thing to keep in mind is that Baby still needs the nutrients that come from whole milk. That means she needs good sources of fat, sufficient protein (the recommended 2 cups of milk provides 16 grams), at least 500 mg calcium, and sources of vitamins A and D.

## 6. BLOOD FORTIFIERS: IRON SOURCES

Baby was born with a fairly good supply of iron, and then her diet of breast milk or formula kept her in good iron status. Once Baby is a year old and no longer taking breast milk or formula as her main source of nutrition, food sources of iron become increasingly important.

*Why?* Iron is required for the production of hemoglobin, the part of the blood that carries oxygen to the body's cells and muscles. Sufficient iron will prevent anemia and support normal brain development.

*How much?* Baby needs 7 mg of iron per day. To give you an idea of what this means, each of these foods provide 1 mg of iron: 1 ounce (2 tablespoons) of beef, 2 ounces chicken, ¼ cup beans, ¾ ounce tofu (about 1 tablespoon plus 1 teaspoon), about ⅔ cup oatmeal, and ⅓ cup cooked spinach. One of the best sources is fortified cereal, providing 4 to 5 mg for every ½ cup of cereal.

### Iron Tips

- If Baby drinks too much milk or eats too many dairy foods, the phosphorus in the dairy food can interfere with her iron absorption, so limit your toddler to no more than 16 ounces of milk each day.
- Iron from meat sources is more easily absorbed than the iron from vegetarian sources. This means that if you rely on vegetable sources of iron, Baby may need more of them.
- Add dried fruit (cut into small pieces) to oatmeal for an iron-rich breakfast. Mix wheat germ into yogurt or applesauce.
- Vitamin C helps the body absorb iron, so serve foods that are rich in this vitamin along with Baby's iron sources. Vitamin C is found in strawberries, oranges, bell peppers, broccoli, potatoes, and orange juice.

## 7. BRAIN BUILDERS: FATS

Many of us get so used to avoiding fat that it's hard to adjust our thinking for Baby's needs. A low-fat diet is recommended only after age two. Until then, Baby needs plenty of fat, so you shouldn't restrict her intake. This doesn't mean your home can become a fatty food free-for-all, though. Don't get in the habit of giving Baby fried foods and fatty snack foods. Choose less processed and more nutritionally dense sources of fat like those listed below.

*Why?* Fats are crucial for healthy development of Baby's brain and nervous system. Her brain is 60 percent fat and growing fast during these early years. Fats also provide a lot of energy and, frankly, they make foods taste better.

*How much?* At least 40 percent of Baby's calories should come from fat. That means about 45 grams a day for a one-year-old who eats 1,000 calories. To give you some perspective, consider that a teaspoon of oil provides about 5 grams of fat. A cup of whole milk provides 8 grams of fat. One quarter of a Florida avocado is 4 grams of fat. And a 1-ounce serving of ground beef (about 2 tablespoons) is about 5 grams of fat. Baby also needs good sources of omega-3 fats, in particular. See side-bar for details.

### Fat Tips

- The healthiest fats (omega-3s) come from fish and from vegetable sources like nuts, avocado, and vegetable oils.
- Avoid sources of trans fats, which are formed when vegetable oils are partially hydrogenated during manufacturing. These fats raise blood cholesterol and are not healthy for babies or adults. Packaged foods like baked goods, snack crackers and chips, candy bars, and fast foods may contain these kinds of fats. Check the Nutrition Facts label under the "Total Fat" section to see if a food contains trans fats. Always look for a trans-fat-free alternative.
- Saturated fats like those found in whole milk, cheese, meat, and eggs are sometimes called bad fats because they can con-

A NOTE FROM DR. BOB

## Don't Let the Label Fool You

Several years ago food makers began to take trans fats out of some foods. But they ran into a little snag: kids and adults who are already used to eating trans fat foods wouldn't eat the healthier options. Trans fats make food taste yummy. They also prolong the shelf life, which cuts down on the cost. Food makers knew that if their products were completely trans fat free, some people wouldn't buy them. So the government compromised with food makers and allowed them to label a food "trans fat free" as long as the amount of trans fat was below 0.5 grams per serving. You will see hydrogenated oils in the ingredients, yet the label on the front will claim "trans fat free." The nutritional label on the back will say "0 trans fat" with an asterisk. That asterisk means there is still a small amount. So, the only way to know for sure that you are avoiding trans fat is to make sure there is no hydrogenated oil in the actual ingredient list.

## ALL ABOUT OMEGA-3S

Omega-3 fats are essential polyunsaturated fats. The word "essential" means our bodies can't manufacture them—we need to get them from our diets. Three omega-3 fats found in foods are alpha-linolenic acid (ALA), eicosapentaenoic acid (EPA), and docosahexaenoic acid (DHA). DHA gets the most attention when we're talking about feeding babies because it is a main structural component of brain and eye tissue and is required for optimal development of these tissues. Many infant formulas and many HAPPYBABY foods are supplemented with this fatty acid to support infant health. People who get plenty of omega-3 fats may have lower risks of degenerative diseases like multiple sclerosis and inflammatory processes like cancer, heart disease, and arthritis. In children, a deficiency of these fats may cause poor school performance, reduced brain development, and vision problems.

*How much?* You won't find omega-3 values on the nutrition label, so we won't burden you with numbers here. The most important thing is to simply serve omega-3 sources to your baby many days of the week. Breast milk and fortified infant formula are sources of DHA; however, once Baby is eating table foods, her breast milk or formula consumption isn't high enough to supply all of her omega-3 needs. The best food sources of omega-3 fats include ground flaxseed or flaxseed oil; cold-water fish like salmon, sardines, and tuna; algae; canola and olive oils; soybeans; walnuts; wheat germ; pumpkin seeds; eggs; beef from grass-fed cows; and fortified baby foods.

## More Fat Tips

- When choosing fish for Baby, be sure to avoid those that are high in mercury, a pollutant that is poisonous and especially dangerous for developing brains.

Fish come in all shades of green:

| The Deepest Green *These fish are healthy and eco-friendly choices* | Lighter Green *These fish are less baby-friendly or eco-friendly options but can be served to Baby, in limited amounts* | Not Green at All *These fish are high in mercury and/or are overfished or caught in a way that detrimentally impacts their habitat* |
|---|---|---|
| Anchovies* | Canned light tuna—limit Baby to an ounce of canned light tuna for every 12 pounds of body weight. Example: If your 2-year-old is 24 pounds, limit him to 2 ounces or ⅓ of a regular-size can, or less per week. (NRDC recommendations) | Mercury-containing: |
| Arctic char, farmed | | Ahi or bigeye tuna |
| Catfish, U.S. | | Albacore/white canned tuna |
| Halibut, Pacific | | King mackerel |
| Mackerel, Atlantic* | | Marlin |
| Mahimahi, U.S. | | Orange roughy |
| Rainbow trout, farmed* | | Shark |

| | | |
|---|---|---|
| Salmon wild,* | Cod, Pacific | Swordfish |
| Sardines, Pacific* | Flounder/sole, Pacific | Tilefish |
| | Sea bass, black | |
| | Sturgeon, white (wild from Washington or Oregon) | Not eco-friendly: |
| | | Chilean sea bass |
| | | Flounder/sole, Atlantic |
| | | Haddock |
| | | Monkfish |
| | | Pompano |
| | | Rockfish |
| | | Salmon, farmed |
| | | Skate |
| | | Snapper |
| | | Sturgeon |

* High in omega-3 fatty acids.

Source: Environmental Defense Fund.[6]

- Sneak in omega-3s by adding a teaspoon of ground flaxseed or wheat germ to foods like oatmeal, applesauce, or yogurt smoothies. (See Recipe on page 259)
- Use olive oil when you cook for Baby (but don't fry in olive oil—it burns more easily than other oils). Organic canola oil is another healthy choice.
- Choose organic milk and meat from grass-fed cows—they contain much higher levels of omega-3 fats than conventional versions.[7]
- See page 216 for information about omega-3 fatty acid supplements that are appropriate for Baby.

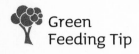

tribute to elevated cholesterol and heart disease in adults. Up until age two, these fats are not a problem for Baby so you don't need to restrict them. Around age two you should gradually transition to lower-fat foods like low-fat or skim milk and low-fat yogurt and cheese in order to reduce your child's saturated fat intake. Don't worry: most children will make the switch easily.

- Nut butters like almond and cashew butter are a great source of healthy unsaturated fats. It's best to delay peanut butter (the most allergenic nut) until two years of age.

## 8. IMMUNE BOOSTERS: PROBIOTICS

Probiotics are "friendly bacteria" that live in our intestines and help the immune system by discouraging the growth of harmful disease-causing bacteria. They provide a boost to the immune system and help to prevent or treat a variety of ailments.

*Why?* Certain strains of probiotics have been shown to reduce colic in infants and also to prevent eczema and allergies. They may help reduce the symptoms of irritable bowel syndrome, prevent all kinds of allergies, help manage lactose intolerance, promote bowel regularity, and prevent infections in the intestines and elsewhere.

*How much?* It's recommended that children (and you, too, Mama) consume probiotics daily for health maintenance purposes. If your child needs to take antibiotics at any time to treat a bacterial infection, consider increasing her intake of probiotic-containing foods or offering a supplement, since the antibiotic will kill off many of the healthy gut bacteria. Extra probiotics will help to bring balance back to her system. For a supplement, the standard recommended dose of probiotics is one billion cells.

### Probiotics Tips

- Probiotics are naturally found in breast milk and fermented foods like yogurt, kefir, aged cheeses, miso, sauerkraut, and kimchi.

- We've added probiotics to our HAPPYBELLIES line of cereals to support immunity and help prevent allergies.
- To find probiotics in foods, look for the words "probiotics" or "live active cultures" on food labels.
- Give Baby yogurt as a snack or with meals. Under age two, use whole milk yogurt and then transition to low fat by age two. She can eat either the plain kind or the kind with fruit. Avoid any yogurts with added artificial colors or flavors, and always go for organic.
- The benefits of probiotics come from continuous long-term consumption, so try to give Baby a good source daily.

A NOTE FROM DR. BOB

## Make Sure Your Baby's Yogurt Is Doing Her Body Good

All yogurts are not created equal. Light yogurts often have an artificial sweetener, a big no-no for babies. Virtually all fruit or flavored yogurt has sugar, even those that are labeled for babies. The healthiest yogurt is plain organic yogurt, with your own added bananas and berries for flavor and sweetness. If you can get your toddler's taste buds used to the healthiest version, great. If not, organic fruit and berry yogurt (with the small amount of sugar to go along) is an OK alternative since the calcium and probiotic content is so healthy. Toddlers who are on the go can have some sugar in their diets—they use it for energy to run around. Parents should be more concerned about snack foods, cookies, candy, soda, and other sweetened beverages.

# DOES BABY NEED A SUPPLEMENT?

There are only two nutritional supplements that offer proven benefits for babies: omega-3 fatty acids and vitamin D.

*Omega-3s:*
- Breast-fed babies: Mama needs to eat good sources of omega-3s or take a supplement of 1000 milligrams of combined ALA, DHA, and EPA each day.
- Formula-fed babies: Choose a formula with added DHA.
- Once Baby is no longer on breast milk or formula: If she doesn't eat any good food sources of omega-3s, consider giving her a supplement. Choose a liquid omega-3 supplement (capsules are choking hazards for babies under age three) that has dosing information for babies more than six months old. It should be a DHA-rich blend made from highly refined fish oil or vegetarian sources that provides 500 to 700 milligrams of omega-3 fats per day. Dr. Bob's dad, Dr. William Sears, has a line of omega-3 supplements called Go Fish, including a liquid that can be given to babies. See www.drsearsfamilyapproved.com for details. Nordic Naturals (www.nordicnaturals.com) and Spectrum (www.spectrumorganics.com) also make liquid omega-3 supplements that are appropriate for Baby.

*Vitamin D:* As discussed in chapter 3, this vitamin is essential not only for Baby's bone health, but vitamin D deficiency has been implicated in so many chronic disease processes that experts now agree that most babies and young children would benefit from a supplement of 400 international units per day. You can purchase over-the-counter vitamin D drops for infants—either combined with vitamins A and C or vitamin D alone. Follow dosing information provided on the package or by your pediatrician.

Don't give Baby other supplements of single vitamins or minerals unless recommended by her pediatrician. As far as a daily multivitamin goes, most babies don't need it. There's no evidence that they make Baby healthier, and besides, artificially manufactured vitamins could never be a substitute for a healthy diet. In fact, most vitamins and minerals in food, as opposed to those in supplements, are absorbed more effectively by the body. So, serve Baby vitamin- and mineral-rich foods or fortified foods instead.

# QUENCHING THEIR THIRST

We've talked a lot about which foods to serve your toddler, but let's not forget her beverages. Here's a quick rundown for you:

- *Breast milk:* Until age one year, this was the recommended beverage for Baby. Once she enters her second year, breast milk can still play a role in her nutrition, but it does take a backseat to food. Give your toddler a beverage in a cup with her meals and keep a sippy cup handy throughout the day. Then breast-feed other times during the day when your child wants a snack or wants to cuddle.
- *Cow's milk:* Whether Baby started on breast milk or formula, at age one start to give her cow's milk to drink. Definitely choose organic (see pages 21–33 for our reasons) and give her about two cups (sixteen ounces) each day. If she drinks less than this, she needs to be getting calcium and fat from other sources. More is not better, though—too much milk can interfere with her iron absorption and put her at risk for anemia.
- *Goat's milk:* If Baby doesn't tolerate cow's milk (or if you prefer to limit her cow's milk intake) goat's milk may be a good alternative. Although goat's milk contains similar proteins to cow's milk, they are easier to digest in the goat's milk, and some children who are allergic to cow's milk tolerate goat's milk much better. Don't switch to goat's milk to get away from lactose, though, as goat's milk contains it, too. With more calcium, vitamin A, B vitamins, and selenium than cow's milk, goat's milk is a very good substitute.
- *Soy milk:* This can be a substitute for cow's milk if Baby doesn't tolerate it or if you don't serve it in your home. Most brands are fortified with calcium and vitamins, often in amounts that make a glass of soy milk equivalent to a glass of cow's milk.
- *Rice milk:* As with soy milk, you need to find a fortified or "enriched" product that provides calcium and vitamins A and D. Rice milk is usually low in fat, so if Baby drinks this instead of whole cow's or goat's milk be sure to include other good sources of fat in her diet. Try to use unsweetened rice milk. The vanilla-flavored versions have a lot of sugar.
- *Almond milk:* This option is a better source of protein and has less sugar than rice milk.
- *Water:* Help Baby get a taste for plain water to foster a preference for this calorie-free fluid. Give water in a cup during the day whenever Baby may be thirsty, like after running around outside (especially in warm weather) or waking up from a nap. Give water with meals whenever Baby isn't drinking milk.

- *Juice:* A small amount of juice can fit just fine into a healthy diet, but it's not at all required for good health. One hundred percent fruit juice usually provides vitamin C, but it also contains a lot of natural sugar. Limit your toddler to less than ¾ cup (6 ounces) per day and dilute it to cut the sweetness.
- *Sugar-sweetened drinks:* Call us the food police, but we say never give a child under age three a sugar-sweetened drink. There's just absolutely no need to introduce such a thing.
- *Artificially sweetened beverages:* This is another kind of beverage that has no place in a toddler's diet. See page 224 for a full discussion about artificial sweeteners.

## RECAP OF FEEDING ESSENTIAL 2: FEED BABY THE GREAT EIGHT

Putting it all together, here's a snapshot of the minimum daily nutrition needs for a twelve- to twenty-four-month old-child, along with two sample menus.

### A Day in the Life of a One- to Two-Year-Old
- 1,000 to 1,300 calories, about 40 percent from fat
- 2 cups milk (or other dairy foods like yogurt and cheese)
- ¾ to 1 cup fruits
- ¾ to 1 cup veggies
- 4 servings bread group (each = ¼ to ½ cup, ¼ slice)
- 2 meats/beans/eggs/tofu (each = ½ to 1 ounce, ½ egg, 1 to 2 tablespoons meat, ¼ to ½ cup beans or tofu)

### *Sample Menu 1*

BREAKFAST
- ½ cup O-shaped cereal
- 1 cup whole milk (some in cereal, some in cup)
- ½ cup strawberries

SNACK
- 4 ounces (½ cup) yogurt
- ½ slice bread or small pancake

LUNCH

- Spinach ravioli
- ½ cup cooked carrots
- Soft peach or pear cut into slices

SNACK

- 3 crackers
- 2 tablespoons chopped avocado

DINNER

- ¼ cup chicken breast, ½ cup broccoli, and ½ cup brown rice—stir-fried with low-sodium sauce, if you prefer
- 1 cup whole milk

*Sample Menu 2*

BREAKFAST

- ½ cup oatmeal
- ½ cup blueberries
- 1 cup whole milk

SNACK

- ½ orange, sliced

LUNCH

- Grilled cheese sandwich on 1 slice whole grain bread
- ½ cup zucchini wheels (zucchini, cut into circles)

SNACK

- 5 pretzels with hummus for dipping

DINNER

- 1 turkey meatball (with or without tomato sauce)
- ½ cup pasta spirals
- ½ cup green beans
- 1 cup whole milk

A NOTE FROM DR. BOB

## Waffles or "Awfuls" for Breakfast

One of the best ways you can shape your baby's young taste buds is to be careful how you present waffles and pancakes. Eating white flour pancakes with syrup is pretty much the same as eating cake. Instead, use whole grain options. And forget the syrup for the first few years. Kids love berries and bananas with whipped cream (unsweetened). My teenager still puts bananas and strawberries on almost every waffle and pancake (along with some maple syrup now) because that's what he's always known.

## Feeding Essential 3: Go for Natural and Whole, Not Artificial or Processed

Plenty of foods technically fall into one of the Great Eight but leave something to be desired nutritionally. Here are some foods to leave off Baby's menu:

### FOODS TO LIMIT: OVERLY PROCESSED (AND NUTRITIONALLY LACKING) FOODS

Processed foods are those that have been treated in some way to be sold commercially. Sometimes, as in canned foods, the foods are exposed to high heat to extend shelf life. Other foods may contain artificial preservatives for the same purpose. Quick-cooking foods like instant rice or instant oatmeal are precooked or altered to cook faster. Just because something is processed doesn't mean it is necessarily unhealthy, of course. Foods like cereals, breads, yogurt, dried fruits, and frozen vegetables are processed but perfectly healthy. So you have to choose your processed foods wisely. The processed foods that contain unhealthy fats, too much sodium, or too much sugar have little redeeming nutritional quality. They don't contribute positively to your child's health, and worse, they actually dull Baby's tastes for fresh healthy foods. Here are some unhealthy processed foods and healthier alternatives:

| Processed Food | Healthier Alternative |
| --- | --- |
| Chicken nuggets | Cooked chicken breast |
| White bread | 100 percent whole wheat bread |
| French fries | Roasted potatoes |
| Apple-filled cereal bar | An apple |
| Hot dog | Sautéed ground beef |
| American cheese slice | Slice of natural cheddar cheese |
| Hot pink "kids" yogurt | Plain yogurt with strawberries on top |

## FOODS TO HIDE: SWEETS, FAST FOOD, AND OTHER JUNK FOOD

These processed foods get a separate mention because they are among the more tempting foods around. While we don't think it's terrible if a toddler has a cookie or potato chips or french fries on occasion, we suggest that you hide these foods from Baby as long as possible. Once Baby gets her first taste, she's going to want more, and none of these foods should make a regular appearance on her plate. And it's not ideal to just tell Baby no all the time, because when a food is forbidden it only increases in appeal. When Baby is older, allowing her "treats" now and then will help to teach her the important lesson of moderation and that you have to make choices about which foods you eat. But as hard as it

# NATURALLY SWEET

It's easy to understand why keeping Baby away from sugary junk food is a good idea. But what about natural sweeteners? Although these sweeteners do tend to contain more vitamins and minerals than refined white sugar, as you'll see below, the end result is the same: they provide unnecessary calories that could displace healthier foods in Baby's diet, they may contribute to dental caries, and they taste sweet, so you could be fueling Baby's sweet tooth by giving them to her. Here's some info about these natural sweeteners, but the bottom line is that Baby shouldn't be eating too many sweets at this stage, regardless of the type.

| Sweeteners | Comments |
| --- | --- |
| Honey | Though not a significant source of vitamins or minerals, honey does contain some B vitamins and even a little iron. As discussed on page 170, honey isn't safe for babies under age one year. |
| Blackstrap molasses | An excellent source of manganese and copper; very good source of iron, calcium, potassium and magnesium; and a good source of vitamin $B_6$. |
| Raw sugar | Despite the promising name, this sugar isn't very different from white table sugar. |
| Stevia | Used as a sweetener in Paraguay and Japan for many years, it was recently approved by the FDA as a food additive. However, we haven't seen too much research on its use for babies and so we wouldn't recommend it for Baby. |
| Agave nectar syrup | A syrup made from the agave plant, it's sometimes used as a substitute for honey (though it is considered safe for babies under age one year). |
| Pure maple syrup | Not to be confused with pancake syrup and other products made of high-fructose corn syrup and other sugars. Real maple syrup is an excellent source of manganese and a good source of zinc. |

will be to teach her these lessons when she's older, it's basically impossible to teach her before age two. Keeping her in the dark about these foods, at least for now, is so much easier.

## FOODS TO AVOID: FOODS WITH ARTIFICIAL ADDITIVES

Foods that contain artificial colors, artificial preservatives, artificial sweeteners, or artificial fats are highly processed and usually lacking in nutritional value. Plus, some artificial additives are not safe or appropriate for babies and toddlers. Even if a food additive is given the label of "GRAS" or "generally recognized as safe" by the U.S. Food and Drug Administration (FDA), you can't assume it was tested on babies. Since we don't know the effects of long-term use of these ingredients on growing bodies, we say avoid them altogether.

### Colors and Preservatives

Recent research found that young children may become more hyperactive when they eat foods that are artificially colored with chemicals like Blue No. 1 or preserved with sodium benzoate. Animal studies have linked some artificial colors and preservatives with an increased risk for cancers. And artificial colors and preservatives may cause allergic reactions in some children, particularly those with allergic conditions like eczema or other food allergies. These ingredients are found mostly in highly processed foods like candy and packaged snack foods. But they also show up in places you may not expect, so check out the food label. We have been shocked to find food coloring in some foods that aren't even colorful, like Blue No. 1 in basic white marshmallows.

It's important to mention that not all colors and preservatives are artificial and some are perfectly benign. For example, annatto extract, beta-carotene, and beet juice are all-natural and safe coloring agents added to some foods. Ascorbic acid and citric acid are natural preservatives that pose no risk for Baby (unless she is allergic or has a sensitivity to the particular ingredient).

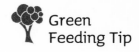
**Green Feeding Tip**

When selecting packaged foods for Baby, look for products packaged with recycled and recyclable materials. Check your local recycling policies and shop accordingly. For example, in New York City we can recycle a glass jar that contained applesauce but not a plastic one. Most communities recycle cardboard egg cartons but not plastic ones.

### Artificial Fats

Two kinds of fake fats that you might find in processed foods are trans fats and the fat substitute olestra (sold under the brand name Olean). Trans fats are created when vegetable oil is made into a more solid fat through a process called hydrogenation. These fats raise levels of the bad LDL cholesterol and lower levels of the good HDL cholesterol. Olestra is an artificial fat that is used in "light" potato chips and other similar snacks. Too much of this ingredient can cause diarrhea. Since Baby needs plenty of fat during her first two years, there's certainly no reason to be buying her light snack chips.

### Artificial Sweeteners

There are many reasons to avoid these ingredients. First of all, some of them have been linked to health problems in animal studies, as we will describe in the following table. True, most studies look at "high" consumption levels, but we have no idea what is considered a safe level of consumption for babies or young children. There's also the basic question of why a baby or toddler would even need to eat products that contain these artificial sweeteners. If there is an occasion to have a cookie or jam or juice every now and then, just give the real thing rather than something with an artificial sweetener. And since artificial sweeteners are anywhere from two hundred to seven hundred times sweeter than sugar, exposing Baby to these foods may only lead to even more of a sweet tooth in the future. Here are some details for you:

| Sweetener | Where It's Found | About Its Safety |
|---|---|---|
| aspartame (NutraSweet, Equal) | The little blue and pink sweetener packets, beverages, gums, other sugar-free foods | FDA's National Toxicology Program found no link to cancer, but other studies have linked high consumption to leukemia, breast cancer, lymphoma, and brain and nerve damage.[8–10] |
| acesulfame potassium (or acesulfame K or ace K) | Diet soda and diet desserts | According to the FDA, there are more than 90 studies that show it to be safe.[11] It's unlikely that any of those studies included babies and toddlers. |

| | | |
|---|---|---|
| saccharin (Sweet'N Low) | Little pink packets and no-sugar-added foods like jams and baked goods, also found in many toothpastes! | Early studies found saccharin to cause cancer in laboratory animals, and at one time it actually carried a warning label stating this. This label was removed in 2001 after the National Cancer Institute determined no cancer link. |
| sucralose (Splenda) | Little yellow packets, in diet sodas and juices, desserts, baked goods | This sweetener is actually made from table sugar but processed so that it has no calories. Of all the artificial sweeteners out there, this one may be safer. However, we're not convinced that we know the long-term effect of a lifetime of consumption so we won't be feeding it to our children anytime soon. |
| sorbitol, mannitol and xylitol | No-sugar-added candies and treats | Generally safe for adults but may have a laxative effect, and in little tummies the effect may be greater. Try to avoid these, too. |
| high-fructose corn syrup (HFCS) | Soft drinks, snack foods, some breads, cereals, sauces like tomato sauce, BBQ sauce, marinades | Fructose is a natural sugar found in many foods. HFCS is made when corn syrup is processed to increase its fructose concentration. It's a substitute for sucrose (table sugar) that is cheaper for food producers and extends the shelf life of foods. A couple of years ago there was much media hype about high HFCS consumption raising the risk of obesity, insulin resistance, and diabetes. However, current research suggests that the risks of eating too much HFCS are actually no different than the risks of eating too much of any type of sugar.[12] The bottom line is that Baby should not be getting too much added sugar in general, so it would be wise to just avoid sources of this ingredient as you would avoid any high-sugar food. |

## Putting It All Together at the Market—Navigating the Aisles and Deciphering Food Labels

Armed with the list of foods to eat and foods to avoid, head to the store. Here are some shopping tips:

- Shop the perimeter of the market to find the healthiest foods for Baby—the produce department, the fresh meats and fish, and the dairy case.
- At least once go to the store with extra time so you can stroll down the aisles and discover products that you may not have seen before. You may spot a grain that you've never tried or an organic option that you didn't know existed.
- For packaged foods, you don't have to guess if a food is healthy for your child—it comes with a guide for you: the food label. Reading food labels will give you all sorts of important information. You can see every ingredient and identify any artificial additives that you want to avoid, determine if the food is organic, and evaluate the nutrient content. Check out the food label checklist below for guidance. And here are some common claims or descriptors you will see on food labels and what they mean:

| Label Claim | What It Means |
|---|---|
| 100 percent organic | Every ingredient in the food meets the definition of organic. |
| USDA Organic | At least 95 percent of the food's ingredients are organic. |
| Made with organic | At least 70 percent of the ingredients are organic and the label will tell you which ones. |
| All-natural | This claim isn't regulated by the FDA, so it could really mean anything . . . or nothing. The only way to determine if something contains all-natural ingredients is to read the ingredient label and look for artificial ingredients. Don't be fooled—there are plenty of "natural" foods that aren't so healthy. Like french fries—just potatoes and oil, right? Natural? Yes. Healthy? No. |
| No added sugar | While it's certainly good to look for foods without added sugar, this claim doesn't actually tell you much about the healthfulness (or sugar content) of the food. For example: Many cranberry and grape juices have "no added sugar," but other ingredients have been added to make them sweeter—either other fruit juices or artificial sweeteners. |
| Made with real fruit | This is a potentially deceptive label claim. Consider how many desserts and processed sweets have raisins or fruit jellies in them. These are "made with real fruit" but may not be the best choice for Baby. |
| Lite/Light | The food has one-third fewer calories or half the fat compared with the regular version of the food. This claim may mean that the food contains a sugar or fat substitute, so read the ingredient list carefully. |
| Low fat | This means the food has 3 grams or less of fat per serving. |
| Reduced fat/sugar | The product contains 25 percent less fat or sugar than regular version of that product. |
| Fresh | This is a claim you may see on meat, fish, and poultry labels. It means that the food is raw, has never been heated or frozen, and contains no preservatives. |

# A Food Label Checklist

Let's say you are holding two boxes of crackers or two boxes of cereal and trying to decide which to buy. And let's just assume for this exercise that the two products cost the same amount so we can take that factor out of the picture. Here's how to use the food labels to figure out which one to serve your baby:

First, look at the ingredient listing to see if it contains any of the following. If it does, think twice about buying it:

- hydrogenated oils (these will also show up as trans fats on the Nutrition Facts label)
- artificial colors (Yellow No. 6, Blue No. 1, etc.)
- artificial preservatives (sodium benzoate, BHT, etc.)
- any allergens that your child must avoid

Then see if either option is made with organic ingredients. Go for the organic one whenever possible.

Finally, look at the Nutrition Facts label and assess the food's nutrient content. Look at the following nutrients and choose the product that wins the nutrient showdown for most of these:

1. less saturated fat
2. less sugar
3. less sodium
4. more fiber (3 grams per serving is a "good" source)
5. more protein, and
6. more of any of the following:
   - vitamin A
   - vitamin C
   - iron
   - calcium

# Taking It Home . . .

Around age one, Baby moves away from baby foods and truly joins the family at the table. Now is your chance to shape Baby's tastes and put her on the path to a healthy and green way of eating. Seize it! We hope our three essentials for green and healthy eating will help you. First, choose organic foods whenever you can. Also, feed Baby a variety of foods to provide her with:

- vitamins, phytochemicals, and fiber from fruits and vegetables
- protein for her growing body
- calcium and vitamin D for her bones and teeth
- healthy fats, especially the omega-3s for her developing brain
- iron-rich foods to prevent anemia
- sources of probiotics for a strong immune system

And finally, steer clear of the foods that have no place in Baby's diet, like overly processed junky foods and foods with artificial sweeteners and colors.

The bonus here is that the whole family benefits when you follow these three healthy eating rules. Of course for the whole family to benefit, the whole family must be eating the same meals. Which brings us to our next chapter, which covers, among other mealtime challenges, how to actually get a healthy dinner on the table in the first place.

# 7

# **The Airplane
and the Hangar**

## Mealtime Challenges and Practical Solutions

You are now an expert on what to feed yourself and your child, but that's only half the battle. Getting your toddler to actually eat the healthy foods is another. Parents may have the best intentions when it comes to Baby's nutrition, but when your mild-mannered baby becomes an opinionated toddler you may experience some challenges at the table. Picky eating and other typical toddler eating behaviors can make mealtimes difficult for parents and kids alike. When the going gets tough you may be tempted to just throw in the towel (or throw out the organic veggies, say). But you've come too far to turn back now. Even if Baby rejects all your best healthy feeding efforts, stay the course! As long as the rest of the family continues with this way of eating, Baby will come around one day. In this chapter, we will provide practical tips and strategies for handling your toddler's behaviors in a way that fosters healthy development and good nutrition.

Finding the time to shop for and prepare healthy meals for yourself and your family is also a challenge. How do you do it all? Well, first, you should let yourself off the hook and realize that for the next year or two, evenings in your home are going to be a little more—how to put this nicely—fun? Active? Total chaos? So, every night doesn't need to be a five-course dinner. Some breakfasts will be quiet and relaxed; others will be quick and a bit rushed while you and Baby run out the door. You will enjoy some peaceful lunchtimes, and some busy days you'll be lucky to eat anything for lunch.

This chapter provides a practical and simple action plan for pulling it all together, including meal and snack ideas for you and your toddler.

## The Typical Toddler at the Table

The toddler stage is known for presenting certain challenges, like temper tantrums, rampant use of the word "no," and the pushing of limits and buttons. And don't be surprised if the "terrible twos" begin well before Baby's second birthday. If only toddlers would just leave all that behind when they sit down to eat. But of course that's not the case. Even the best eaters can give parents a run for their money at times. It's not uncommon for toddlers to refuse to eat new foods or foods that they once enjoyed, to be almost militant about which plate they use at mealtime or how their food is cut, or to dissolve into a weepy mess if their foods touch each other on the plate or if they see a food they don't like.

When you first started feeding Baby solids, there may have been some times when Baby was less than enthusiastic. Perhaps you turned to a classic baby-feeding trick: sending the spoon toward the open mouth of your delighted child while exclaiming, "Zoom, zoom, here it comes!" It didn't take much to get over that bump in the road, right? As Baby becomes a toddler, you may soon be nostalgic for those simple times.

If your toddler starts with challenging mealtime behaviors, she isn't just being "naughty" or trying to manipulate you. Developmentally there is a lot going on at this age that will influence behavior. It may help you to understand what's going on behind the scenes:

Your baby's weight tripled in the first year, but in the second she'll gain only about five pounds. This growth slowdown leads to changes in her appetite, too. She may not feel so hungry anymore.

Toddlers have a growing sense of independence ("I do it myself" may become a common refrain) as they are increasingly able to explore their world on foot and express themselves through language. Some picky eating is just a child's way of asserting her newfound independence.

Toddlers tend to fear new things, so if they are given a food that looks unfamiliar, it can be scary to them. This is one reason toddlers like to eat the same foods over and over.

Sometimes teething can make a toddler's mouth feel sore and can make food seem unappealing.

Most toddlers are easily distractible and may not have the attention span to last through a long meal.

Toddlers like to test limits in order to understand them better. They want to see what happens, for example, if they refuse to eat their meal or if they throw food on the floor.

Of course, just because it's normal for toddlers to be picky or difficult doesn't mean you should give up and give in to their every whim. Now more than ever it's important to help shape your child's healthy eating habits. Mamas and dads are challenged to stay the course of healthy eating while negotiating the toddler table obstacle course.

## How Not to Serve the "Chicken Nugget Diet"

A wise person once said, "You can lead a horse to water but you cannot make him drink." This saying would make a great mantra for parents of toddlers. As the Mama, you need to decide which foods to serve your child. There are nutrients that she needs, and the only way she'll get them is if you make sure they are available to her. It's your job to choose all-natural and organic foods, create nutritionally balanced meals, make them look appealing, tell her the food is yummy, and eat a big forkful with a smile on your face . . . but at the end of the day, you can't (and shouldn't) force her to eat it. Not only will you create a mealtime battle of the greatest proportions, but you'd be missing the point: we want to *teach* our children healthy habits, not literally shove them down their throats.

If you accept this premise of toddler feeding, you can see that it leaves you with two basic options: (1) you can just give up and serve your toddler what you know she will eat every night (the chicken nugget diet), or (2) you can serve her what you know she *should* eat, with certain accommodations to encourage her to actually do so.

Option 2, of course, is what we're here to help you with. It's entirely appropriate to jump through a few hoops to encourage your toddler to eat well, but the goal is to keep the dinner table from becoming a full-blown circus. You can tell if the situation with your toddler is out of control if the following phrases sound familiar. Accommodations like these may make mealtimes less stressful in the short term, but they foster bad eating habits that may stay with your child for many years to come:

· "The only way she'll eat is if I put her in front of the television"
· "I have to chase her around the house with the spoon—she won't sit in her high chair"
· "I just give her chicken nuggets and carrot sticks every night because it's all she will eat"

The good news is that it's never too late to get back on the right track. Strategies for encouraging healthy eating for your toddler include managing mealtime behaviors effectively, setting up a positive eating environment, and selecting and presenting foods in a toddler-friendly way.

## MANAGING MEALTIME BEHAVIORS

As Baby becomes a toddler you've probably noticed that your job as a parent keeps getting harder! All of a sudden you're thinking about how to get her to be well behaved, and you're forced to find the balance between being overly permissive and being an inflexible dictator. Here are some ways to work together to manage challenging mealtime behaviors:

- *Don't become a short-order cook or enter into negotiation with your child about what she will eat.* The best thing you can do is put a meal on the table, and if there are protests, tell her that she doesn't have to eat everything on her plate if there's something she doesn't like. What if she doesn't eat a thing? That probably won't happen if you follow our next tip.
- *Offer a sure-thing food with each meal.* This is something you know your child likes and will eat, even if she refuses everything else. For example, put some whole grain bread on the table or serve a favorite fruit as a side dish. Be careful to keep any second helpings of this favorite out of sight, so when your child wants more, you can honestly say it's all gone. She'll have to try something else on her plate if she's still hungry.
- *Try, try again.* You hear a lot of parents lament that their kids don't like vegetables or other healthy foods, but we think sometimes parents give up on them too soon. You need to serve your child a food at least fifteen times before you decide she's not going to eat it. And even then, remember to put that vegetable back into the meal rotation in the future (kids change their minds, you know). This means that even if you are certain your child won't eat a particular vegetable you should probably serve it to her anyway. It sends an important message about your expectations, and quite often you will be surprised when she gobbles it up behind your back.
- *Offer choices.* Toddlers like to feel like they are in control, so give yours reasonable choices to make at mealtime. Don't offer yes-or-no choices. For example, instead of asking, "Do you want broccoli?" ask, "Do you want green beans or broccoli?" or "Are you having an apple or a pear?" Let her pick the pasta shape or the kind of dipping sauce she wants.

- *Don't punish Baby if she doesn't eat something that you serve her, and don't reward her if she does.* Making too much of what she's eating can lead to a power struggle at the table as Baby will learn that she has the ability to make you really upset or really happy as a result of what she eats. Be supportive and offer praise about her behavior—"You ate your lunch so nicely" or "I like that you tried something new today"—but don't focus on the food itself. ("Yay, you ate the green beans!" or "If you don't eat your carrots, I'm going to take away your doll.")
- *Have a routine.* Give Baby her meals and snacks around the same time every day. When Baby knows what to expect she feels more secure and may be more open to trying new things.

| Toddler Eating Behavior | What Could Be Behind It | Strategies for Handling |
|---|---|---|
| Refusing to eat, eating like a bird, etc. | • Growth slows, so she's not so hungry<br>• Teething pain makes eating uncomfortable<br>• She's distracted by all there is to do and the skills she's learning | Don't force feed. Offer healthy foods and allow toddler to decide how much to eat. |
| Refusing to eat something that you know that she likes | Growing independence and limit-testing | Nonchalance. "I think you like it because you ate it last week. But if you don't like it, just leave it on your plate." |
| Wanting the same foods at every meal or refusing to try anything new | Fear of new things | Always offer 1 thing you know she likes, eat new foods together, don't force the issue, but continue offering new things up to 20 times. |
| Misbehavior and tantrums at the table | • Limit-testing<br>• Inability to sit still for too long<br>• Asserting independence | Avoid making mealtime a battle of wills. Instead, stay calm, communicate your table rules in brief toddler-friendly statements (e.g., "We don't throw food"), and simply end the meal if Baby's behavior is not acceptable. |

# Reverse Psychology—
# Works Every Time (Almost)!

A creative and effective way to get a picky eater to eat is to act as if you don't want her to eat. Everyone sits down for a meal, you put Baby in the high chair, and you and your spouse start eating, talking, and having fun together. Don't even put any food in front of Baby. Act as though you aren't even wondering if she's going to eat. Most toddlers will feel left out. They'll decide, "Hey, I'll show them. I'm going to insist on eating!" But don't suddenly put a whole plate of food down in front of your child. This may be overwhelming. Act as if you are reluctantly putting some food on a plate and allowing Baby to eat it. Don't make a big deal of it. Don't watch Baby eat. Don't really say anything about eating. Engage Baby in conversation about other topics. Include her in the family fun.

## SETTING UP A POSITIVE EATING ENVIRONMENT

Because every child is different, we can't tell you exactly how to make your child behave during mealtime, or to what extent you should even be trying to make him behave. In our mind, the most important behavioral concept to teach your child is that eating is a positive experience. But you and your child may have different ideas of what a positive meal is. To you, it may be sitting quietly at the table, neatly taking bite after bite, while talking and smiling together until all plates are empty. I've heard that children who behave this way do exist, and if you have one, you can just laugh at the rest of us and read this section for fun.

For those of you with "normal" toddlers, your child's idea of a positive eating experience may be walking around the room, playing with toys, while coming up to you for a bite every few minutes. It may be sitting in a high chair and eating, but pretending he's the drummer in a rock band the whole time. Or it may be sitting on your lap, eating your food. And of course there's the all-time favorite—not eating anything at all!

All of these scenarios are normal, and your child's preferences may change from day to day. You have to decide whether you just want to go with the flow and let your child eat on his own terms (as long as those terms are reasonable to you), or try to impose some semblance of order and boundaries at mealtime. You know your child best. This is one area where we can't tell you what to do. We suggest that you learn, through trial and error, what your child needs and wants. Be flexible and make changes as you go. Be consistent with the boundaries you set, but if this causes too many battles, make a change. For example: it's nice to teach a toddler to sit in the high chair for meals. While teaching this, you wouldn't want to sometimes let her get down and run around, then walk up to the table for a bite. You'd want to calmly and happily say, "We take bites sitting down," and allow eating only when your child complies. You can let her get down if she insists, then let her change her mind and get back into the high chair for more food. Consistency helps a child feel more stable.

But if teaching such a boundary creates weeks of frustrating tantrums during every meal, that's not good either. You'd need to sense when a change in routine should be allowed. For example, move the high chair into the garage and let your child become a standing-up eater, as long as things don't get messy and out of hand. Don't chase her around the room with bites. Let her come up and ask.

You may feel that you are letting your child have her way by being too permissive, but you are also letting her take charge, making a decision for herself, and keeping meals positive. That can be a good thing. And you can avoid letting her realize she's gotten her way by allowing such changes in between meals. Don't give in during a mealtime tantrum and say, "OK, you can get down and I'll give you bites while you run around." Wait for the next meal when the high chair is out of sight and it's a new day.

There are, perhaps, a few boundaries that are nonnegotiable. Throwing food is one—when the meal starts flying, it's time to get down. Spitting out food onto the floor while running around is probably another. Purposefully dumping out a bowl of food or a drink may get too messy. Of course, these things are fun to watch during the first few months of starting solids, and you must get pictures, but over age one is probably a little old for this.

### Toddler-Friendly Tools

Imagine your kitchen and dining area as a restaurant. You are not only the chef, but also the maître d'. Part of your role is to create an environment where Baby is comfortable and has everything she needs to eat successfully.

- Serve food at a table. Don't ever chase Baby around the house with a spoon, and don't let her wander around with food in her mouth either. First of all, it's messy and it's not polite. More important, it's a choking hazard.
- It's not realistic to expect a toddler to sit patiently and wait for very long. Bring your toddler to the table once his meal is at his place and ready to go. Then, when he's finished eating, let him be excused or give him a toy to keep him occupied while the others finish.
- Make sure Baby has the right utensils for the job. Here's when you might expect Baby to be able to use common utensils:

| Age | Skills |
| --- | --- |
| 9 months | Finger feeding, holding empty spoon, banging empty spoon |
| 12 months | Drinking from open cup (with spilling) |

| 12–14 months | Bringing full spoon to mouth, but spilling most |
|---|---|
| 15–18 months | Scoops food and brings full spoon to mouth, spilling some |
| 24 months | Brings full spoon or fork to mouth successfully |
| 2½ years | Full self-feeding with spoon and fork with little spilling |

- Remove distractions so Baby can focus on her food. Get toys or books off the table and turn off the television.
- Eat with your child. You are a very influential role model for your child, in all facets of your lifestyle, including eating habits. Seeing you eat something may help your toddler get over a fear of new things, and her desire to be just like you may override her desire to avoid a new food.

## SERVING TODDLER-FRIENDLY FOOD

There's a difference between foods that are appropriate and appealing for toddlers and young children, and "kids' food." Think about the kids' menu at a local family restaurant. Chances are there are chicken fingers, grilled cheese, and macaroni and cheese on the list of offerings. These foods are fine every once in a while, but the goal is to avoid falling into the kids' food trap and having a child who eats only these foods. Instead, make your healthy family meals more appealing to your toddler so he learns to eat a broader variety of foods:

- Offer Baby foods that are healthy *and* tasty. We tend to assume babies and toddlers want bland foods. It may or may not be the case. Try seasonings like herbs and mild spices, and cooking methods like roasting and sautéing to bring out the best flavors in foods.

# GREEN FEEDING

## Choosing Safe Bowls and Plates for Baby

Once Baby can start to learn to feed herself it's helpful to have tableware that's an appropriate size for her tiny hands and small portions and that are eco-friendly, which means they are free of any harmful chemicals.

| Material | Pros | Cons | Bottom Line |
|---|---|---|---|
| Melamine resin—made from melamine and formaldehyde | Won't break, heat resistant. | The National Toxicology Program found that melamine plates and bowls can leach elemental melamine if they come in contact with hot, acidic foods. No safe level of intake of melamine has ever been determined. And the other ingredient, formaldehyde, is a known carcinogen that you probably don't want Baby to ingest. Plus, melamine dishes aren't recyclable. | Not the safest option. If you do use melamine plates, hand wash them and don't use them to serve hot foods. |
| Stainless steel | Dishwasher safe, won't break. | Retains heat, so use caution when serving hot foods. Not microwave safe because they're metal. Most difficult to find. | One of the best options, if you can find them. (Tip: restaurant supply stores often sell small stainless bowls and plates used for prepping meals in the kitchen.) |

| | | | |
|---|---|---|---|
| Plastics | There are many BPA-, phthalate-, and PVC-free options available. Won't break. | Even though most manufacturers state that their products are dishwasher safe, we recommend against using high heat on plastic tableware for Baby. Same is true for microwaving. | A fine option if you choose wisely. Read labels or ask manufacturers about the types of plastic used, and avoid anything that's not BPA free. Don't microwave in plastic, and for added safety, don't machine wash, either. |
| Ceramic | Usually microwave and oven safe, dishwasher safe. | Breakable. Some glazes used to color ceramics contain lead, and it may be difficult for you to determine the safety of a ceramic dish, especially if it's imported from a country with less stringent safety rules. | Skip the ceramics for now, and revisit the idea when Baby is old enough not to throw her plate to the floor. |
| Bamboo | Made from sustainable bamboo plants. Biodegrades 4 to 6 months after disposal. | Not microwave or dishwasher safe. If you leave items soaking in the sink, the bamboo could start to break down. | A safe and eco-friendly option. Although bamboo dishes are typically disposable, be sure to hand wash and reuse as much as possible. |

*Sampling of safe tableware:* Skip Hop's Palette Plate (www.skiphop.com), Bambu Kids bamboo tableware (www.bambuhome.com), Thinkbaby's Stainless Steel Feeding Set (www.thinkbabybottles.com), Sassy's Less Mess Toddler Bowls (www.sassybaby.com), bowls and plates by Boon (www.booninc.com), and Green Sprouts cornstarch-based tableware by i play, available at www.thesoftlanding.com.

- Be realistic about quantities. A typical toddler serving size is only one-quarter of an adult serving size. That means if you'd eat a cup of mashed potatoes, Baby may eat only a few tablespoons. Serve portions that are small and you won't overwhelm your toddler. If she wants more, you can always serve seconds.
- Consider the shape of Baby's foods and try different things. For example, your twenty-month-old may prefer to gnaw on a whole piece of fruit instead of little pieces. Or maybe she would like thin slices instead. And don't be surprised if she changes her mind daily about it. You can even get creative and cut foods into different shapes like sweet potato circle "wheels" or a red bell pepper cut into the shape of a heart.
- Consider the textures of Baby's foods and cater to her preferences if you can. If she likes crunchy foods, give her cucumbers, bell pepper strips, celery, carrots, and raw broccoli. If she prefers soft, serve cooked veggies instead.
- Pay attention to the temperature of the foods. Toddlers usually don't like things too hot. Some prefer all their food to be cold or room temperature. (Note: Just be sure to properly heat any food that needs to be cooked for safety, such as raw meats and fish, eggs, etc. You can always cool it back down after cooking.)
- Let them eat dip! Many toddlers enjoy dipping foods into sauces. That's why we created Secret Sauces for our HAPPY-BITES toddler meals. Other good dips include pureed vegetables, bean dips, or guacamole. Strips of bread, pita triangles, whole grain crackers, carrot sticks, bell pepper strips, and chicken strips all make perfect dippers.
- Make (healthy) food fun.
  - Use cookie cutters to cut sandwiches, tofu slices, even chicken breasts into fun shapes.
  - Find foods that are your child's favorite color (but stick to naturally colorful foods like blue potatoes and blueberries or orange slices and cubes of sweet potato).
  - Arrange the meal on the plate in the shape of a smiley face or other shape. A family favorite: turkey burger fire

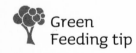

## Green Feeding tip

. . . . . . . . . . . . . . . . . . . .

If Baby likes to dip foods in ketchup, choose an organic variety. Besides lacking pesticides, it doesn't contain high-fructose corn syrup.

# SWEET TREATS

As you'll likely see, once Baby is a little older and socializing with other children at parties, in school, and in your community, sweets are everywhere. In some studies, a child's sugar intake, particularly from sugar-sweetened beverages like soda and fruit-flavored drinks, is linked to her risk for being overweight.[1] Too much sugar isn't good for Baby's teeth, either. That sugar causes young children to be hyper is highly disputed by scientific studies.[2] Some children will be more affected than others. It may just be that parties and holiday celebrations cause hyperactive behavior—not the treats served at them. The food coloring and preservatives found in some sugary treats may also be to blame for that hyperactivity.[3]

Perhaps the most important reason to limit sweets, though, is that sugary treats and junk food usually replace healthier foods in a child's diet. During the years when you're trying to form healthy eating habits for your child, it's important that she get the good stuff, not fill up on sweets. On the flip side, we know that when a food is forbidden, it becomes more enticing and children have a harder time controlling themselves when presented with the rare opportunity to eat it (like at school or a birthday party). So here's a good plan:

1. Hold out as long as you can before introducing sugary treats to Baby. Babies under two certainly don't need dessert and would have no reason to even expect such a thing unless they were exposed to it.

2. Once Baby understands that the ice cream truck cometh (probably close to age two or older), take a smart and moderate approach: don't keep junky sweets like candy and highly processed bakery items around, and don't serve Baby sugar-sweetened beverages. Never use sweets as a reward for good behavior. But try to relax if she goes to an occasional birthday party or holiday celebration and partakes of a cupcake or ice cream or candy. At home, focus on making the "treats" that you serve her as healthy as possible:

   - Frozen 100 percent fruit bars or frozen fruit slices
   - Other fruit desserts, such as baked apples topped with oats and brown sugar
   - Fruit and yogurt parfait
   - Homemade or all-natural cookies or minimuffins (See page 263 for a recipe)
   - Banana or strawberry bread
   - Graham crackers, wafer cookies (remember to avoid trans fats and artificial colors or sweeteners. See the list on page 224 for a refresher.)

trucks—rectangular burgers (made with spinach and carrots ground in with the meat), smeared with ketchup to make them red, with sweet potato "wheels"—baked sweet potato cut into circles.

## Confronting the Biggest Challenge of All: Getting a Healthy Meal on the Table

With all the challenges that come with feeding babies and toddlers, the ultimate may be actually getting the meal on the table in the first place. Three meals a day, seven days a week . . . there's no rest for the weary!

Sometimes the task of getting dinner on the table is so daunting that families give up altogether and resort to picking up their meals at fast-food or take-out places. We know that about half of the food consumed by U.S. families is eaten away from home, and about 40 percent of this is fast food.[4] For older children and teens, the more fast-food meals they eat, the worse their eating habits become and the higher their risk of becoming obese. Think about your goal—it's not just to get food into Baby so he doesn't starve. It's to get healthy food into him so he develops and thrives and learns a preference for these wholesome foods.

The best tip we can share with busy families is to get organized and plan ahead. Healthy, balanced, and varied meals don't usually just appear on the table. Some moms may be able to whip up healthy and delicious meals every night without any forethought, but that isn't the case for most of us. If it's five o'clock on a weeknight and you don't already know what's for dinner, you're in trouble.

By age one, Baby has worked his way through new foods, learned how to deal with all kinds of textures and flavors, and can join you at the family table. Ideally, you should be able to prepare only one dinner, most nights of the week, for the whole family. Sure, you might need to alter it somewhat for Baby, but you shouldn't have to create an entirely separate menu for him. The key to keeping it all together and making it work: plan, plan, plan.

Let's take you through our process for planning healthy meals:

## STEP 1: INVENTORY

Check out the pantry and fridge to see if there's anything you need to use up. If so, plan meals that incorporate those ingredients. This is a great way to make sure food doesn't go to waste in your home and to save money, too. We call this fridge management, and it's almost like a game, figuring out how to plan around the food we have so that we never have to throw something away because it went bad before we got around to using it.

## STEP 2: MENU DEVELOPMENT

It can take about fifteen or twenty minutes a week to plan what the family will eat. First, map out your schedule for the week so you can create a realistic meal plan. Are there any nights when you won't be home at dinnertime? Anything going on that will make time particularly tight for certain meals? For your busy nights you can plan the most simple and least time-consuming meals possible.

*Breakfast:* We know that most people don't actually plan breakfast in advance. You'll probably just keep various options on hand to make on a whim. Here are some toddler-friendly breakfast ideas for the whole family:

- Dry cereal (whole grain, low sugar) with milk and fruit on the side or in the bowl
- Fruit and yogurt smoothie (see Recipes)
- Whole grain or multigrain toast with cream cheese and jelly
- Freezer waffles or pancakes (for Oatmeal Pancakes, see Recipes) with fruit puree for dipping
- Bagel with spreadable cheese or nut butter
- Eggless banana minimuffin (see Recipes), slice of cheese, piece of fruit
- Berries, yogurt, and dry cereal
- Oatmeal with fresh or frozen fruit thrown in, cup of milk on the side

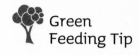

**Green Feeding Tip**

. . . . . . . . . . . . . . . . . . . .

Did you know that almost 15 percent of the food that Americans throw out in their homes is unopened packaged food?[5] What a waste! Planning ahead can help you avoid having food around that nobody gets around to eating.

A NOTE FROM DR. BOB

## Flexibility Is Key at Breakfast Time

Toddlers can be a challenge when it comes to breakfast. Some will wake up in a great mood and be ready to eat anything. Others will be grumpy and unlikely to be thrilled about eating. Some may prefer to have choices, and others may do better if you just make some time and sit down together to eat it. Your child's preferences may change day to day. Learn to read your child's moods and be ready to be flexible. We suggest you don't start off the day with any battles. Keep the first meal of the day positive, which may mean serving your child breakfast on her own terms.

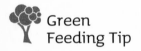 Green Feeding Tip

· · · · · · · · · · · · · · · · · · · · · ·

When packing a meal for Baby, use an insulated lunch bag and add a small freezer pack to keep the food fresh. Avoid bags made of PVC—a type of vinyl that may contain chemicals called plasticizers, which are known to interfere with hormone function. Instead, opt for nonvinyl bags like those made by Built NY and ACME, both available at www.reusablebags.com, and the lunch bags from L.L.Bean (www.llbean.com) and Lands' End (www.lands end.com), among others.

- Eggs—scrambled or hard-boiled
- HAPPYBITES Breakfast Pocket

*Lunch:* Consider if you'll be home at lunchtime or if you'll need to pack, because some meals pack better than others. The easiest lunch possible might be the leftovers from the dinner you served the night before, but only if you'll be somewhere you can easily heat up your food and sit at a table with Baby. If you'll be on the go, finger foods may be a better choice. As you're planning, include ingredients for Tiny Finger Sandwiches for Baby (see Recipes), fruit that you can easily cut up and place into a covered container, whole grain crackers and cheese slices or sticks, and vegetables that Baby can eat raw, like cucumber or zucchini, or steamed, like broccoli florets or carrots.

*Dinner:* When figuring out a menu for dinner, aim for the meals to be balanced. That basically means including foods from a few different food groups, a nice array of nutrients, and in the right proportions. For example, don't serve just pasta with sauce (only starch and vegetable) or chicken with rice (protein and starch). Baby may decide to only eat one or two of the food groups on his plate, but a well-planned dinner includes representatives from the vegetable, protein, and starch groups. A quick method for creating a balanced and well-proportioned meal with these three types of foods is to imagine a dinner plate that's divided into four equal sections. For one section, choose a food that provides protein, such as chicken, beef, beans, tofu, pork, cheese, or fish. The next section is for the starchy food. This could be bread, pita, pasta, rice, barley, potatoes, couscous, or corn. Then choose vegetables to fill up the remaining two sections of the plate (half the plate). Pick one or several types of veggies, such as green beans, broccoli, tomatoes, zucchini, asparagus, mushrooms, lettuce, carrots, etc. This is just a rough guide, of course. Not every meal will fit perfectly into this mold. But if it's close enough, your meal will be pretty well-balanced. The food groups that are missing—fruits and perhaps dairy foods—can be served on the side or as dessert (or with other meals or snacks).

This is not to say that your eighteen-month-old will eat a dinner of half vegetables, but remember the premise here: you are planning the meal for the whole family. Expect your toddler to select one, two, or three of the foods on the plate to eat. Some of them will be gobbled up entirely; others will be left untouched. The important thing is to offer a balanced varied menu to Baby.

If you want to serve a meal that isn't quite going to work for your toddler, try to adapt the ingredients in a way that allows you to still not make two meals. For example, if you are making spicy taco salad, you may have to keep some of the taco meat aside for Baby before you add the spices. Baby may not eat Cobb salad, but he can certainly eat the hard-boiled egg and avocado along with a cooked vegetable and a dinner roll.

Here are some toddler-friendly dinner ideas (which can also double as lunch menus):

- Finger Food Dipping Platter (see Recipes)
- Multipurpose Roasted Chicken (see Recipes) with rice and steamed broccoli

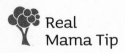
. . . . . . . . . . . . . . . . . . . . .

"If you reserve a little pasta
before you add that put-
tanesca sauce, or save some
chicken before covering it
with the chili spice rub, you
can work less in the kitchen,
serve your baby healthy and
varied meals, and still eat
like a grown-up yourself."

—April, Arlington, VA

- Leftover roasted chicken soft tacos
- Hidden Veggie Burger (see Recipes) on a bun with carrot and celery sticks
- Baked fish fillet or Easy Salmon Cakes (see Recipes) with a small baked potato and green beans
- Pasta with ground beef or chicken cooked in Throw Together Tomato Sauce (see Recipes)
- Grilled pork chop with mushrooms and barley with grilled or steamed asparagus
- Quick Tofu Stir-Fry (see Recipes) with broccoli, cauliflower, and carrots served with brown rice
- Mix-and-Match Quesadillas (see Recipes) served with baby carrots on the side
- Breakfast-for-Dinner Quiche (see Recipes) with baked sweet potato fries
- HAPPYBITES Mac + Cheese with Red "Monkey" Sauce
- HAPPYBITES Salmon Stix with White "Bear" Sauce
- HAPPYBITES Breakfast Pocket
- HAPPYBITES Veggie Tots with Orange "Cheetah" Sauce

A NOTE FROM DR. BOB

## Taking a Fast Food Break? Make It a Sandwich

When you find yourself and Baby stopping somewhere for a fast lunch, try to go to a sandwich shop. The whole grain bread and healthy turkey-and-cheese sandwich are so much better than the fried food you'll find elsewhere. Delay the discovery of french fries as long as you can!

- HAPPYBITES Fish Bites with Green "Roo" Sauce
- Tiny finger sandwiches (see Recipes)

*Leftovers:* When planning, think about making extras to freeze for the future or to use for other meals during the week. Or, make enough to serve for lunch the next day. Some families aren't into leftovers, but that doesn't mean you have to waste food. Figure out how to repurpose leftovers smartly. Here are some examples:

| *A Leftover . . .* | *. . . Becomes a New Meal* |
| --- | --- |
| Steamed broccoli | Put into a broccoli and cheese quiche |
| Vegetable side dish | Puree and add to pasta sauce or chop and make a vegetable soup |
| Roasted chicken | Shred for chicken tacos or quesadillas |
| Hamburger patties | Crumble and put into a noodle casserole |
| Fish fillet | Flake and make into fish cakes |
| Baked potato | Cube, brown in a pan, and serve with eggs |

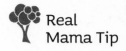

## Real Mama Tip

"I save money by planning meals around the same ingredients. For instance, if I'm buying fresh basil and Parmesan cheese that week, then I'll make pasta one day, basil-lemon rice with Parmesan-crusted fish on another day, Italian meatloaf on another, etc. That way nothing goes to waste and I save money!"

—*Ximena, San Diego, California*

A NOTE FROM DR. BOB

## It's Better with Butter

As adults we need to limit our butter intake because of the cholesterol. But for toddlers, natural sources of cholesterol are fine. When they were younger, my kids would almost always eat their veggies when we melted a little butter over them.

# ABOUT HIDING VEGETABLES

Do you feel that hiding vegetables in Baby's foods is kind of sneaky? It is! And we're all for it. It's kind of like giving Baby a vitamin supplement hidden in her food, but much tastier. Actually, the concept was the premise for our HAPPYBITES meals for toddlers—each has a ton of hidden veggies inside and in the dipping sauces. At home, there are many opportunities to hide fruits and vegetables in Baby's meals. You can add applesauce to your muffin recipe, add pureed squash to your spaghetti sauce, add chopped or pureed spinach to your burger patties (see our recipe for Hidden Veggie Burgers, page 264). If you want to go all out and make your own veggie purees to cook with on a regular basis we recommend checking out *Deceptively Delicious* by Jessica Seinfeld for some recipes and ideas. There's just one important rule to follow here: If you're hiding vegetables in Baby's foods, you still have to serve him a vegetable that he can see. Hiding a vegetable is a great way to get the nutrients in, but seeing it on the plate is also important for him learning that there's an expectation that he eat vegetables with his meal.

*Snacks:* Toddlers are on the go from sunup to sundown. To help them make it through, they need one to three healthy snacks in addition to their meals. So as part of your meal plan, factor in snacks. Serve your child his snacks at around the same time each day, at the table whenever possible. Snack time is a prime opportunity for providing some of the vitamins and minerals that your child needs, so try to think of snacks as minimeals instead of as treats. Here are some ideas:

- *Fruit:* apple, pear, plum, apricot, peach, nectarine, kiwi, pineapple, berries, banana, cantaloupe, watermelon, honeydew melon, papaya, mango, applesauce, cut grapes.*
- *Grain snacks:* whole grain crackers, toasted bread with fruit preserves, pretzels, oatmeal, cold cereal (dry or with milk), puffed cereal, homemade minimuffins.
- *Veggie snacks:* choose Baby's favorite vegetable and let him dip in HAPPYBITES Secret Sauces, hummus, salsa, nut butter, or guacamole. Try carrot sticks, red or yellow bell pepper strips,

jicama slices, and broccoli florets (call them "trees"). If raw vegetables are too hard for Baby to chew, steam them lightly to soften them, and then serve warm or chilled.

- *Dairy snacks:* yogurt, yogurt and fruit smoothie, cheese and crackers, cheese with apple slices (choose low fat or nonfat dairy products for toddlers age two and up)
- *Protein-packed snacks:* hummus or black bean dip (See page 266 for a recipe.) with pita triangles, crackers, or sliced veggies; half a peanut butter** sandwich

  * Choking hazard. See page 169 for details.

  ** Potential allergen. See page 167 for details.

## STEP 3: LIST-IN-HAND SHOPPING

Once you have a plan for what your family will eat over the next several days, make a shopping list. Keep in mind that inventory you did in step 1. If you'll be following a recipe for a particular meal, check to see how much you need of each ingredient. Then, list in hand, head to the store. Shopping from a list serves so many purposes. First of all, you won't forget something that you need for a particular meal. Second, you will control impulse buying. Plus, it's faster. If you have the "pleasure" of grocery shopping with your toddler (most Mamas find few things less fun), you'll be grateful that the decisions have been made and all you need to do is find the item, throw in the cart, and move on to the next. Wandering up and down the aisles aimlessly waiting to be inspired is a little cumbersome with Baby in tow. Plus, when you buy only what you know that you need, not only do you minimize kitchen waste but you spend less, too!

## STEP 4: PRE-PREPPING

After you get the grocery items home from the store, there's still a long journey between the fridge or pantry and the dinner table. When you're a busy person (and if you have a toddler, you automatically qualify) it's important to avoid procrastination and always seize the moment to get

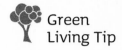

## Green Living Tip

. . . . . . . . . . . . . . . . . . . . .

Planning a menu for several days at a time will help you make fewer trips to the grocery store, which will mean less gasoline spent getting to and from the market. Consider this: even if your store is just five miles away, each round trip requires about a quarter of a gallon of gas. Another way to use less gasoline is to try to combine all your car errands into one trip. Just put a cooler in the trunk to keep your refrigerated items cold if you're not going straight home after the grocery store.

# BEYOND THE SUPERMARKET

## Community-Supported Agriculture

A community-supported agriculture group, or CSA, is basically a buying group for fresh farm products. A group of people in a community buys a share of a farmer's crops. When the farmer harvests his crops, he brings them to a distribution location, where the CSA members pick up their share. It's a wonderful way to support local farmers, many of whom use organic farming and other sustainable practices. It's also a great way for your family to get fresh and in-season produce throughout the year, especially if you live in an area where it isn't always available (like some urban neighborhoods). Depending on the farm and the CSA setup, you may be able to buy a share of just the fruit harvest or vegetables alone. Sometimes you can purchase meat or eggs through a CSA. Some CSAs even provide other fresh products, such as cheeses, herbs, and honey. For more information about CSAs and to find one in your area, go to www.localharvest.org/csa/.

started on any preliminary preparations for that (or the next) night's meal. Deciding in advance what your meals are makes it easy to figure out which steps you can pre-prep. If you have time in the morning to chop some ingredients for dinner, do it. Maybe the stir-fry vegetables can be chopped while Baby naps. Or you could mix the ingredients for a meatloaf early in the day while your toddler plays on the kitchen floor, so when it's crunch time later in the afternoon you just have to throw the meatloaf into the oven. If you're a Mama who works outside the home, pre-prep plans may need to get creative. One amazingly organized mother, who is a teacher during the day, told us she makes dinner for the next night each night after her baby is in bed. Then, when she gets home from work, she can serve the already prepared dinner right away, and she's able to have the whole family sit down together at the table. Other Mamas we know cook every Sunday afternoon and freeze meals for the whole week. Look at your schedule and your lifestyle to decide how you could squeeze in some pre-prep to help you with the dinnertime rush.

# How to Get Through Unhappy Hour!

If your child is like most, you've already discovered that the late afternoon and early evening hours are the crankiest of the day—not the easiest time to balance making a gourmet meal with a needy toddler. On nights when you can't pre-prep (as suggested above), here are some ways you can entertain your toddler while you throw the meal together:

- *High chair snack:* Move the high chair into the kitchen and sit your child down with a snack you know he'll enjoy for ten to fifteen minutes. So what if it ruins her dinner—she's under two.
- *Strike up the band:* Pull some pots and pans out of the cupboard, turn on some music, and let your child bang away while you cook (keep him well away from the stove top, of course, so nothing hot splashes his way).
- *Bouncing time:* Purchase a baby jumper seat, hang it in the kitchen doorway, and let him bounce around for a while. Music may help here as well.
- *Baby sling:* We never recommend cooking on a stove top with a baby in arms, but for all the rest of your prep time "wear" Baby around the kitchen.
- *Baby's kitchen:* If your toddler is into his own baking, set up a toy kitchen nearby and talk him through the steps you are taking to make dinner. Give him some real veggies and other nonmessy items to "cook" with.

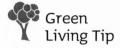

## Green Living Tip

It's estimated that Americans use 100 billion plastic grocery bags a year.[6] Not only do these bags require oil for manufacture and transport, but they also fill up our landfills or become litter that can endanger wildlife. Paper bags aren't much better. They require more chemicals and energy to produce, and create more solid waste than plastic bags. Your best bet: Bring a reusable bag to the store. Many stores sell them, sometimes for one dollar or less. Keep your reusable bags in your car or stroller for impromptu shopping trips. If you are stuck without your own sack, try to recycle whichever bag you end up with. Go to www.plasticbagrecycling.org to find a drop-off center near you.

When you make meals ahead, freeze in containers that are intended for the freezer—it will say on the label or packaging. Although zip-top freezer bags are fine for short-term freezer storage, they don't prevent freezer burn as well as tightly sealed containers, and they create more waste. Instead, pick up a few freezer containers made from glass or BPA-free polypropylene plastic (sometimes labeled with recycling code 5) with well-fitting covers. You'll find options at stores like the Container Store (www.containerstore.com), Bed Bath & Beyond (www.bedbathandbeyond.com), or Wal-Mart (www.walmart.com).

## GROCERY SHOPPING IN ALL SHADES OF GREEN

*The palest green:* Plan a few meals at a time so that you don't have to run to the store each day or resort to less-than-healthy convenience or takeout foods. Bring reusable bags to the market.

*A little greener:* Try to plan a week's worth of meals and do one shopping trip per week. Use reusable shopping bags. Avoid single-serve packaged foods—individually wrapped cheese slices and single-serve applesauce cups, for example—in order to reduce packaging waste.

*The deepest shade of green:* Plan a week or more of meals at a time, and manage your pantry and fridge resources effectively so nothing ever goes to waste. Do one big grocery shop every week to ten days, and always use reusable shopping bags. Never buy individually wrapped packaging and when possible, buy foods in bulk to minimize packaging waste. Choose products that are packaged in recyclable and recycled materials, and buy from food stores and companies who use environmentally responsible practices.

## STEP 5: FINAL PREP AND SERVE

The last step, of course, is to complete the preparation of the meal and get it on the table. Be realistic about how much time you need because nothing is more stressful than having a hungry toddler fussing and clinging to your legs as you scurry to get his meal on the table. If your schedule is too tight to get dinner ready before Baby gets hungry for it, consider doing what one smart Mama we know does: serve Baby his vegetable as an appetizer.

## MORE TIPS FOR MAKING IT WORK

- Keep a menu calendar in the kitchen. Write your menu and any important notes (for example, "take chicken out of freezer") so you can refer to them quickly to figure out "what's for dinner?"
- If you do a lot of cooking and freezing, especially if you keep things in a freezer in your basement or garage, keep a running list of what you have frozen and post it on the fridge.
- Keep a little notebook of ideas—if you have a meal that's a big hit, write it down. If you get a great idea from your sister-in-law, write it down. If you read a toddler-friendly food idea in a magazine, write it down. Then, if you get stuck or need ideas, refer to your handy list!
- Always keep standard staples in your pantry, such as whole grain cereals, whole wheat pasta, canned or dry beans, olive oil, dried herbs and spices, canned or jarred tomatoes or sauce. A quick throw-together meal is easy if the basics are on hand.
- Talk to other Mamas and share ideas! I've gotten some of my best meal-planning tips and recipes from friends and family.
- Seek out resources for meal planning like family-friendly food magazines and the *Six O'Clock Scramble* online newsletter (www.6oclockscramble.com) or the cookbook of the same name.

A NOTE FROM DR. BOB

# Dad to the Rescue!

Nothing makes us husbands feel more useful than making dinner for the family (while the tired Mama/wife relaxes in a hot bath). And what could be easier than pasta? A couple of times each month I'll offer to prepare dinner. My wife jokingly says, "Great! What kind of spaghetti will you be making?" She knows that's about the only thing I can throw together (well, that and fish sticks, of course). So, always keep some pasta and canned sauce on hand for those days that you need Dad/husband to come to the rescue. And I apologize for the wife-always-makes-dinner stereotype. That's just how it is in my family, with Cheryl being such an awesome chef and all.

## TIME SAVERS

Although some "convenience" foods are lacking in the healthy and all-natural departments, you can take some shortcuts in the kitchen to save time without sacrificing appeal and health.

*The freezer is your friend:* Frozen fruits and vegetables are just as nutritious as fresh, if not more. And they can make life easier because they are always on hand, they rarely go bad before you can eat them, etc. (That's why HAPPYBABY chose to do frozen baby food.)

- Buy frozen organic fruits and vegetables to have in the freezer. Frozen berries are great for adding to smoothies or hot cereal at breakfast time. Frozen peaches and mangos defrost well and can be a stand-alone snack. Frozen veggies go with almost any meal—soups, stir-fry dishes, casseroles, meat-and-potato-type meals, and pasta dishes.

- Frozen waffles are a good breakfast staple, and you can find all sorts of varieties these days—multigrain, gluten-free, eggless. . . . Check out your freezer case.

*Let someone else do the work:* At most grocery stores you can find a variety of pre-prepped vegetables and other ready-to-cook foods. You may pay a premium, but for some families it may be worth it.

- Peeled and cubed butternut squash
- Carrot and celery sticks
- Bagged salad mixes
- Cut fruit for fruit salad
- Sliced pepper rings
- Ready-to-cook vegetable combos for stir fries, soups, and pasta dishes
- Baking mixes—you can find all-natural brands and multigrain mixes
- Marinated chicken or beef—head to your natural foods market to find organic varieties
- Boxed rice or grain mixes—look for low-sodium all-natural versions (and recycle the cardboard box!)

# Recipes

The recipes featured here are easy, relatively quick, and sure to please Baby, older siblings, and even the grown-ups in the family. They aren't gourmet and not necessarily what we'd serve at a dinner party, but these dishes are perfect for real Mamas who are busy and juggling Baby's care, housekeeping and other work, and getting meals on the table.

Many of these recipes have prep steps that can be done early in the day—during naptime perhaps. And many feature cooking short-cuts that save you time without sacrificing good nutrition. Although we don't mention it in every recipe, of course we recommend choosing organic ingredients whenever possible. Enjoy!

## OATMEAL PANCAKES
## (WITH FRUIT PUREE FOR DIPPING)

Makes 20 silver-dollar-sized pancakes or 12 adult-sized ones.

1¼ cups quick-cooking oats

1 cup plain nonfat yogurt

1 cup whole milk

1 teaspoon sugar

¼ cup all purpose flour

¼ cup whole wheat flour

1 teaspoon baking soda

1 teaspoon salt

2 large eggs, beaten

1. Combine the oats, yogurt, milk, and sugar in a large bowl.
2. Stir in the flours, baking soda, and salt.
3. Add the eggs and mix well.
4. Heat a large non-stick skillet or griddle over medium heat.
5. For each pancake, spoon ¼ cup of the batter onto the hot pan. Cook for a couple of minutes, until the pancake starts to bubble and the bottoms are brown. Flip and cook the other side until lightly browned.
6. Repeat until all the batter is gone.
7. Serve cut into strips with unsweetened applesauce or thawed HappyBaby Wiser Apple or Paradise Puree for dipping.

## FRUIT AND YOGURT SMOOTHIE

Makes about four 4-ounce servings

There's no added sugar in this basic smoothie recipe because Baby doesn't need any! Although we've suggested banana and strawberry, feel free to use one cup of any fruit that you have on hand. And if the smoothie seems too thick for a sippy cup add more milk or use less yogurt. Ground flaxseed or wheat germ is added for an extra nutrition boost: ground flaxseed is a source of omega-3 fatty acids; wheat germ provides iron and B vitamins.

1 cup milk

¾ cup plain yogurt

1 small banana (about ½ cup fruit)

6–7 fresh or frozen strawberries (about ½ cup fruit)

2 teaspoons ground flaxseed or wheat germ

1. Place all ingredients into a blender. Blend until smooth and serve.

## MULTIPURPOSE CHICKEN

If you've never roasted a whole chicken before you're going to be surprised how easy it is to do. Plus, it's inexpensive and one chicken provides the whole family with dinner and then leftovers for lunches or snacks for days. Use in quesadillas, mix into pasta dishes, add to soup, use as a soft taco filling, or find your own favorite uses.

1 whole organic chicken (3½ to 4 pounds)

1–2 tablespoons olive oil

½ teaspoon kosher salt

⅛ teaspoon pepper

1 lemon, quartered

3 sprigs fresh rosemary (or other herb like parsley, thyme, or sage)

(continued on next page)

1. Preheat oven to 425°F.

2. Unwrap the chicken from its packaging and reach into the neck cavity to remove the bag of giblets. Rinse chicken well, inside and out, and pat dry with paper towels.

3. Place the chicken, breast side up, on a rack inside a roasting pan or on a broiling pan (with drip pan beneath). Insert the lemon and fresh herbs into the cavity of the chicken. Rub the outside of the chicken with olive oil. Sprinkle most of the salt and pepper on the outside of the bird and throw the final dash inside the chicken cavity with the lemons and herbs.

4. Roast chicken in the oven until the juices run clear and a meat thermometer inserted into the thickest part of the thigh reads 180°F, between 60 and 90 minutes. After the first 30 minutes, baste the chicken with the pan juices and repeat every 15 minutes until chicken is done.

5. Remove the chicken from the oven and let it rest on a cutting board or a platter for 15 minutes before carving. If you've never carved a chicken before, don't be intimidated. Do a Google search to find simple instructions and perhaps even pictures to guide you. And once you do it one time, you'll be a pro.

## BREAKFAST-FOR-DINNER QUICHE

Makes 8 slices

Neither of Amy's children were particularly keen on broccoli as toddlers, but when disguised in this cheesy eggy quiche with its tasty flaky crust they gobbled it up. For busy Mamas a store-bought pie crust may be more realistic than homemade—look for a crust with no partially hydrogenated oils in the ingredient list.

1 9-inch pie crust

1½ cup broccoli, chopped in bite-sized pieces (you may use fresh or frozen)

1 teaspoon olive or canola oil

½ cup red onion, chopped

1 garlic clove, minced

¾ cup swiss or cheddar cheese, shredded

3 eggs

1½ cup whole milk (you may substitute low fat or nonfat milk)

½ teaspoon salt

¼ teaspoon pepper

1. Preheat oven to 375°F.
2. *If using raw broccoli:* Place the chopped broccoli in a medium sauté pan with ⅛ to ¼ cup water. Cover and steam over medium-high heat for 5 minutes or until the broccoli is tender but before it gets gray-green and mushy. Drain and transfer into a bowl.
   *If using frozen broccoli:* Cook according to package directions. If needed, chop the cooked broccoli into small pieces.
3. While the broccoli cooks, crack the eggs into a medium bowl and beat well. Add the milk, salt and pepper. Set aside.
4. After broccoli is transferred into a bowl, using the same pan, heat oil over medium heat. Add the red onion and garlic. Cook until onions are translucent and tender, about 4 minutes, stirring occasionally. Turn off the heat, add the broccoli back into the pan and stir to combine.
5. Sprinkle cheese in the bottom of the pie crust. Add the cooked vegetables in an even layer. Then, pour the egg mixture on top until the crust is filled.
6. Carefully place the quiche in the oven on the center rack. Cook for 40 minutes or until the quiche is set. (Note: If you use low fat or nonfat milk, cooking time will increase to 55–60 minutes.)
7. Remove from oven and let cool for 15 minutes before serving or freeze for up to 6 months.

# THROW-TOGETHER SPAGHETTI SAUCE

Makes about 4 cups

This simple sauce is nice and smooth, making it appealing for picky toddlers. Plus, you'll hide onions and carrots or squash in this sauce, and Baby will never know. If you prefer to avoid canned goods make your own crushed tomatoes from fresh using the recipe that follows.

¼ cup olive oil

½ cup onion, grated or pureed in a blender or food processor (1 small onion)

3 cloves garlic, crushed

1 28-ounce can crushed tomatoes

⅓ cup pureed carrots or winter squash (or 3 cubes HAPPYBABY carrots or squash, thawed)

1 tablespoon fresh oregano, chopped (or 1 teaspoon dried)

1 tablespoon fresh basil, chopped or thyme (or 1 teaspoon dried)

¼ teaspoon salt

⅛ teaspoon pepper

1. Heat the oil in a saucepan over medium heat. Add the onion and garlic. Cook for 3 minutes, stirring occasionally.
2. Add the tomatoes, pureed carrots or squash, herbs, salt and pepper. Bring to a boil and then reduce the heat to medium-low and simmer for 25 to 30 minutes.

## FRESH CRUSHED TOMATOES

Makes about 3 to 4 cups crushed tomatoes,
equivalent to one 28-ounce can crushed tomatoes.

*6–7 round tomatoes (or 12 roma tomatoes)*

1. With a knife, etch an "x" into the end of the tomatoes. Drop tomatoes into a pot of boiling water. Boil for about a minute and transfer tomatoes to a bowl of ice. Once cool enough to handle the tomatoes remove their skin—it should slip right off.
2. Cut tomatoes in half or quarters and squeeze out the seeds and excess water using your clean hands. With a knife, remove any tough parts of the tomato like the core or particularly tough pieces of flesh.
3. Add the prepped tomatoes back to the pot. Cook over medium heat, gently simmering and squishing the tomatoes with a wooden spoon until they are fully crushed, about 8 to 10 minutes.

## EGGLESS BANANA MINI MUFFINS

Makes 24 mini-muffins or 12 standard muffins

These muffins are an alternative to store-bought baked goods for Baby—they are relatively low in sugar, full of whole grains, and free of saturated and trans fats. Broken into small pieces they make a perfect finger food for 9 to 12 month old babies who aren't yet eating egg whites. Plus, they freeze well. Thaw a frozen muffin in the fridge or by heating in the microwave for about 15 seconds.

*(continued on next page)*

¾ cup all purpose flour

¾ cup whole wheat flour (if unavailable, substitute all-purpose flour)

1 cup rolled oats

½ cup brown sugar, unpacked

2 teaspoons baking powder

1 teaspoon baking soda

¼ teaspoon salt

¾ cup skim milk

¼ cup vegetable oil

½ teaspoon vanilla extract

1 cup mashed bananas (about 2 medium bananas)

1. Preheat oven to 400°F. Prepare the muffin pan(s): lightly grease cups with the vegetable oil and dust with the flour.

2. In a large bowl combine the flours, oats, brown sugar, baking powder, baking soda, and salt.

3. In a small bowl mash the bananas. Add the milk, oil, and vanilla and combine well.

4. Stir the banana mixture into the flour mixture until just combined.

5. Spoon the batter into the prepared muffin pans. Bake the mini-muffins for 12 to 15 minutes or until lightly golden brown. Full-size muffins will take about 20 to 25 minutes. When done, cool in the pans on a wire rack for 5 minutes. Then, gently remove muffins from the pan and set muffins on the wire rack until completely cool.

6. Muffins may be served immediately, stored in an airtight container in the pantry for two to three days or in a freezer-safe container in the freezer for several months.

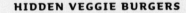

## HIDDEN VEGGIE BURGERS

Makes 2 toddler-sized burgers and 3 adult-sized burgers

Some toddlers shy away from meat and chicken because of its texture but ground meats tend to be more acceptable. Adding vegetables to these burger patties not only piles on the vitamins and minerals, but the moisture helps extra lean meats like ground turkey breast or ground chicken stay juicy when cooked.

1 pound organic ground meat (lean beef, turkey, or chicken)

¼ cup pureed vegetable of your choice—we recommend spinach, carrots, or mushrooms

2 teaspoons Worcestershire sauce*

A dash of salt and fresh ground pepper

1. In a bowl mix the meat, vegetable puree, Worcestershire sauce, and a dash of salt and pepper.
2. Form two small handfuls of the meat mixture into toddler-sized burger patties. With the remaining meat, create three larger adult-sized burgers.
3. Cook the burger patties on the grill or in a non-stick pan on the stove-top. Cook for 4 minutes on the first side, then flip and cook for 5 more minutes or until meat is done (no pink left in the meat).
4. For babies and toddlers, serve the burger broken up into bite sized pieces for finger-feeding. For adults, serve on a whole grain hamburger bun with lettuce, tomato, onion, or other favorite burger toppings.

*Allergen warning: Worcestershire sauce contains fish (anchovies)

## FINGER FOOD DIPPING PLATTER

This isn't a recipe so much as a serving suggestion. Simply make a platter with a bunch of dippers and a few different dips. It's a great idea for older toddlers who enjoy feeding themselves and dipping their foods. And it's also a great way to use up leftovers like cooked chicken, veggies, etc.

DIPPER IDEAS (CHOOSE TWO OR MORE):

- Chicken strips—Bake or sauté a chicken breast, cool, and then cut into strips.
- Tofu cubes or strips—Drain water from the tofu package and cut into the desired shape. No need to cook—eat as is.
- Carrot sticks, broccoli florets ("trees"), bell pepper strips, sliced mushrooms—Use raw if Baby can bite into them or steam veggies in a small amount of water until just tender.

(continued on next page)

- White or sweet potato sticks—Peel and cut potatoes into french-fry shaped pieces. Toss in a little olive oil and bake on a baking sheet at 425°F for about 25 minutes or until done.
- Bread strips—Remove crusts for younger toddlers.
- Cooked pasta—Try dippable shapes like penne, rigatoni, or ziti.

DIP IDEAS (CHOOSE TWO OR MORE):
- Black bean dip (see recipe below)
- Guerilla Greens Guacamole (see recipe below)
- Baby Ganoush eggplant dip (see recipe on page 183)
- Plain yogurt seasoned with a dash of garlic powder and dill
- Store-bought hummus
- Organic ketchup

## BLACK BEAN DIP

Makes 2 cups

As Baby approaches age two she may enjoy dipping foods. This bean dip will up the nutrient content of any meal or snack and tastes great with pita bread strips, crackers, raw or cooked vegetable sticks, or strips of chicken.

15-ounce can black beans, rinsed and drained (or 1½ cups cooked beans)

½ cup jarred organic or fresh mild salsa

2 tablespoons lime juice (about 1 lime)

3 tablespoons plain yogurt (or sour cream)

1. Combine all ingredients in food processor bowl. Blend until smooth, about 20 to 30 seconds.
2. Transfer to a small bowl. Dip something in and enjoy!

## GUERILLA GREENS GUACAMOLE

*(Courtesy of Nirit Yadin, Whole Foods Market Princeton, New Jersey)*

Makes about 2 adult portions plus 2 to 3 baby-sized portions.

Some veggie-phobic toddlers are willing to accept greens in the form of guacamole. You can use the green background of the avocado to sneak in other green vegetables like green beans and finely chopped leafy greens.

4 ripe Haas avocados

3 tablespoons fresh lemon juice

4 dashes Tabasco sauce (optional)

½ cup finely chopped red onion

1 large garlic clove, minced

1 teaspoon kosher salt

1 teaspoon freshly ground pepper

1 medium tomato, seeded and finely chopped

¼ cup HappyBaby pureed peas or green beans or chopped leafy greens

1. Put the lemon juice, Tabasco sauce, onion, garlic, green vegetables, salt and pepper in a food processor and chop very finely.
2. Halve and pit the avocados, then scoop the flesh into a bowl. Add the onion mixture along with the tomatoes and mash with a potato masher or fork until almost smooth.
3. Taste and add more salt, pepper or olive oil to taste.

## QUICK TOFU "STIR-FRY"

In a true stir-fry the ingredients are cooked in very hot oil until the vegetables are just crisp-tender. For toddlers, this stir-fry recipe takes some shortcuts and cooks the vegetables to be a little more tender for easy chewing. Baking the tofu in the oven gives it a nice texture and while tofu cooks you

*(continued on next page)*

can prep the veggies and sauce. For a super easy throw-together meal, bake the tofu up to a day in advance and use leftover cooked vegetables.

1 14-ounce package tofu, drained of any liquid

½ cup broth

3 tablespoons low-sodium soy sauce

2 teaspoons cornstarch

1½ tablespoons water

1 tablespoon oil

3 cloves garlic, minced

1 tablespoon ginger, grated or minced

2 cups broccoli or green beans, chopped

2 cups carrots, thinly sliced

2 cups mushrooms (any type), chopped

¼ teaspoon chili paste with garlic (find in the Asian section of your market)

Cooked rice or Asian noodles

1. Preheat the oven to 350°F. Gently squeeze the block of tofu to remove any excess water. Chop into cubes. Place on a lightly oiled baking sheet and put in the oven until lightly browned, about 35 minutes.
2. Mix the broth and soy sauce in a medium bowl. Set aside.
3. Mix the cornstarch with water in a separate small bowl. Set aside.
4. Heat the oil in a large sauté pan or wok over medium-high heat.
5. Add garlic and ginger. Cook 1 minute, stirring constantly.
6. Add other vegetables. Cook about 5 minutes, until just tender.
7. Add sauce to the pan and bring to a boil. Then, reduce heat to medium and add cornstarch and water mixture. Stir as the sauce cooks and thickens, for about 2 minutes.
8. Add the tofu cubes and toss well to coat with the sauce and mix with the veggies.
9. After you portion off some stir-fry for Baby, add the chili paste to the grown-ups' portion.
10. Serve over rice or Asian noodles.

## EASY SALMON CAKES

Makes 8 salmon cakes (Adult serving is 2 cakes, toddler serving is ½ to 1 cake)

The most eco-friendly and healthy type of salmon is wild (as opposed to farmed). Fresh or frozen wild salmon is ideal—they make the best patties. However, if fresh or frozen isn't available or if it's too expensive, canned is fine too—it's typically wild, not farmed. Tip: Grating the onion in this recipe helps to camouflage it so that Baby won't be able to feel it on her tongue. Use the same trick in your favorite meatball or meatloaf recipe.

1 pound fresh salmon or 15 ounces canned salmon, drained

1 cup breadcrumbs

2 large eggs, beaten

½ cup onion, grated (about 1 small onion)

1 teaspoon lemon zest (about 1 small lemon)

½ teaspoon dried dill or 1½ teaspoons fresh dill

1. *If using fresh salmon:* Preheat oven to 350°F. Place the salmon fillets or steaks into a baking dish. Bake for 15 to 20 minutes. Fish should be flaky. Let cool. Flake apart with a fork, discarding any skin or bones. (Flaked salmon can be stored in the refrigerator for a few hours or overnight in a sealed container. Or, move right along to the next step.)

   *If using canned salmon:* Drain any liquid and remove any bones. Place in a large bowl. If needed, flake apart the salmon with a fork.

2. Increase oven temp to 450°F. Prepare a baking sheet by lining with parchment paper or misting with a little oil to prevent sticking.

3. In a large bowl, combine the salmon, breadcrumbs, eggs, onion, lemon zest, and dill. Mixture should stick together when pressed into a patty but not be too wet. If it's too wet add more breadcrumbs.

*(continued on next page)*

4. Add 2 teaspoons of the olive oil to a sauté pan and heat over medium heat. Form the salmon mixture into patties and lightly brown them in the pan for 2 minutes on each side.

5. Transfer the patties onto the prepared baking sheet. Cook at 450°F for 15 minutes.

## MIX AND MATCH QUESADILLAS

Makes 4 quesadillas; Each serves 1 adult or 2 toddlers.

Quesadillas—basically cheese-filled tortillas—are a great way to use leftovers. Mix and match whatever vegetable and protein foods you have in your house. Though best when hot off the stove-top, you can cook these in advance and re-heat for Baby if need be.

4 6-inch flour tortillas

1 cup grated cheese (Monterey Jack or Cheddar work well)

¼ cup mild salsa or finely diced tomatoes

1½ cups additional fillings (mix and match):

- 1 cup chopped vegetables— spinach (frozen or fresh), cooked broccoli, cooked green beans

- ½ cup protein food—black beans (either canned, drained and rinsed, or cooked from dry beans), shredded cooked chicken, cooked ground beef, or finely chopped tofu

1. Place 1 tortilla into a non-stick pan (or use a regular pan with ½ teaspoon oil to prevent sticking).

2. Add the toppings to the tortilla, spreading them out to cover the whole surface. For each, use ¼ cup cheese, 2 tablespoons salsa or tomatoes, ¼ cup vegetables, and 2 tablespoons protein (for example, ¼ cup spinach plus 2 tablespoons beans). Place another tortilla on top.

3. Cook over medium heat for about 5 minutes. Flip the quesadilla over and cook another 3 minutes, until second side is lightly browned and cheese is melted.

4. Cut into bite-sized pieces for Baby or into two or four wedges for older children and adults. (Tip: Instead of a fork and knife, use a pizza cutter for easy slicing.)

5. Serving suggestion: Serve with extra salsa and Guerilla Greens Guacamole (see recipe above).

## TINY FINGER SANDWICHES

Serves 1 toddler

Sandwiches are the classic lunch choice and pack well for on-the-go families. For Baby, make his sandwich and then cut it into bite-sized pieces—we recommend using a pizza cutter for super-easy slicing. Alternatively, an older toddler may be able to hold a crustless sandwich in her hands and bite or gnaw off small bits for herself, but supervise this closely as many toddlers will take way more than they can safely chew and swallow.

1 slice whole grain sandwich bread, crusts cut off

Choose a filling:

- 2–3 tablespoons egg salad
- 2–3 tablespoons salmon salad
- 1 tablespoon cream cheese with 1 teaspoon jelly
- 1 slice cheese
- 2 tablespoons hummus and 1 slice cheese

1. Cut the bread into 2 halves.

2. Spread filling onto one half of the bread and cover with the other half.

3. For Baby, smush the sandwich to make it flatter and cut before serving.

# Taking It Home . . .

The toddler years are an extra nutritional challenge. You and your baby can thrive and enjoy these times by approaching mealtimes by:

- Patiently managing mealtime behaviors
- Setting up a positive mealtime experience and being flexible to your baby's needs
- Presenting foods in a toddler-friendly way
- Teaching the picky eater how to enjoy foods

You can also manage your mealtime preparations and shopping, and minimize waste and strain on the environment by:

- Keeping an inventory
- Planning menus ahead of time
- Being a green shopper, including visiting local farmer's markets and tapping into community-supported agriculture
- Having realistic expectations of what you are capable of with an active toddler and adjusting your life accordingly

Mealtime, especially dinner, doesn't have to be total chaos. You can find plenty of ways to enjoy this age, even at the dinner table. Yes, it will be draining from time to time, but you can turn these years into a positive experience as you understand, guide, and thrive with your toddler.

## PART THREE

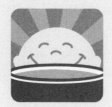

# The Green
# and
# Happy Home

# 8

# Kid Stuff

## Green and Healthy Products for Your Happy Baby

How can someone so small require so much stuff! Diapers, wipes, bottles, toys, bedding . . . babies acquire more household products than newlyweds at a bridal shower. Though there are many considerations when choosing products for Baby, health and safety come first. And as we've seen before, healthy choices are often the most green, too. This chapter provides a straightforward tutorial on the baby and toddler gear that require the greatest scrutiny. We will show you how to weigh the risks and find safe and green options, and share ways to minimize waste and keep Baby's "footprint" as small as her tiny feet.

How much does this matter? Well, the choices you make now are the building blocks you can use for teaching your child about green living as she grows. You want her planet to be a better place in fifty years. It all starts now, with you and her (and millions of other parent-child pairs around the world). It has to start somewhere. Your child will also be watching how you raise her younger siblings green, so the lessons will really start to sink in. And it's not just for the planet. Your natural choices are good for her physical health as well. We'll show you how to minimize your baby's exposure to chemicals in all the everyday items you will be using for many years to come.

# Diapers and Wipes

Perhaps because they are the most essential of baby gear items, many of us don't even give the "diaper dilemma" any thought—we just buy the newborn-size disposables and go along our merry way for the next two to three years. At some point, though, perhaps you've realized how many hundreds and thousands of diapers you're sending to the landfills and how many disposable wipes you use each day. Follow these thoughts far enough and you may start to consider using cloth diapers. Or maybe you've already made the switch. They've got to be better for the planet, right? Well, it's not so simple. Since cloth diapers seem like the holy grail of eco-friendly and healthy baby care, you may be surprised to learn that there are some concerns about the amount of energy that's required for the production and laundering of cloth diapers. Studies show it may be 13 to 27 percent more than the energy required by disposables.[1] How does the energy required for cloth compare to the waste created by disposables? And how do other considerations like Baby's health come into the picture? It can be hard to figure it all out. Instead of declaring one type of diaper the absolute eco-winner, let us share with you more info about your options, plus some facts about disposable diaper wipes and an I-can-actually-picture-myself-doing-that discussion about eco-friendlier compromises and alternatives.

## DISPOSABLE DIAPERS

It's not hard to figure out why disposable diapers are the most common choice of American Mamas (it's estimated that more than 90 percent of American baby bottoms are covered with them). They are so convenient, reliable, and easy that many of us don't even wish to think about the downsides. Indulge us, then, for a moment, as we explain the disposable diaper's darker side.

The materials used to make disposables vary depending on the brand, but most include a variety of plastics and elastic materials. The absorbent core is made partly of wood pulp and usually a superabsorbent polymer (SAP) that absorbs liquid and becomes a gel-like substance. Perhaps you've seen SAP—if you leave a wet diaper on Baby too long, sometimes it oozes out of the core and you find it crystallized and on Baby's bum.

The SAP in most disposable diapers make them very good at keeping Baby dry, but you still need to change them every few hours. If she averages about eight diapers a day over her first year, Baby will end up using almost three thousand diapers—possibly up to seven thousand in total before she's eventually potty trained. That means that the babies born this year will use more than 10.8 billion diapers in total. Add older babies, and the American disposable diaper use is estimated to be between 18 and 23 billion a year! That's a lot of diapers. So, here's where we get to the eco-effects of all these disposables:

- *Tons of waste.* Every year about 3.7 million tons of diaper waste (not even including the messes made in them) goes into American landfills.[2] And the diapers aren't biodegradable—mostly because of the materials they are made of, including some of the plastic parts and the SAP in the diaper's core. Even ingredients that are technically biodegradable can't really break down once they get to landfills because so little light and air reach them.
- *Resource drain.* You probably don't think about this, but production of most disposable diapers requires petroleum, a non-renewable resource—3.5 billion gallons a year[3] to be precise. And we cut down 250,000 trees each year to provide the wood pulp used in the absorbent core.[4]
- *Pollution.* Many components of typical diapers may be bleached with chlorine, which sends dioxins—carcinogens that accumulate and persist in the environment—into our air and waterways. Plus, when poopy diapers land in landfills, the leaching of feces into the surrounding land is a real concern for human health.

Meanwhile, disposable diapers are not without health impacts:

- *Irritated lungs.* VOCs (volatile organic compounds) are found in some disposable diapers, along with perfumes—the artificial baby "fresh" scent that smacks you in the face when you open the package. Both may irritate Baby's lungs. They could even exacerbate asthma.[5]
- *Issues down below.* For boys, disposable diapers may hold in too much heat and lead to increased scrotal temperature, theoretically impacting Baby's sperm development.[6] And some people worry that the chemicals in the diapers aren't healthy for Baby's skin.

It's not a terribly pretty picture, but we're not trying to make you feel bad if you choose disposables. Let's end on a positive point. Besides the obvious ease of use and convenience, some babies who are prone to diaper rashes may actually do better with disposables, probably because the SAP used in the core is really good at sucking moisture away from Baby's skin.[7] And SAP, though not so great for the planet and frowned upon by antidisposable folks, does appear to be perfectly safe to use as a diaper ingredient.[8]

## If You Choose Disposables, Reduce Their Impact on Baby's Health and the Planet

- Choose a brand with no chlorine bleach, no perfumes, and less of the nonbiodegradable SAP:
- Seventh Generation diapers (www.seventhgeneration.com) use less SAP than the standard national brand diapers and are chlorine free and fragrance free, too.
- Earth's Best TenderCare diapers (www.earthsbest.com) are chlorine free and perfume free.
- Nature Babycare diapers (www.naty.com) contain no oil-based plastics, are fragrance and chlorine free, and the wood pulp used for their absorbent core comes from sustainable forests.

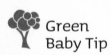

**Green Baby Tip**

If you're in the market for a diaper bag, check out one by Wee Generation (www .weegeneration.com) made of 100 percent postconsumer recycled plastic bottles, or look for other PVC-free bags like those by Fleurville (fleurville .com), Skip Hop (www.skip hop.com), Petunia Pickle Bottom (www.petuniapickle bottom.com), and many others.

- Whole Foods 365 Everyday Value brand diapers are chlorine free and fragrance free and contain wood pulp from sustainable forests.
- *Use the least absorbent type possible:* Let's say that you try the low-SAP brands mentioned above, and they don't keep Baby as dry overnight. Instead of abandoning them altogether, just use them during the day and use a more absorbent diaper like a standard Pampers or Huggies brand diaper for overnight.
- *Flush the flushable stuff:* When Baby poops, take her diaper over to the toilet and shake it out and flush it down. Solid waste belongs in the sewage treatment system, not in landfills, where

## BETTER DIAPER CREAMS

The best way to avoid a diaper rash is to change Baby's diaper frequently (every couple of hours). If Baby looks like she's on her way to a rash, sometimes a layer of diaper cream can help by serving as a barrier to the moisture. Both the Environmental Working Group's cosmetic safety database, Skin Deep (www.cosmeticdatabase.org), which focuses on health hazards, and GoodGuide (www.goodguide.com), which also takes eco-consciousness into account, rate the following creams as good choices:

- Vaseline Petroleum Jelly
- Badger Diaper Cream (www.badgerbalm.com)
- Aquaphor Baby Healing Ointment (www.eucerinus.com)
- Burt's Bees Baby Bee Diaper Ointment (www.burtsbees.com)
- Terressentials 100% Organic Terrific Tush Treatment (www.terressentials.com)
- California Baby Calming Diaper Rash Cream (www.californiababy.com)

For tough rashes, a medicated zinc oxide product like Triple Paste Medicated Ointment (www.triplepaste.com) may work best. If nothing seems to work, ask your pediatrician if an antifungal cream may be needed.

it may leach out to the surrounding land and waterways. (Note: This may be more practical once Baby is on solid foods, with more solid messes.)

- *Open Baby's window:* Occasionally let some outside air in to circulate any gases emitted from the disposable diapers stored in her room.
- *Change every few hours:* This will protect Baby's tush.

## NOT YOUR MAMA'S CLOTH DIAPERS

On the other side of the diaper spectrum are cloth diapers. If you've never used them before, you may not be familiar with how they actually work, and maybe you can't imagine that you would use them. Or maybe cloth diapers conjure up images of ultrahippie families that aren't like yours. Only a small percentage of American homes use cloth diapers, but we think you'd be surprised how mainstream they can be. New styles and tools have made it easier than ever to use cloth, and there are plenty of good reasons to do so. These aren't your mother's cloth diapers. Here's a crash course to get you acquainted with the different types of cloth diapers you can choose from:

1. *Diapers that you use with diaper covers.* These go under a water-proof outer cover that protects baby's clothes, your furniture, your lap, etc. Covers may be made of wool, vinyl, polyester, laminated fabrics, and/or cotton. If you're picturing diaper pins like those in the olden days—it's not like that anymore. Diaper covers are made with Velcro or snap clasps so no pins are required. You'll find covers made by Thirsties (www.thirstiesbaby.com), Bumkins (www.bumkins.com), and Bummis (www.bummis.com), among others. The absorbent diaper that goes under this outer layer comes in a few styles:
- *Prefolds.* This is your most basic and economical choice. Picture what you're using as a burp cloth—it's probably a prefold cloth

diaper. You fold it into the right shape and stuff it into a diaper cover.

- *Contoured.* Like prefolds, these go inside a diaper cover. Unlike prefolds, which can be a little bulky, these are cut and shaped to fit around Baby's body. Kissaluvs (kissaluvs.com) and Tiny Tush (www.tinytush.com) both make a variety of organic and nonorganic contour cloth diapers.

- *Fitted.* These diapers look like diaper covers because they are fully fitted to cover Baby as a disposable would, and they snap or Velcro shut to stay in place. But they aren't lined with a waterproof material, so you still need a diaper cover on top. Kissaluvs, Tiny Tush, and Thirsties all make a fitted diaper.

2. *Diapers that don't require a separate diaper cover.* These cloth diapering systems have the waterproof layer built right in, so there aren't as many pieces to deal with. Some Mamas use these for when Baby is with a babysitter or in day care for hours at a time, so they don't have to ask their child care provider to figure out the other cloth diaper contraptions.

- *All-in-ones.* This is the most disposable-like cloth diaper in that it's a one-piece diaper that has the absorbent layer and the waterproof outer layer all in one. Bumkins and bumGenius (www.bumgenius.com), Swaddlebees (swaddlebees.com) and Dream-Eze (www.thenaturalbabyco.com) are popular brands of all-in-ones.

- *Pocket diapers.* These are basically all-in-ones that have a pocket where you slip in an absorbent liner. Since the liner comes out when you launder it, these have the benefit of drying faster after washing. Plus, you can switch the absorbency of the liner, depending on your needs. For example, you can use more absorbent liners at night and then lighter ones during the day, if that makes sense for your baby. Try the ones by FuzziBunz (www.fuzzibunz.com) or Wahmies (www.wahmies .com).

To any of the diapers, you can add an additional liner (also called doublers) to protect against leaks. Some Mamas do this only overnight or, if they have a big-time pee-er, all the time. You can find organic cotton or hemp doublers by Baby Greens (available at www.softcloth bunz.com) and doublers by Tiny Tush, Kissaluvs, and Thirsties, too. There are even disposable liners that help with particularly messy cleanups. Kushies makes a flushable one, and you can find other varieties at any cloth diaper store.

Of course, you don't have to use one type all the time. Lots of families have different diapers for different needs. Many cloth diaper stores will sell you variety or sample packs so you can try out different styles. Even if you need a few different types and buy some all-in-ones and pocket diapers, which are the most expensive options, you're going to spend only a couple hundred dollars on your diapering system. So, compared with the thousands of dollars you could spend on disposables, cloth diapers are extremely affordable.

For many new Mamas, the idea of cleaning the cloth diapers is what keeps them from making the switch. The reality is that yes, it's more work than throwing out a disposable, but it's not as bad as you're imagining. Messy diapers get emptied into the toilet and rinsed off before going into the diaper pail or bag. There are even tools to help with this. The Mini-Shower Spray Wand (www.minishower.com) and the bum-Genius Diaper Sprayer (available on www.diapers.com) actually hook up to your toilet, and you simply spray messy diapers off so you don't have to rinse or soak them before washing. Then the diaper goes into a diaper pail or a waterproof laundry bag until laundry day. Wet diapers just go straight into the pail or bag.

When it's time to do the laundry, most cloth diaper experts recommend doing a cold water presoak to prevent stains from setting in. Then you wash with hot water (at least 140 degrees), rinse with cold, and do an extra rinse cycle to really make sure there's no odor left. You can add one-half cup white vinegar to the rinse to help whiten and freshen the fabrics. Then you dry—either with an automatic dryer or on a clothesline in the sun. To keep the smells and stains to a minimum, it's best to do the laundry every two days or so. Many Mamas find that once they are in the routine of cleaning the diapers, it's not a big deal at all. It's just like any other household task.

So it's actually doable, if you are willing to do the extra work. And if you're willing, there's a big payoff: health for Baby and the planet. Here are some of the benefits of cloth:

- There's 100 percent less landfill waste than with disposables.
- Baby's skin comes in contact with far fewer chemicals, especially if you choose organic fabrics and safe laundry soaps (see next chapter for suggestions). For some sensitive babies, this may lead to fewer diaper rashes.
- Unlike disposables, there's no off-gassing of hazardous toxins for Baby to breathe in.
- Cloth-diapered babies tend to potty train earlier than disposable diaper wearers, probably because the cloth can't wick moisture away from Baby as effectively, so Baby eventually learns that she feels uncomfortable when she goes in her diaper and is motivated to stop doing it.

A NOTE FROM DR. BOB

## Cloth Is Nicer to Baby's Bottom

As a pediatrician I obviously see a lot of diaper rashes in my office. In my experience, diaper rash seems less common with babies who wear cloth diapers. If you find yourself constantly fighting diaper rash and going through tube after tube of diaper cream, give cloth diapers a try.

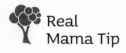

## Cloth Diapering for the Hesitant Mama

· Choose a cloth-disposable combo method (discussed later in this chapter) until you're fully comfortable with cloth. (Or do a combo method until Baby is toilet trained.)

· Use all-in-ones or pocket diapers because they are so easy.

· If it's the laundry and mess that have you avoiding cloth, use a diaper service so you don't have to deal with it at all. Go to www .diapernet.org to find a diaper service near you. Green bonus: industrial laundries use less water and less power than home laundering.

· Visit cloth diapering Web sites and blogs like www.softcloth bunz.com and www.clothdiaperblog.com to learn more and ask your questions.

## Cloth Diapering for the Gung-ho Green Mama

· Use prefolds or contour cloth diapers with covers. After Baby has outgrown them you can use the diapers as rags for cleaning.

· Choose diapers made from organic fabrics like organic cotton, and consider trying sustainable fibers like bamboo or hemp, as well.

· Air-dry instead of machine dry to reduce carbon emissions and use less electricity.

### THE DIAPER HYBRID—GDIAPERS BRAND DIAPERS

For Mamas who don't feel great about their disposable diapers but can't commit to cloth, meet the gDiaper (www.gdiaper.com). If you've never heard of this innovative diaper brand, head to your local natural products market and check it out. These hybrid diapers consist of a disposable inner snap-in liner, made with a little SAP to effectively prevent leaks, and then a reusable cover they call 'little g' diaper pants. The best part is that the liner isn't just disposable—it's flushable and compostable (when only peed upon—you can't add poopy liners to your compost pile). The diapers become compost in 50 to 150 days, depending on the conditions. Although they do contain some SAP, they have far less than typical disposables, and since they get flushed and not thrown out, gDiapers are considered to be one of the most eco-friendly options on the market. And since they are part disposable, part reusable, they may be perfect for Mamas who don't love the idea of disposable diapers but can't commit to cloth.

## ANOTHER OPTION: COMPROMISE!

Just as with other aspects of baby greening, you don't have to choose an all-or-nothing approach to diapering. There are lots of combo methods and compromises that may work for your family, mitigate the health effects and waste of disposables, and minimize the hassle and laundry that's required when you go 100 percent cloth. Here are a few ideas:

- Use cloth when you're home, disposables when you're out.
- Use cloth during day, disposables at night.
- Use gDiapers at home, disposables when you're out.
- Use a less absorbent gel-free disposable during the day and a regular one at night.
- Use disposables on your breast-fed newborn, and start with cloth after Baby starts solid foods (and her poops become less explosive).

A NOTE FROM DR. BOB

## **Baby Girls and Baby Wipes**

Baby's vaginal area can be especially sensitive to soaps and chemicals in wipes. It's best to avoid using a baby wipe anywhere inside the outer labia. If you need to clean out any poop or dirt from the inner vagina, first rinse out the wipe with warm water or use a burp rag with warm water.

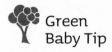

## Green Baby Tip

. . . . . . . . . . . . . . . . . . . .

If you buy one of those odor-resistant dirty diaper pails for disposables, in two years you'll have a huge piece of plastic that you no longer need, not to mention the special plastic bags you'll be buying and throwing away until then. We've yet to find a pail system that fully removes the dirty diaper odor anyway. Instead, take dirty diapers directly out to the trash. Or use a basic covered trash can to store dirties until you can make it to the garbage. Occasionally sprinkle some baking soda in the bottom of the pail and on top of the diapers to help absorb odor. Then you can continue using the pail as a trash can long after Baby is out of diapers.

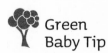

## Green Baby Tip

. . . . . . . . . . . . . . . . . . . .

When you buy diaper wipes, skip the hard plastic tub. To create less plastic waste, choose the refill packs instead.

In the end (no pun intended!) you have to make the right choice for your family and for your baby. Here's a simplified list of the pros and cons of both types of diapers to help you make your decision. If you can't decide one way or the other, at least follow some of the numerous compromises mentioned above.

| Disposable Diapers | | Cloth Diapers | |
|---|---|---|---|
| Pros | Cons | Pros | Cons |
| · Easy and convenient | · Expensive | · Cheaper | · More work |
| · No laundry-related electricity and water use | · Millions of tons of landfill waste | · No chemicals exposed to Baby's skin and lungs | · Laundry-related electricity and water use |
| · Fewer diaper rashes for most babies | · VOCs and other chemicals exposed to Baby's skin and lungs | · Fewer diaper rashes for chemical-sensitive babies | · Do not keep Baby's skin as dry—require more frequent changing |
| | · Later potty training | · Earlier potty training | |

# Diper Wipes

The companion to the diaper, wipes are yet another essential baby care product. While most of us tend to just reach for the closest bin of big brand name disposables, you do have other options. You can make your own or you can select healthier and greener wipes if you know what to look for. Plus, if you use disposables you can be conscious of how many you use and try to use fewer. Think about what shade of green your diaper wipe habits are now and how can you be greener.

*The palest green: don't use as many as you used to.* We know that Mamas use diaper wipes not only at the changing table, but for wiping dirty hands, wiping off toys, even cleaning furniture! Disposable wipes are so convenient that many of us don't give any thought to the fact that they are made from trees and other natural resources. And when we throw them away they land in our landfills. Just being more conscious of how many wipes you use may help you stop before reaching for more. For small messes tear one in half. For household cleanups use some of the green cleaning tips we provide in the next chapter. For dirty hands and faces there's good old-fashioned soap and water. There is one situation where it's best not to scrimp, though: when wiping a baby girl, use a clean wipe for the vaginal area rather than the same one you wiped the poop with. That can risk giving your little girl a bladder infection.

*A little greener: skip the icky chemicals.* If you really look at the ingredient list for most disposable wipes, you start to question whether you really want to be wiping Baby's skin with such things! Typical wipes contain things like bis-PEG/PPG-16/16, PEG/PPG-16/16 dimethicone, sodium hydroxymethylglycinate, disodium EDTA, and other chemicals considered to be potentially hazardous. Even some wipes designed for "sensitive" skin contain chemicals that are considered to be hazardous to human health. You may be wondering why they're even allowed to be in baby things. Well, that's a very good question.

Rather than memorize a list of not-so-good-for-baby wipe ingredients, just look for disposable wipes from all-natural brands such as Nature Babycare and Seventh Generation that contain ingredients like aloe gel, glycerin (a vegetable-oil-derived softener), and potassium sorbate, an all-natural preservative. In general, the fewer ingredients there are in your wipes and the more ingredients that you can recognize and pronounce, the more likely the product is to be a safer option. The Environmental Working Group's list of safe baby wipes (those with "low" hazard ratings) includes wipes from Tushies, TenderCare, Seventh Generation, Avalon Organics, and Inspiration Vibration. Visit www.cosmeticdatabase.com for current lists of recommended wipes. Many of these brands also provide the added benefit of being slightly better for the planet since they aren't bleached and don't send more chemicals into the environment.

*The deepest shade of green: make your own!* Of course you could skip disposable wipes and just make your own if really want to minimize waste. This would also be the best way to guarantee that the materials and substances touching Baby's skin are safe and pure. You can either buy unbleached cotton cloths to use as wipes (bumGenius makes a twelve-pack, www.bumgenius.com), or if you have cotton T-shirts or flannel shirts or sheets that you would otherwise throw out, cut them into strips to use as wipes. After use, rinse and throw them into a diaper pail to await laundry day. Wash on hot, just as you would cloth diapers. To moisten the wipes, you can either use water alone; heavily diluted all-natural baby wash like the body washes by California Baby (www.californiababy.com) or Burt's Bees (www.burtsbees.com); an all-natural wipes solution like the ones by bumGenius or Kissaluvs; or an au naturel blend of essential oils and water—an Internet search will provide several recipe options.

## Nontoxic Baby Bath Care

Just like the diapers and wipes you choose, the bath and other body care products that come into direct contact with Baby's skin deserve special scrutiny. The unsettling thing about baby care products like body washes, shampoos, diaper creams, and lotions is that they aren't closely regulated by anybody. Testing of the products is voluntary and can be done by the manufacturers themselves. With just a few exceptions, there's no systematic testing of the ingredients found in these products. When you're picking out products for Baby, here are some ways to minimize any potential risks:

1. *Use less.* Think about how many products you use on Baby's hair and skin, and ask yourself if you could get by without some of them. For example, most babies who don't have eczema or another skin condition don't need any body lotion. Some babies don't even need diaper cream on a regular basis. Mamas of these tough-skinned babies may reach for the diaper cream

only when some redness or irritation appears. And then once it's passed, the cream goes back into the drawer for several days or weeks.

2. *Be sensitive.* If a product has been formulated for sensitive skin, there's a good bet that it's a decent choice for Baby. But don't necessarily take the label's word for it. Make sure the ingredient label backs up the claim and shows the product to be fragrance free, artificial preservative free, and made without petroleum-based chemicals, which can be rough on sensitive skin.

3. *Read the labels.* Look out for ingredients that we know are health concerns including:

   • *Fragrance.* Not only are some synthetic fragrances irritating to Baby's nose and lungs and may cause allergic reactions or sensitivities, but when you see fragrance

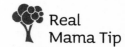

**Real Mama Tip**

"Instead of diaper creams or baby lotions that contain chemicals, I use olive oil. It's very healing to my baby's skin when she gets a minor diaper rash or a little patch of dryness."

—*Sepi, Great Neck, New York*

A NOTE FROM DR. BOB

## Natural Care for Rashes and Cradle Cap

Many babies develop some dry red patches on their skin. These eczema areas are harmless (unless widespread and itchy), but most Mamas like Baby's skin to be smooth and perfect. Instead of using regular moisturizing lotions that contain various chemicals, try a natural skin softener like jojoba oil, cocoa butter, or shea butter. You'll also notice your baby's scalp gets a little (or a lot!) crusty from time to time. This cradle cap is harmless, but you can minimize it by using a baby shampoo with tea tree oil. California Baby makes one, and you can find others with a quick online search or at your local health food store.

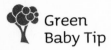 Green
Baby Tip
. . . . . . . . . . . . . . . . . . .
To see how your favorite
baby care products
measure up, check out
the GoodGuide at www
.goodguide.com. You will
see how products are rated
based on the health and
safety of their ingredients,
their environmental impact,
and even the social responsibility of their manufacturer.

on the label, it may indicate that the product contains
phthalates to help the fragrance last longer. Phthalates
are known to disrupt the hormonal system in the body.
Studies show that baby boys in particular are at risk for
reproductive development problems when exposed to
phthalates in the womb.[9,10] To avoid phthalates in baby
care products, choose products that contain no synthetic
fragrance and are unscented or scented with natural oils
only. You can also look for "phthalate-free" on the label.

- *Parabens.* These chemicals are preservatives used in
some bath and body products. Like phthalates, they are
known to interfere with reproductive hormones.[11] They
may also be a skin irritant. Parabens are easier to spot
than phthalates because they're listed right on the ingredient label as methylparaben, butylparaben, propylpara-
ben, etc.

- *Sodium laurel (or laureth) sulfate, DMDM dydantoin, and
PEG (polyethylene glycol) compounds.* Studies have found
that these chemical ingredients in body care products
may be contaminated with carcinogenic substances,
though it's unclear to what extent.[12]

4. *Choose organic and plant-based ingredients.* It's no absolute
guarantee, but if a product contains organic ingredients and is
also labeled as being all-natural and nontoxic, chances are, it's
on the safer side of the spectrum. We like some of the organic
and all-natural baby care products by Avalon Organics (www
.avalonorganics.com), JASON Baby (www.jason-natural.com),
Weleda Baby (usa.weleda.com), Burt's Bees (www.burtsbees
.com), and California Baby (www.californiababy.com).

# SUNSCREEN

## A Baby Care Necessity

Sunlight, though great for forming vitamin D, is also a cause of skin cancer, which affects about one million Americans each year.[13] Bad sunburns during childhood increase Baby's cancer risk, so it's important to always protect her when she's playing in the sun for extended periods. Of course, since babies do need some sunlight, don't worry when walking to the car or taking a short fifteen-minute stroll. Sunscreen shouldn't be an everyday treatment for babies. We don't know everything we should about all the chemicals used in sunscreens. Here are some ideas to follow:

- When Baby is younger than six months, her skin is thin and can't produce melanin, a pigment that is protective against certain UV rays. She's also apt to be sensitive to some of the chemicals that could be found in sunscreens. So, until she's six months old, rather than use sunscreen to protect her, use protective clothing, umbrellas, and shade as shields if Baby's exposure will be more than fifteen minutes during the heat of the day.
- After six months of age, whenever Baby is in the sun for extended periods, use a nontoxic sunscreen that blocks both UVA and UVB rays. Choose mineral-based sunscreens containing zinc oxide and titanium oxide, which are physical sunblocks—they actually deflect UV rays away from the skin, rather than absorb them. We like Badger SPF 30 Sunscreen (www.badgerbalm.com), California Baby No Fragrance SPF 30+ Sunscreen Lotion (www.californiababy.com), and Avalon Organics Baby Natural Mineral Sunscreen SPF 18 (www.avalonorganics.com).
- Avoid chemical sunscreens made with oxybenzone, a possible carcinogen and hormone disrupter.
- Apply Baby's sunscreen about thirty minutes before leaving the house, and don't forget to reapply after a couple of hours or if Baby gets wet splashing in the pool or playing in the sprinkler.
- Hats, beach umbrellas, and protective clothing are still essential, even if Baby is lathered in sunscreen. Don't leave home without them. And stay in the shade when you can.

# Choosing Green and Healthy Furnishings

Baby will spend lots of time asleep during her first year or two (let's hope!), so the furnishings in her room, or yours if she sleeps with you, play a role in her overall health. Your furniture and other decor choices also contribute to your household's overall environmental impact. As you read through this section, know that we're not trying to make you feel that danger is lurking around every corner, even though it's going to read like a laundry list of hazards. This is about making better choices whenever you have the option. And we even have some tips for you if you've already picked out furniture and nursery gear that are less green or health-conscious options.

## CRIBS AND OTHER WOOD FURNITURE

The first step to furnishing a healthy and green nursery is to select healthy and green furniture. Baby furniture—cribs, dressers, changing tables, toy boxes—may be made with different types of woods and with various kinds of finishes, some healthier than others. The best option is furniture made from solid wood and with nontoxic finishes (stains, lacquers, etc.). If it's not solid wood, it's probably made with some kind of pressed wood product. Certain types of pressed wood, including plywood, particleboard, and medium-density fiberboard (MDF), are made from wood chips that are glued together with resins that contain solvents, including formaldehyde. Yes, as in the embalming fluid. The formaldehyde and other solvents used in the production of this furniture may escape into the air in Baby's room. These off-gassed VOCs are inhaled and may irritate Baby's lungs. Many of them are also known or suspected cancer causers. If you find furniture that has pressed wood components (often found as shelving and tops and backs of pieces of furniture), find out if it's a low-VOC or VOC-free product and if the finishes are nontoxic. Just ask the manufacturer directly by contacting their customer service department.

If you want your nursery to be green, the wood should come from a

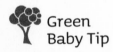

## Green Baby Tip

When looking for sustainable wood furniture for Baby's room you should know that many eco-experts find the Sustainable Forestry Initiative's certification to be less than meaningful because SFI is a paper industry group, not an environmental organization.

well-managed, sustainable forest. Instead of clear cutting, which can destroy animal and plant habitats and lead to erosion and pollution runoff, sustainable forestry practices help to protect and preserve forests while still harvesting the wood for our use. The Forest Stewardship Council and Rainforest Alliance certify wood products as being from sustainable forests. You can go to www.certifiedwood.org and www.fsc-info.org to find manufacturers that use FSC-certified wood. Some of the companies that we've found who are making safe and eco-friendly baby furniture include Ikea (www.ikea.com), Ecotots (www.ecotots.com), Pacific Rim (www.pacificrimwoodworking.com), Dwell Studio (www.dwellstudio.com), and Baby Miró (available at www.babyearth.com).

## Hand-Me-Down Crib Safety

Using an antique or hand-me-down is certainly an eco-friendly way to go because no new trees have to be cut down, but be sure to think about basic crib safety, too. New cribs (post 2000) are required to meet all current federal safety standards set by the Consumer Product Safety Commission. If you're using a used crib at home (or if Baby sleeps in one at Grandma's house or the babysitter's), first make sure it hasn't been recalled. Go to www.recalls.gov to look it up. Then carefully inspect it for safety:

- There should be at least 26 inches between the mattress support at its lowest position and the top of the adjustable side rail when it's at its highest position.
- There should be at least 9 inches between the mattress support at its highest position and the adjustable side rail at its lowest position.
- There should be no more than 2⅜ inches between the slats, spindles, and corner posts.
- The mattress should be flush against the sides. If you can fit two fingers or more along the side, the mattress is too small, and Baby risks getting stuck and hurt.
- The drop side should lock and require some pressure to release and to lower.

- Panels should not have decorative cutouts. These could trap an infant's head.
- Corner posts shouldn't stick up past the top of the side rails and sides of the crib. (Corner posts that stick up—picture a four-poster bed—pose a strangulation hazard.)
- There should be no missing hardware—even one missing or loose screw can put Baby's safety at risk.

## CRIB MATTRESSES

Once you have a crib, you need a mattress. The soft filling that you'll find in a typical crib mattress and in most upholstered furniture is made of polyurethane foam, which is a nice cushiony material but unfortunately very flammable. To protect consumers from these furnishings going up in flames, manufacturers add flame retardant chemicals. If you're like us you prefer Baby's things not to ignite, but . . . the problem with these synthetic chemicals is that they act a bit like volatile compounds in that they do escape into the air. Once in the air, they can stick to dust particles and can be inhaled into Baby's lungs.

One particular class of flame retardants called PBDEs have been linked to problems with brain development, hormonal function, and immune system health.[14] After being banned in Europe for several years, a 2003 study showed that American women had up to 75 times as many PBDEs in their breast milk than European women. This was evidence of a far greater exposure to PBDEs than scientists had previously thought.[15] By 2005 production of certain PBDEs was banned in the U.S.

If you have a crib mattress or upholstered furniture made after 2005 it's not treated with PBDEs, however there may be other synthetic flame retardant chemicals added in order to meet mattress safety standards. And flame retardants aren't the only toxins found in conventional mattresses—any number of solvents that emit VOCs may be in conventional mattresses including formaldehyde and toluene, among others.

Organic and natural mattresses are a good alternative to conventional mattresses not only because they contain fewer toxins, but also because they are made with natural fibers instead of non-renewable petroleum-based materials. The tricky thing, though, is that even organic mattresses may be treated with flame retardant chemicals. The exception is an organic mattress made with untreated wool—the lanolin that coats a lamb's wool is naturally flame resistant so manufacturers aren't required to add additional flame retardants. If Baby is sensitive to wool and you want a completely chemical-free cotton mattress you may need a prescription from your pediatrician to purchase one.

You may now be wondering, "Does *my* Baby's mattress contain chemicals?" Unless you sought out an all-natural mattress labeled as chemical-free, it's almost guaranteed that your crib mattress and changing table pad contain some chemicals. If it's too late to return it to the store, don't panic—see below for some tips on minimizing your mattress's impact. If you're on your way to the store to pick one up, here's how to avoid toxic mattress ingredients:

- Look for chemical-free mattresses and upholstered furniture. Alternatives are typically made with natural latex, cotton, and untreated wool. Check out the healthy crib mattress offerings from Ecobaby (www.ecobaby.com), Vivetique (www.vivetique

.com), and Naturepedic (www.naturepedic.com), among others.

- Don't forget about other upholstered items like changing table pads. Look for chemical-free versions. Check out www.our greenhouse.com and www.ahappyplanet.com for some options.
- If you have furniture in your home with exposed foam cushions, have them reupholstered or replaced to minimize the release of PBDEs and other chemicals.

## CARPET AND THROW RUGS

Having some kind of carpeting in Baby's room or play space provides padding for Baby's inevitable trips and spills. Conventional carpets are made with synthetic fibers that are derived from nonrenewable petroleum and may off-gas formaldehyde and other solvents that are used in the glues and finishes. The fumes give floor coverings that "new" smell, and they also irritate eyes and lungs. Wall-to-wall carpeting can also trap dust and other allergens that can exacerbate respiratory problems like asthma. If you have wall-to-wall, don't rip it up (unless you were already planning to lay down something new)—just be sure to vacuum regularly, with a HEPA-filter vacuum if possible. And open Baby's windows whenever you can to circulate fresh air. If you are still deciding what will cover Baby's floor, choose from these healthier alternatives:

- Look for rugs labeled as nontoxic and made from all-natural fibers instead of petroleum-based materials. Ikea carries a variety of natural fiber rugs, as does Pottery Barn (www.pot terybarn.com). Check your local rug and carpet vendors for more options.
- If you have a choice, consider carpet tiles or small area rugs that you can take outside, shake out, and easily wash, such as the carpet squares by Flor (www.flor.com), which also come in natural fibers like wool.
- Skip carpet stain-repellent treatments. Yes, Baby will probably stain something sooner or later, but the perfluorochemicals

(PFCs) used in some of these treatments have been linked to birth defects, developmental problems, and cancer.[16]

## PAINTED WALLS AND PAINTED FURNITURE

Painting Baby's room is a common home improvement project for new moms and dads. When picking out paint you can avoid those that contain VOCs and other toxic chemicals. If your room or furniture is long since painted (we're talking forty years ago or more), you'll want to think about lead and how to protect Baby from exposure.

### Lead

This heavy metal is found in paints that were manufactured before 1978, when lead was not yet banned as an ingredient. If you have antique painted furniture, antique painted toys, or an older home, you can probably assume that you have lead paint around. Health issues arise when lead-based paints flake off or dissolve into dust and can be swallowed or inhaled by Baby. Ingesting a lead-based paint chip just one square inch in size can cause lead poisoning, as can ingesting smaller amounts over a longer period of time. Lead poisoning leads to mental impairments like learning disabilities, intestinal problems like nausea and diarrhea, kidney problems, and reproductive problems. What to do about lead paint:

- If you have home improvement projects that require scraping pre-1978 paint, call trained professionals to do it. They specialize in dealing with the paint dust and reducing your family's exposure to it.
- If you have walls in your home that you suspect have lead paint but the paint is intact—no chips coming off—it's probably best just to let them be. Be sure to dust regularly with a wet rag, and use a high-phosphate cleanser on windowsills and other areas where there is wear and tear.
- If you have older furniture or toys that you suspect were painted with lead paint, get rid of them.

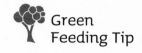

**Green Feeding Tip**

Deficiencies of certain nutrients, such as iron, zinc, and calcium, may actually increase lead absorption in the body, so there's yet another reason to feed Baby right and take your prenatal vitamin if you're nursing.

Ask your pediatrician about lead testing. It's mandatory in some states.

### VOCs

In conventional modern paints, solvents are added to help the paint perform better—to help it spread evenly, dry evenly, and last longer. But as the paint dries, and for months (or even years) afterward, these solvents emit volatile organic compounds—VOCs. These fumes give paint its odor and can cause headaches and respiratory problems. They're also linked to kidney and liver problems. Luckily, it's really easy to avoid VOCs in paint these days. Federal regulations limit the VOC content of paints, and even mainstream paint manufacturers have introduced low-VOC or no-VOC paints in the past year or two. Here's what to look for:

- Paints labeled "Low VOC" may have fewer than 250 grams of VOC per liter of paint. Better are paints that are certified with the Green Seal GS-11 standard, which will have less than 50 grams of VOC per liter for flat paints, and less than 150 grams per liter for nonflat paints.
- "No-VOC" paints will have less than 5 grams of VOC per liter of paint.
- For completely VOC-free and nontoxic paints, look for brands made from naturally derived plant oils, tree resins, natural waxes, natural pigments, and mineral dyes.
- VOCs aren't the only toxins that may be present in paints, so look for water-based paints that are formaldehyde free, in addition to being low in VOCs.
- Check out eco-home sites like www.thegreenguide.com/home -garden, www.eartheasy.com, and www.greenhomeguide.com for paint recommendations.

## QUICK GUIDE TO HEALTHY GREEN NURSERY FURNISHINGS

| Type of Furnishing | Concerns | Advice |
|---|---|---|
| Cribs and wood furniture | Sustainability of the wood<br><br>VOCs and formaldehyde emitted from plywood, particleboard, or MDF | Choose furniture made with solid wood harvested from managed forests and treated with the least toxic finishes.<br><br>Avoid plywood, particleboard, and MDF constructed with formaldehyde-containing glues. |
| Mattresses and upholstered furniture | Petroleum-derived ingredients, synthetic flame retardants, formaldehyde and other solvents | Choose chemical-free alternatives made with wool and other fabrics instead of polyurethane foam fillings. |
| Painted walls and furniture | VOCs emitted in their production and use<br><br>Pre-1978 lead-based paints | If you're painting either before or after Baby arrives, choose VOC-free or low-VOC paints.<br><br>If Baby is around pre-1978 paint, take steps to minimize her risk of lead poisoning. |
| Carpets and rugs | VOCs emitted in production and use, petroleum-derived ingredients | Choose natural fiber rugs that aren't treated with toxic chemicals.<br><br>If you can't find a natural fiber rug, fully air out any synthetic fiber rugs before bringing them into Baby's room.<br><br>If Baby has new carpeting, have her sleep in another room at least until the new carpet smell has gone—about a month.<br><br>Choose small rugs or carpet tiles that can easily be washed. |

# I CAN'T SWITCH OUT ALL MY BABY FURNITURE, CRIB MATTRESS, AND CARPETING. WHAT NOW?

If you're not in a position to start from scratch and buy all-green furniture, mattresses, and carpet, all is not lost. There are things you can do to minimize Baby's exposures to the potentially toxic chemicals that may be emitted from the materials in her room:

- *Deal with dust:* In addition to being an allergen that can irritate Baby's nasal passages and lungs, dust can contain many of the chemicals that are released in the home.
  - Vacuum regularly, preferably with a HEPA (high-efficiency particulate air) filter vacuum cleaner that can trap fine dust and allergens.
  - Consider purchasing a HEPA filter air purifier for the room where Baby sleeps.
  - Dust regularly with a rag wet with a mild cleaning agent. (For green cleaning tips, see chapter 9)
- *Ventilate:* When possible, open Baby's windows and air out her room. This will allow some of the toxic gases to escape.
- *Wash off the chemicals:* Whenever you buy new bedding, throw rugs, stuffed animals, or window treatments, wash them well before you put them out in Baby's room.
  - If you purchase furniture made with particleboard or plywood, air it out before bringing it into Baby's room. Putting it outside where air can circulate around it will allow many of the chemicals to off-gas outside.

## Safe Toys—into the Mouths of Babes

It's hard to find good statistics on how many toys the average American baby has at her disposal, but we're pretty sure the number is large. And whether it's a rattle, a bath toy, a building block, or a doll, almost all of them will double as a teether at some point or another. Under the assumption that Baby will be licking and chewing all the toys in your toy bin, look for nontoxic and age-appropriate toys for Baby. While you're at it, you can find some eco-friendly options, too!

## GENERAL TOY SAFETY

In the United States, toys are monitored by the Consumer Product Safety Commission. This agency sets standards for safe materials for toys, determines labeling requirements, and disseminates recall information. After the Consumer Product Safety Improvement Act was passed in 2008, the CPSC has stricter lead rules than we used to have, requirements that will allow for easier tracking of recalled items, and they've banned certain chemicals in toys and baby gear. But even despite the rules, regulations, and monitoring, unsafe substances can still get into Baby's toys, especially if they are manufactured overseas. Whatever kinds of toys you choose for Baby, be sure to stay up-to-date on toy recalls. You can sign up for recall email alerts at www.recalls.gov or www.cpsc.gov.

It's also important to choose toys for Baby that are suited to her age. Sometimes, age guidelines provided by toy manufacturers have to do with the developmental skills Baby will need to get the most out of a particular toy. But for the most part, when you see a warning that says a toy is only for kids ages three and up, this guidance has to do with the size of the pieces and whether they pose a choking risk. Until Baby is about three years old (the age when she'll stop putting everything in her mouth) anything that is smaller than 1.75 inches (4.4 centimeters) in diameter is considered to be unsafe. Things like marbles, small balls, coins, wheels that may detach from toy cars, eyes on stuffed animals, board game pieces, and any other small toys should be saved until she's older. Clothing with buttons sewed on may not be a good idea; if the thread loosens, Baby can pull the button off and choke on it. Good rule of thumb: if something fits through the hollow of a toilet paper roll, keep it away from Baby. While we're on the subject of choking, be careful with things like coins, batteries, refrigerator magnets, and other household items that are choking hazards. Keep these safely out of Baby's reach at all times.

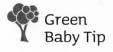

### Green Baby Tip

If Baby has a battery-powered toy that she can't get enough of, consider switching to rechargeable batteries. One rechargeable battery can replace up to three hundred regular batteries!

### Green Baby Tip

. . . . . . . . . . . . . . . . . . . .

The most eco-friendly thing you can do about Baby's toys is to buy fewer of them. Besides creating less waste, you'll probably be helping her develop a rich imagination and avoid the path toward materialism and greed.

## Rubber Ducky Danger?

Polyvinyl chloride (PVC) is soft vinyl material found in some rubber ducks, raincoats, kids' backpacks, and other baby gear. To make it soft and pliable, manufacturers add chemical plasticizers, like phthalates. These chemicals can leach out of the PVC and are believed to be harmful to the reproductive system, especially for baby boys, and may cause damage to the liver and kidneys as well. Phthalates have been banned in Europe and Japan, and recently, a few types have been banned from baby gear in the United States. Even before these new rules were in place, Wal-Mart, Babies "R" Us, and other large retailers agreed to stop selling toys and other baby gear with phthalates as of January 2009. Another concern about PVC is that when it's produced or incinerated, dioxins are released into the atmosphere. Plus, according to Healthy Toys.org, toys made from PVC also may contain traces of cadmium, mercury, and lead—heavy metals you don't want Baby ingesting.

## SAFE TEETHING TOYS

When you're buying toys that you intend Baby to suck and chew on, look for safe options:

- Look for "PVC free" on the label of any plastic teether (if it's not on the label, visit the manufacturer's Web site to investigate the ingredients before you buy it). The online emporium the Soft Landing (www.thesoftlanding.com) has many BPA- and PVC-free options by brands like Sassy, Nûby, and Natursutten.
- As far as we know, EVA (ethylene vinyl acetate) is a safer substitute for PVC. It's found in some plastic teethers, for example, the ones by Natursutten,.
- If you want to err on the extra safe (and eco-friendly) side, skip plastic altogether and go for solid wood teething toys made from unpainted solid hardwoods or ones made from natural rubber. Vulli, a French company, makes many natural rubber teether toys. You can find wood and rubber teethers on www.amazon.com and at many small toy stores.

The great news is that many toy manufacturers are phasing out PVC and phthalates. You may see "PVC free" on labels now. If you're looking at a vinyl-like item for Baby—waterproof bibs or toy backpacks, for example—look for "PVC free," and if you don't find it on the label, contact the manufacturer to be sure.

Some products that used to be made with PVC may now be made with EVA—ethylene vinyl acetate. You'll find this as an ingredient in plastic teethers and some waterproof bibs. So far, EVA appears to be safe for babies, and we know that it doesn't contain phthalates or other plasticizers. (See box for more on safe teethers.)

## Proper Paint

The paint used in baby toys should be nontoxic, of course. Some toys, however, may contain lead-based paint and are dangerous for babies because they can lead to lead poisoning. Antique toys like blocks or painted train sets may contain lead-based paint. If you have these toys in your possession, don't let Baby play with them. Unfortunately, it's not just antique toys that may contain lead. It's not allowed as a toy ingredient anymore, but it could still show up. A couple of years ago 1.5 million sets of Thomas the Tank Engine train figurines were recalled due to lead paint. And this was only a few months after a recall of a million painted toys manufactured by Fisher-Price. To keep Baby safe from lead paint, it may help to look for toys that are manufactured in Europe or the United States, and be sure to get on the CPSC's recall notification list (www.cpsc.gov) so you'll be alerted if any of your baby's toys are found to contain lead paint.

## ECO-FRIENDLY PLAYTIME

There are so many ways to go green in the playroom. Besides avoiding PVC and lead as mentioned above, look for other great toys that are eco-friendly.

- Toys made from solid wood taken from sustainable forests (certified by FSC or Rainforest Alliance) are a great choice.

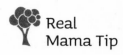

### Real Mama Tip

"If you have older children around the house, keep their toys separated from the baby's. We found it easier to keep the baby safe when we made it a rule that certain of our older child's toys are only brought off the shelf when the baby is safely in her high chair or crib."

—Amy, Rockville, Maryland

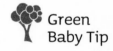

### Green Baby Tip

When you're greening Baby's toy chest, take a look at your pet's toys, too. Not only could the chemicals in your pet's toys enter Baby's play space, but Baby can't tell the difference between her PVC-free rubber ducky and Spot's squeaky chew toy. It's a good bet that at some point that chew toy will end up in Baby's mouth.

# A GREEN WISH LIST

With a new baby at home, chances are you'll be getting some gifts: at her birth, at her baptism or other religious ceremony, for Baby's first birthday, and Baby's first Christmas or Chanukah. Loved ones are likely to shower the new baby with presents. But how do you avoid getting piles of stuff that you don't want or need? Or stuff that you don't want Baby to have, for example, unsafe plastic toys? Here's how to keep it green:

- For pregnant Mamas: Register for green baby gear. Even baby superstores have a broad selection of organic bedding and clothes, all-natural baby care products, and solid wood furniture.
- At holidays and for birthdays make a wish list to share with close family or others who ask you what Baby "needs." It's not bossy (if you're tactful about it)—most people will welcome the suggestions.
- In lieu of gifts, ask for donations to worthy causes in Baby's honor. HAPPYBABY's charity of choice is Project Peanut Butter (www.projectpeanutbutter.org), which feeds hungry children in Africa. Choose an organization that means something to you.
- When you give Baby gifts, don't use wrapping paper. Old newspapers are just as fun for her to rip open and not as wasteful.
- When you get a gift that you can't use, don't throw it out or let it collect dust in the corner of the closet. Donate it to a local shelter or collection center for a family in need.

Many of these are completely untreated and unfinished or finished with nontoxic stains or paints. Check out the wooden toys by Selecta (available at www.Amazon.com) and HABA (available from a number of retailers, including Oompa.com).
- Stuffed animals, dolls, and "lovey" toys made from organic cotton, wool, or hemp. Under the Nile (www.underthenile.com) makes organic stuffed toys and several different lovey toys. Baby may also like the Green Sprouts Organic Blankie Animal by i play (www.iplaybabywear.com) or MiYim's Lovie Blankees (www.miyim.com).
- Toys made from postconsumer recycled materials. Green Toys (www.greentoys.com) makes tea sets, sand toys, and play

kitchen toys from old milk jugs. You can also find stuffed toys made from old sweaters and blankets (or make your own).

· Nonelectronic toys that don't require batteries. Batteries may leach mercury, lead, and other heavy metals into the ground after they are thrown away.

# Healthy Fabrics for Baby

Onesies, footie pajamas, bedding, cloth diapers, towels, swaddling blankets, slings . . . Baby is snuggled and cuddled by fabric twenty-four hours a day. On the health and safety side, when you're selecting fabrics for Baby's bed or body, think about which chemicals are used in the processing and whether they are produced with sustainability in mind. Here's a rundown of the different options available to you:

## COTTON

By far the most common fabric used for baby clothes and gear, cotton is a soft, lightweight, and strong fabric that breathes well. Organic cotton clothes and bedding are becoming ubiquitous—you can find them at eco-chic boutiques and big-box stores alike. The reason that organic cotton is becoming such a staple for green parents is that conventional cotton is particularly damaging to the environment and the workers who grow it. It's estimated that 25 percent of the world's insecticides and 10 percent of the world's pesticides are used on conventional cotton crops.[17] And according to the EPA, seven of the nineteen most common pesticides used for cotton are possible, likely, probable, or known carcinogens.[18]

Organic cotton, of course, is grown without any synthetic pesticides. Organic cotton clothes for Baby will likely be free from other toxic chemicals as well. According to Global Organic Textile Standard (GOTS) restrictions, organic textiles must not be treated with formaldehyde, the dyes must be nontoxic, and any zippers or other accessories on the fabrics must be safe, too—PVC free and nickel free. Some cotton

A NOTE FROM DR. BOB

## Eczema or Other Rashes—
## Try Organic Cotton

As a pediatrician, I see eczema and other infant rashes quite frequently. The first step in treatment is to switch Baby over to organic cotton clothing. That often corrects the problem.

connoisseurs say that organic cotton is even a better quality than non-organic because the softness and strength of the fibers are not compromised by chemical pesticides and fertilizers. Look for adorable organic cotton creations from manufacturers like Under the Nile (www.underthenile.com), Sage Creek Organics (www.sagecreekorganics.com), Cotton Monkey (www.cottonmonkey.com), Speesees (www.speesees.com), Baby Greens (www.babygreensorganics.com), and even more mainstream vendors like BabyGap (www.babygap.com).

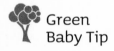

### Green Baby Tip

Plastic bibs are great for messy eaters because you can give them a quick rinse in the sink after the meal, but look out for ones that indicate that they are PVC-free, like the waterproof bibs by Bumkins, Mimi the Sardine (www.mimithesardine.com), and Kiddopotamus.

### THE SYNTHETICS

Besides cotton, typical textiles used in baby clothes include polyester, nylon, and acrylic, all made from crude oil, a nonrenewable resource. The processing of petroleum into textiles requires using a lot of energy and some pretty powerful chemicals that put workers' health at risk and create pollution. From Baby's perspective, polyester and other synthetic fibers won't breathe as well as natural fibers and may not be a good choice for babies with sensitive skin. Are synthetic fibers *dangerous* for Baby? Probably not. But if you're going green, go for natural, organic, nontoxic fabrics instead.

## RENEWABLE FIBERS

Even at its organically grown best, cotton is still a crop that is fairly taxing to the land. It requires significant water resources and takes a lot of space. Even greener options are textiles made from renewable fibers such as bamboo, hemp, and even soy. Usually mixed with cotton or other fibers, these materials will up the eco-ante of Baby's wardrobe:

- *Bamboo.* Grown with very few pesticides, bamboo grows so quickly and so easily that it's considered the most renewable type of wood. Bamboo fibers are naturally antimicrobial and likely won't cause an allergic reaction in Baby. Check out the Bamboosa (www.bamboosa.com) and BabyBam Collection (www.babybamcollection.com) Web sites for some cute (and quite affordable) bamboo duds. Kiddopotamus also makes a bamboo SwaddleMe adjustable infant wrap (www.kiddopotamus.com).
- *Hemp.* This is a durable fiber that comes from the fast-growing hemp plant. Like cotton, hemp fabrics breathe well. Most of the hemp you'll find for Baby will be in the cloth diaper world. BabyKicks (www.babykicks.com), and Swaddlebees (www.swaddlebees.com) make hemp-based cloth diapers.
- *Soy.* Soy fiber is made from pulp left over from the production of tofu, soy milk, and other soy products, so it's a very sustainable textile fiber. The finished product is soft and durable. To our knowledge, Babysoy (www.babysoyusa.com) is the only company using this thread to make baby clothes.

## AVOIDING FABRIC CHEMICALS

The chemicals used to treat and process certain fabrics can put Baby's health at risk and muck up the environment, too. Here's a quick guide to avoiding chemicals in Baby's wardrobe:

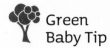

**Green Baby Tip**

You can find recycled polyester made from PET plastic beverage bottles (the ones with recycle code 1). Pixel Organics brand (www.pixelorganics.com) uses this recycled polyester as a filler in their organic cotton crib bumpers and quilts.

| Chemical to Avoid and Where It's Found | Why It's a Concern | Ways to Avoid It |
|---|---|---|
| Chlorine bleach, used to whiten cottons | Releases dioxin, a potent cancer-causing chemical | Choose unbleached cottons when they are available. |
| Flame retardants, found in some sleepwear for babies older than 9 months | Accumulate in fatty tissue and breast milk, may affect brain and nervous system development | Choose organic cotton sleepwear, or make sure you choose the tight-fitting cotton PJs offered by nonorganic brands.<br><br>You'll know there's no flame retardant if you see a bright yellow warning label that says, "For child's safety, garment should fit snugly. This garment is not flame resistant. Loose-fitting garment is more likely to catch fire" or "Not intended for sleepwear" printed on the clothing label. |
| Antimicrobial agent triclosan, found in some socks | Endocrine disrupter; may be contributing to antibiotic-resistant bacteria problem | Skip any clothing or fabric gear that is treated with triclosan (it will be on the label). |
| Harsh dyes and other toxic chemicals | Variety of potential health effects, including skin irritation and toxicity to various organs | You can look for a label that indicates the product has Oeko-Tex Standard 100 certification, which means that the fabric is free of the 100 substances commonly used in textiles that are known to be harmful to human health. You can also read labels to find nontoxic pigments and dyes. |

# Taking It Home . . .

## THE HEALTHY BABY CARE AND GEAR SUMMARY

| Gear | Green and Health Options |
|---|---|
| Diapers | Organic cloth diapers or eco-friendly disposables like gDiapers, or low-SAP bleach-free diapers from Seventh Generation, Nature Babycare, Tushies, and Whole Foods 365 Everyday Value. |
| Wipes | Make your own out of organic cotton strips or cloths, or buy chlorine-free, fragrance-free brands and use fewer. |
| Bath and body products | Look out for concerning chemical ingredients, and choose all-natural and organic products whenever you can. |
| Furniture | Choose solid wood when you can. If you buy pressed wood, look for low-VOC and formaldehyde-free products with nontoxic finishes. |
| Mattresses | Choose all-natural mattresses made with wool, natural latex, and organic fibers instead of traditional mattresses that contain synthetic flame retardants. |
| Rugs | Opt for small all-natural fiber throw rugs instead of wall-to-wall carpet or large synthetic rugs. |
| Toys | Avoid PVC and paint that could contain lead. Opt for safe plastics or all-natural materials like solid wood with nontoxic finishes, natural rubber, organic fabric toys. |
| Clothes and bedding | Choose organic cotton, bamboo, or hemp. Look for nontoxic processes and fabric dyes. Avoid polyester pajamas treated with flame retardants. |

# 9

# A Happy Home

*Making a Clean and Green Home for Baby*

I n the last chapter we focused on baby *stuff*. Now we will expand your green efforts for the rest of the house. Remember way back in chapter 1 when we discussed the importance of limiting chemical exposures during infancy in today's world? Baby's brain is growing and her immune system is developing. It's critical to keep her body as clean as possible during these early years. So much of what you do around the house can affect Baby's health. We will show you how to make your daily cleaning and living routine greener to decrease Baby's exposure to cleaning chemicals and other household dangers.

But remember, this isn't all just about Baby. We all have a responsibility to the planet. Now that you are asking the planet to support another life, you can give back to the earth in many ways. We will show you how to reduce your baby-related waste and make your home more energy efficient and environmentally responsible as you take good care of your family.

We know that you've been learning so many new ideas throughout this book. The lessons we'll share with you in this chapter are fairly easy (. . . ish). It's going to take some effort, but your baby will grow up living these changes. That means her family will do all this and more when she grows up. OK, we just jumped ahead a little. Let's back up and talk about changes you and Baby can make starting today.

## Green Cleaning

Before we launch into the gloomy tale of how your conventional cleaning products are dangerous for Baby and how the air in your home may be a hundred times more polluted than the air outside,[1] we'll give you the good news: Green cleaning is probably one of the easiest green changes you can make after Baby arrives. It's just a matter of picking out some green cleaning products (store bought or homemade), learning some new techniques, and then using them. There's nothing you need to update as Baby gets older, and there aren't a lot of complicated situations to navigate. It's a do-it-and-forget-it kind of thing.

It's actually ironic that the cleaning we do to keep Baby away from dirt and germs could actually harm her. The fact is that conventional cleaning supplies are a smorgasbord of toxic chemicals, such as chlorine compounds, phosphates, and solvents. And we don't know about your baby, but ours love to lick and chew on things they aren't supposed to—windowsills, toys, and the floor. If you use harsh chemicals to clean something in your home, Baby could be right behind you, ready to put it into her mouth.

Then there's the pollution issue. Lots of conventional cleaning products are made with petroleum-based ingredients, production of which causes emissions of carbon dioxide and release of toxic chemicals into the environment. When you use these products in your home, they pollute your indoor air with volatile organic compounds (VOCs), synthetic fragrances, and other chemicals that can irritate Baby's lungs. And if the cleaning products aren't disposed of properly, chemicals could leach into your community's groundwater or get into rivers and streams and hurt aquatic life.

Fortunately (or maybe unfortunately), it doesn't mean you have to stop cleaning. You just have to clean in a healthier and greener way. We know you're busy with the whole new baby gig right now and maybe you don't feel up to doing a complete cleaning overhaul. To make it easy we've broken green cleaning down for you into four different shades of green. Pick whichever shade you're feeling right now, and then come back once you're ready to do more.

## THE PALEST GREEN CLEAN: AVOID THE REALLY BAD STUFF

Take the smallest step toward greener cleaning by not buying the things that are most dangerous—the ones containing the most toxins and poisons that are dangerous if touched, even potentially lethal if ingested. Some cleaning chemicals are solvents that irritate the lungs and skin. Others, like synthetic perfumes and dyes, can be allergens. And still other cleaning chemicals are hormone disrupters, like the alkylphenol ethoxylates found in some laundry detergents. It puts Baby's health at risk even to have many of these nasty chemicals around the house.

It would be so much easier if we could give you a list of specific ingredients that we know are harmful and you could just take it with you to the store. Well, if we gave you the ingredient list it wouldn't really do you much good. You won't find cleaning product ingredients listed on the labels because manufacturers don't have to disclose them (what's up with that?). It's a shame, too, because some of these ingredients are kind of scary! Since you can't look for specific ingredients on labels, use these tips to find safer options to replace the worst cleaning chemicals:

| Product or Ingredient to Avoid | Why? | How to Find a Safer Option |
|---|---|---|
| Anything that has "Danger" or "Poison" on the label | The product contains a toxic or corrosive chemical. | Choose a product that doesn't have this kind of warning on the label. |

| | | |
|---|---|---|
| Conventional drain cleaners | These are highly corrosive and harmful or fatal if swallowed. Also highly irritating to the skin and eyes. | Pouring boiling water into the drain may help clear a grease-based clog. Or try enzyme-based cleaners like Biokleen's Bac-Out (biokleenhome.com) or Earthworm Family-Safe Drain Cleaner (acleanearth.com). |
| Conventional oven cleaners | These emit irritating vapors and are highly corrosive. | Use baking soda: Make a thick paste with baking soda and water. Apply to any spots that need cleaning. Leave on overnight. Clean off the paste and rinse off any white residue. |
| Colorants, dyes, and synthetic perfumes—used in laundry soaps | Certain types of these chemicals can cause adverse reactions, including allergies, and they may even be carcinogens. | They won't be on the labels, so look for products that specifically say "Dye free" and "Fragrance free" or one that specifies all-natural scents only. |
| Dishwashing detergents containing phosphates | Phosphates get into waterways and lead to algae blooms, which kill fish and other aquatic life. | Choose one labeled "Phosphate free." |
| Chlorine bleach | Irritates eyes, skin, and lungs; responsible for thousands of poisoning incidents in children each year; creates harmful chloramine gas when mixed with ammonia from other cleaning products. | Look for nonchlorine bleach products. Most are made with hydrogen peroxide, a nontoxic bleach. |
| Antibacterial hand soaps containing triclosan | Triclosan contributes to the rise of antibiotic-resistant bacteria and doesn't even clean better than regular soap. | Use regular hand soap instead and wash properly—rub sudsy hands together for at least 15 seconds before rinsing. |

## A LITTLE GREENER: DO MORE TO MINIMIZE THE EFFECTS OF YOUR CLEANING

If you want to take green cleaning a little further, take steps to minimize the effects of your conventional cleaning products and techniques on Baby's health and on the environment. Whether you're using all-natural or synthetic products, here are some green cleaning best practices:

- No matter how "safe" a cleaning product is, keep it away from Baby. Store cleaning products—even homemade and all-natural ones—on a high shelf or in a locked cabinet.
- Because so many household chemicals contain volatile organic compounds (VOCs), make sure to properly ventilate the house when you're cleaning. Open windows and/or turn on a fan to circulate the air.
- Use fewer products. If something can be wiped away with some water on a sponge, don't spray a harsh disinfectant on it.
- Wear gloves. Even nontoxic cleaners can still be tough on the skin.
- After you use any cleaning product that contains chemicals, do an extra swipe with a clean wet rag to remove any remaining chemical residue.
- When you throw away a chemical product, dispose of it properly. Check out www.earth911.org for instructions.
- For cleaning products that you use regularly, choose the largest package available. Bulk packaging is typically cheaper for you and better for the environment because it requires less plastic and fewer trips to the store.
- Look for products packaged in recycled and recyclable packaging.
- If you're cleaning with conventional products, it's best to use only one at a time—especially in small spaces like bathrooms. Be particularly careful not to mix products that contain bleach (like certain laundry products and some bath and kitchen

## Don't Give Baby a Chemical Bath

Before giving Baby a bath in the tub, give it a quick rinse to wash away any residue left over from when the tub was last cleaned. You know Baby is going to be drinking some of that bath water, so this precaution limits what she swallows in addition to decreasing chemical exposure to her skin.

cleaners) and ammonia (found in glass cleaners and some dishwashing liquids) because the mixture creates a gas called chloramine, which irritates the lungs and can cause coughing and choking.

## EVEN GREENER: MAKE THE SWITCH TO GREEN CLEANING SUPPLIES

Go a little further down the green path and make the switch to all-natural green cleaning products and practices. Greener cleaners are made from plant-based and all-natural ingredients instead of petroleum-based ingredients. These products should be dye free and fragrance free or contain fragrances made only from essential oils and not synthetic perfumes. Take a closer look at your cleaning tools, too. Paper towels are definitely the easiest to reach for, but most paper towel brands are made from virgin paper, which in essence means that trees were cut down just to make the product. Plus, most white paper products like standard paper towels are bleached, causing the release of toxic chemicals into our environment. Instead of buying bleached virgin paper products, use paper towels made from recycled unbleached paper instead. According to the Natural Resources Defense Council, if every

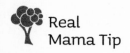

### Real Mama Tip

. . . . . . . . . . . . . . . . . . . . . .

"Instead of using chemicals on my tile floors I use a steam cleaner. The steam cleans the dirt and sanitizes the floor. My baby can crawl on the floor and I don't have to worry."

—*Yvonne, Phoenix, Arizona*

household in America switched *just one roll* of their virgin paper towels for a roll of towels made from 100 percent recycled paper, 544,000 trees would be saved.[2]

Here are some key things to look for when you're choosing better cleaning supplies:

- If there's no "warning," "caution," "poison," or "danger" warning on a product's label, the federal government doesn't consider the product to be hazardous to your health. (Depending on your level of skepticism toward our government regulators, this may or may not make you feel better, but at least it's a start.)
- Choose products made from vegetable-based and organic ingredients (with the absence of the harmful ingredients highlighted above).
- Choose paper products made from recycled paper. One hundred percent postconsumer recycled paper is the greenest option.
- Buy from companies who are committed to the environment. To learn about a cleaning product company's environmental track record and practices, you can visit www.goodguide.com.

There are so many brands and types to choose from, whether you go to a natural market or a mainstream one. Here are some of the products that have fared best in product tests by journalists, evaluations by the EPA, and label reviews by us:

| Cleaning Product | A Selection of Top Green Cleaning Products |
| --- | --- |
| Laundry detergent | Planet laundry detergent (www.planetinc.com)<br>Seventh Generation Free & Clear (www.seventhgeneration.com)<br>Method 3X Concentrated Detergent (Free & Clear) |
| Laundry stain remover | Shout Trigger Laundry Stain Remover (www.shoutitout.com) |

| | |
|---|---|
| Dryer sheets | Nellie's Dryerballs (www.nelliesallnatural.com) |
| Wood floors and furniture cleaner | Murphy Oil Soap (www.murphyoilsoap.colgate.com) |
| Glass and surface cleaners | Seventh Generation Natural Glass & Surface Cleaner |
| | Earth Friendly Products Window Kleener with vinegar (www.ecos.com) |
| | Green Works Natural Glass & Surface Cleaner (www.greenworkscleaners.com) |
| Tub and sink cleaner | Bon Ami Polishing Cleanser (www.bonami.com) |
| | 20 Mule Team Borax (www.20muleteamlaundry.com) |
| Toilet cleaner | Method Lil' Bowl Blu (www.methodhome.com) |
| General cleaners | Earth Friendly Products Orange Plus Ready-to-Use Surface Cleaner |
| | Seventh Generation All-Purpose Cleaner |
| | Green Works Natural All-Purpose Cleaner |
| | Method All-Surface Cleaner (Go Naked) |
| | BabyGanics All-Purpose Household Cleaner (unscented) (www.babyganics.com) |
| Granite countertop cleaner | Method Daily Granite polish |
| Paper towels and napkins | Seventh Generation 100 percent recycled unbleached paper towels |

Sources: EPA's Design for the Environment program-recognized products in "How 'Green' Cleaners Measure Up," *Washington Post*, April 19, 2007, http://www.washingtonpost.com/wp-srv/artsandliving/homeandgarden/features/2007/green-cleaners-041907/chart.html; and Sarah Van Schagen, "I Don't Want No Scrub: A Test of Eight Green Bathroom-Cleaning Products," *Grist*, March 25, 2008, http://www.grist.org/advice/products/2008/03/25/).

## THE DEEPEST SHADE OF GREEN: HOMEMADE CLEANING PRODUCTS AND DROPPING THE DISPOSABLES

The final stop on our green cleaning tour is making homemade cleaning supplies and avoiding all unnecessary cleaning-related waste by

# How Clean Does Baby's Environment Have to Be?

You will probably be surprised to learn that the everyday germs that Baby may be exposed to around the house are probably harmless. Yes, you can let your baby lick the floor. Of course, I can never get any first-time parent to trust me on this, and you're probably no exception. It's funny watching various parents in my office. I can always tell the first babies from a third or fourth baby. First-time moms are very protective, with Baby wrapped in a blanket and a box of disinfectant wipes ready to use in case Baby touches something outside the blanket. Veteran moms have learned not to worry about this—I actually see some let their baby roll around on my office floor, licking away! There's no right or wrong level of germ protection. The main germs you *should* try to minimize are cold and flu viruses that may float around in public areas. So be as careful as you want to be when you are out. Just don't feel that Baby's home life has to be sterile, and don't let it be a source of stress for you.

using reusable tools instead of disposable ones. Homemade all-natural cleaning solutions are like home remedies for your house. It's so much easier than you may think to make them and so much cheaper, too. Plus, you can take a breath of fresh air and relief in knowing you're keeping chemicals out of Baby's reach and out of the ecosystem.

Simple homemade cleaning solutions contain one or more of just a few key ingredients: white vinegar (just your basic vinegar—like what you might use to make salad dressing), baking soda (not baking *powder*), and water (from the tap is fine!). To boost the cleaning power of these ingredients many recipes have you add a little liquid castile soap. And if you really crave pleasant scents, you can also add a drop of your favorite essential oil (eucalyptus, lavender, etc.) to many of the solutions. If you're ready to go all out with the homemade and all-natural cleaning solutions, check out Annie Berthold-Bond's classic book *Better Basics for the Home*.

To start cleaning with some basic homemade mixtures you'll need to buy a few spray bottles, a large container of distilled white vinegar, and a box of baking soda. You may want to get started with a batch of all-purpose cleaner and/or glass cleaner to just keep in the cupboard. Other solutions can be made up on the spot, so to speak. Here are some specific recipes you can use:

## Vinegar: For All-Purpose Cleaning, Making Things Sparkle, and Even Killing Germs

| *Cleaning Need* | *Vinegar Recipe* |
| --- | --- |
| Baby's new toy has a sticky spot where the price tag used to be. | All-purpose cleaner: Mix equal parts vinegar and water. Add a drop of castile soap for added cleaning power. |
| Oops! Baby stained the carpet. | Stain remover: Mix 1 teaspoon vinegar, 2 cups water, 1 teaspoon castile liquid soap in a bowl. Apply to the stain and scrub with a brush or rag. Rinse with wet towel and blot dry. Repeat until stain is gone. Dry with a fan or blow dryer. |
| Baby kissed her reflection in the window, and now there are spots. | Glass cleaner: Mix ¼ cup vinegar and ¾ cup water in a spray bottle. Spray on window. Wipe off with rag or newspaper. |
| The no-wax floor under Baby's high chair is disgusting! | Floor cleaner: Mix ½ cup vinegar, ½ gallon warm water in a bucket, and mop away! |
| The play group is coming over, and the toilet is less than sparkly. | Toilet bowl cleaners:<br><br>Spray with straight vinegar and brush vigorously.<br><br>Add 3 cups of vinegar to the bowl. Let sit for 30 minutes. Flush. |

## Baking Soda: For Getting Rid of Odors and Scouring

| The Smelly or Grimy Thing You Need to Clean | How to Use Baking Soda to Do It |
|---|---|
| Baby's crib, changing table, or high chair; the kitchen counter, bathtub, and sinks | Sprinkle baking soda on a wet sponge or rag. Scrub. |
| Smelly diaper pail | Occasionally sprinkle baking soda into the bottom of the pail or on top of the diapers themselves. (And empty the diaper pail every day or so to avoid odors.) |
| Smelly carpet or rug | Sprinkle baking soda on the smell. Let sit 15 minutes and then vacuum. |

### Beyond Wipes and Paper Towels

It's pretty darned easy to reach for a premoistened cleaning wipe or grab a paper towel for a quick cleanup. But it's also pretty easy to reach for something else, if it's readily available. So outfit your cleaning closet with some of these eco-friendlier options:

- *Natural sponges:* Avoid synthetic materials and sponges treated with antibacterial chemicals. Instead, try all-natural sponges like the EcoSponge by Pacific Dry Goods (www.pacificdry goods.com) or natural cellulose sponges by Twist (www .twistclean.com) or Casabella (www.casabella.com), among others. Since sponges will hold onto bacteria that could grow mold or mildew, clean them regularly either on the top shelf of the dishwasher or microwave the wet sponge for one to two minutes—steam should be coming off it.
- *Rags:* Rip up old T-shirts (if you're not using them for diaper wipes!) and use as cleaning rags. Or buy reusable cloths made from microfiber. Yes, they're made from a petroleum-based fabric (nylon and polyester), but using them instead of paper towels will save so many trees that it's a worthy tradeoff. If you

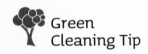 **Green Cleaning Tip**

When a homemade cleaner recipe calls for castile soap, it's not referring to a particular brand of soap. Castile soaps are natural soaps made mostly from olive oil. You can find a variety of brands at a good natural food or home store.

# CLEANING UP THE SUPER-YUCK

## Disinfecting Tips

With a baby in the house you're going to be confronted by truly yucky messes: Poop that has escaped the diaper. Vomit. Goopy sneezes. Ick. In these situations you might feel the urge to reach for the bleach and disinfect everything in sight. But just because you need to really kill the germs doesn't mean you need harsher chemicals.

- Use tea tree oil, a natural disinfectant, to disinfect hard surfaces. Mix two teaspoons of tea tree oil with two cups water in a spray bottle, shake to blend, and then spray. Don't rinse. This mixture also works well to kill mold. (Beware: Tea tree oil is perfectly safe for humans but it's toxic to cats.)
- Another simple disinfecting method: Put 3 percent hydrogen peroxide (the basic type you can find at the drugstore) in one spray bottle and undiluted white vinegar in another. Spray the two on whatever needs disinfecting, one right after another. Lab tests show this combo kills salmonella, shigella, and *E. coli* just as well as harsher chemicals.

really prefer natural fabrics, choose cloths made from bamboo by Pacific Dry Goods or Twist (Web sites noted above).

## MORE CLEANING TIPS

In addition to choosing greener cleaning supplies, here are more ways to keep Baby's home clean safely:

- Adopt a no-shoe policy. Many of the chemicals, dirt, allergens, and germs in your home are tracked in on your shoes. Removing shoes at the door is one of the best ways to cut Baby's exposure.
- Remove unnecessary clutter. Not only does a clutter-free home help you clear your mind, it's also a good way to cut down on dust, so it's good for Baby's lungs.

# DON'T BE GREEN-WASHED
# BY GREEN LABEL CLAIMS

| *Claims that Sound Nice but Don't Mean Much* | *Claims that Sound Nice* and *Mean Something* |
|---|---|
| "Biodegradable": Misleading because most ingredients are biodegradable, but it doesn't mean we want the breakdown by-products floating around our rivers and streams.<br><br>"Natural": There's no official definition of what this means.<br><br>"Nontoxic": Not meaningful because there's no regulated definition. | "Green Seal Certified": This seal indicates that the product meets certain health and environmental standards, including being nontoxic and made in an eco-friendly facility. It's a very reputable seal but not too common yet, so it shouldn't be your only gauge of safety.<br><br>"Phosphate free" or "Contains no phosphates": Look for this label on dishwashing detergents. (All laundry soaps in the United States are phosphate-free.)<br><br>"Organic": If a product is made with organic ingredients, they will be clearly stated on the label, and the product may or may not bear the USDA Organic seal. |

Source: *Consumer Reports*, www.greenerchoices.org.

- To avoid mildew and mold in the bathroom, open a window or use a fan to ventilate the room, and wash your towels and bath mat regularly.
- Always clean from the top down. Dust high shelves and work your way down to the floor. Allow dust to settle before you vacuum.
- Don't let people smoke in your home. Secondhand smoke from a cigarette contains thousands of chemicals that pollute your air.

- Use a vacuum outfitted with a HEPA filter. It's most effective at trapping allergens like dust and other tiny particles that can pollute your indoor air.
- Skip the air fresheners. These products emit VOCs into the air. In one large study, infants in homes where an air freshener was used regularly had more diarrhea and earaches than infants in other homes. The Mamas who used air freshener also reported having more headaches.[3] To deal with odors, open a box of baking soda and set it in the smelly area. Or scent the air with a natural room spray like Method's Aroma Spray or fragrance oil diffuser reeds.
- Choose candles wisely. If you use candles to set the mood or to scent the air, be aware that most household candles are made with paraffin wax, which emits toxic solvents like benzene and toluene into the air. Instead, choose candles made from soy or beeswax and scented with natural oils. They're safer, not to mention that they are more eco-friendly than paraffin candles, which are made from petroleum—a nonrenewable resource.

## Greening the Rest of the House: Waste Reduction and Energy Conservation

Here's a question for you: What have you thrown in your garbage today? A few disposable diapers and wipes, some paper towels, a cereal box, an empty diaper cream tube? The average American throws away about 4.5 pounds of waste per day. If you're like us, your garbage pails fill up faster now that you have a baby under your roof. This is partly because Baby requires you to have more stuff, like diapering supplies, toys, extra food, etc. Disposable diapers and wipes definitely take up some trash can space, but even if you never use a single disposable product you're still generating more packaging waste than you did before. You may also be eating and entertaining at home more than you did before, leading to yet more garbage.

So, here's where we come to the well-known green living mantra:

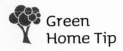

"Reduce, reuse, and recycle." If you take a good look at your purchases and household behaviors and begin to live by this credo, the benefits are great—for the earth, for you, and for Baby:

- You'll send less garbage to our overflowing landfills
- There will be less trash from your home that can escape from the pail, truck, or landfill and become litter
- Your household will drain the planet of fewer natural resources
- You'll be protecting wildlife and their habitats from the effects of unchecked household waste
- By not overindulging Baby with unnecessary stuff you'll be discouraging materialism

There are probably hundreds of ways to reduce, reuse, and recycle when it comes to raising a green baby. So far in earlier chapters we've talked about minimizing food waste, choosing reusable bags instead of plastic bags at the market, buying recyclable food packages, buying fewer toys, and buying certain products in bulk, just to name a few ideas. Here are even more ways for you and Baby to lighten the planet's load, starting at home.

## REDUCE

In an era where every company is trying to win the hearts of green consumers—especially the ones with new babies—and there are green products for every need and every occasion, we can lose track of a basic tenet of green living, which is to consume less. It's not about finding green products to buy; it's about buying less to begin with! When you reduce your consumption of stuff, you reduce your impact on natural resources and your contribution to the stream of waste that ends up in landfills and incinerators. According to Annie Leonard's wonderfully informative film *The Story of Stuff* (www.storyofstuff.org), to make and transport the stuff that would fill up one garbage can in your home, about seventy garbage cans worth of waste was created further upstream.

In order to reduce how much you're throwing out, you have to be more careful about what you buy and skip the things you don't need. Some baby-related products are clearly unnecessary—like the diaper wipes warmer. I'm pretty sure Baby will survive a room temperature wipe. Or the bottle warmer—you can warm a bottle in a bowl of hot water just as easily. Remember that most of the things that you bring into your home will eventually be discarded, so think twice before bringing them in in the first place.

## Reduction Tips

- *Buy less plastic for Baby:* Of all the materials to reduce consumption of, plastic is a good one. The production of many plastics requires petroleum, a nonrenewable resource. Plastics production also releases toxic pollutants and greenhouse gas emissions into the atmosphere, and the disposal of plastics leads to piles of trash that will never biodegrade and the potential leaching of chemicals from our landfills. Choose wooden toys, stainless steel sippy cups, and glass jars of food instead of their plastic counterparts.
- *Fend off junk mail:* After Baby arrives, the catalogs start showing up in the mail. How did they even find out that Baby joined the household? Who knows? While you can certainly recycle magazines and catalogs, it's even better to go straight to the source to stop them from showing up at all. Call the company and ask to be removed from its mailing list. Or go to Web sites like www .catalogchoice.com and www.dmachoice.com to register as a person who doesn't want the direct marketing mail. You'll have to log in, give your name, and provide some information from the mailing label of the catalog you no longer want. After several weeks you'll start to notice a drop in catalog mail.
- *Visit the library:* Some books are worth having for your personal collection, but sometimes it makes more sense to just borrow one from the library. You can even browse recent parenting magazines and borrow movies from your local library.
- *Think twice about disposables:* Pack Baby's lunch in a reusable

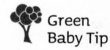

**Green Baby Tip**

Consider skipping the baby birth announcements or at the very least pick one made from 100 percent postconsumer recycled paper and printed with eco-friendly processes. Better yet, send designed e-mails to alert everyone of your special delivery.

## Cloth Napkins Instead of Paper

With three boys to feed, you can imagine how many paper napkins we would go through and recycle every day. So a few years ago we stopped using paper napkins in our house and pulled out all those cloth napkins that had been sitting in our dining room hutch for years. This is a perfect example of where it's better to *reduce* than to recycle. Half the time the kids don't even use their napkin (their shirt or pants work just as well for wiping their hands, right?). And when this happens we just throw the cloth napkins back onto the clean pile to use again.

container instead of plastic bags. Use real plates instead of paper ones, real bibs instead of single-use disposable ones. Choose rags and cloth towels instead of paper ones.

- *Fix rather than replace:* Put an iron-on patch on a pair of play pants with a holey knee instead of buying a new pair. When Baby's sippy cup loses a valve, search online for a replacement instead of buying a whole new cup.

### REUSE

Here's a good habit to get into: before you throw anything away, ask yourself if you could use it for something else, or if someone else could use it instead. Baby will outgrow shoes, toys, and clothes so fast it will make your head spin. If you think you may have another baby one day, save anything that's in good shape so it can be used again. If you don't have the storage space or a future need for the stuff, pass it along to a younger niece or nephew, a friend, or donate it to needy strangers.

In your town there are probably several collection centers for toys, clothes, and other household items. Ask around at schools, synagogues, churches, mosques, and hospitals for suggestions.

You can also tap into your Mama network to make the most of Baby's stuff. Whether you want to get rid of outgrown things or toys or clothes that you're tired of, chances are that someone in your group of friends would want it. Host a toy exchange or clothing swap. Or ask friends and family for hand-me-downs instead of new things for Baby's birthday or holidays. If you'd rather make some money off the stuff (nothing wrong with that kind of green!), get a bunch of families in your neighborhood together for a big yard sale or sell your things to a consignment shop or on eBay.

Make the most of other people's old stuff, too. If you need something, especially something that you'll only need for a short time (e.g., an infant swing or a stationary play center), ask around to see if you can borrow it. It's not so hard to find people who are looking to get rid of the things that you need. Join a network like Freecycle (www.freecycle.org) or visit community bulletin boards (real ones or the online variety like www.craigslist.org) to find what you need.

Some items in your home won't be so obviously reusable, but you can often find new uses for your garbage:

| What's Old . . . | . . . Is New Again |
| --- | --- |
| Outgrown cloth diapers and burp cloths | Cleaning rags |
| Old socks | Fill with potpourri and use as drawer fresheners |
| Baby food jars | Storage for small items like rubber bands, sewing supplies, craft supplies, nails and screws |
| Shoe boxes | Gift boxes, school art projects for older children |
| Stained discarded baby clothes | Cleaning rags |
| Discarded paper from the mail or from work | Scrap paper for Baby to draw on with crayons or for your grocery lists |

# Should You Reuse Shoes?

When our first child was born, the salesman at the baby shoe store told us we shouldn't hand down our child's shoes to the next child because the shoe specifically molds to the child's foot. I thought that was very clever—we'd have to come back to buy new shoes for each child. Well, we didn't buy it. Reusing shoes is just fine for infants and toddlers. As our kids got older, though, we found they were wearing out their shoes faster than they would outgrow them, so we eventually had to put each child in new shoes. But one way we found to save a bundle of money (and conserve resources) is to reuse soccer, baseball, and football cleats. Our kids outgrow them every year or two, and they still look barely used. I take great joy in pulling out a pair of used cleats from our cleat box for the younger kids, not just because I save seventy-five dollars, but also because I'm putting less manufacturing strain on the planet. I know your baby isn't quite at this point yet, but when you get there be sure to save those cleats.

Another way we reuse shoes is in my pediatric office. We have a big box in which we collect used shoes from patients. Every month one of our staff members goes down to Mexico to do charity work for kids and families, and she takes that big box with her. What a great way to reuse shoes!

## RECYCLE

Even if you *have* to bring it into your house (i.e., you can't reduce) and you can't find a way to reuse it, sometimes you can at least recycle it. When we recycle we prevent the need for the extraction of virgin materials to make new products from scratch, and we reduce the flow of trash to the landfills and incinerators. Recycling saves natural resources and reduces pollution. The materials we recycle are used to make consumer products like paper goods, packaging, beverage containers, plastic bottles, furniture, and even innovative building materials. Americans are recycling more than ever before and reaping the benefits:

- Keeping plastics and other materials out of the landfill prevents the leaching of chemicals into nearby groundwater sources and soil.
- Keeping plastics out of incinerators prevents the release of toxic chemicals into the air.
- It's estimated that in 2007 American recycling saved the equivalent of more than ten billion gallons of gasoline.[4]
- The seven million tons of metal (e.g., aluminum and steel cans, metal hangers) we recycled in 2007 provided a reduction in greenhouse gas emissions equivalent to taking 4.5 million cars off the road.[4]
- Every pound of paper we recycle eliminates four pounds of $CO_2$ emissions.[5]

Many towns and cities these days have curbside pickup recycling programs, and most others have drop-off centers (so there's really no excuse for not doing it). Recycling policies vary from place to place, and some programs actually fine you if you break the rules, so it's important to know how your town's recycling program works. For example, some programs take any plastics with certain numbers on the bottom, others recycle only plastic beverage containers (New York City, for example, recycles plastic bottles and jugs but not wide-mouth plastic containers like margarine tubs and yogurt cups). Most recycling programs won't take bottle tops, spray tops, or other covers and request that you rinse out your recyclables and separate the different types of materials. To figure out what you need to do, call your town's public works or sanitation department.

Besides recycling discarded items from your home, try also to buy

A NOTE FROM DR. BOB

## Recycling in the Home Offers Many Teachable Moments

In our kitchen we have a blue trash can (for recycling) and a white one (for trash). Our kids constantly ask us, "Blue or white?" whenever they throw something away. This gives them the opportunity to get used to what items can be recycled and what can't, so it gets ingrained in them early on. It also allows us to make comments like, "Yeah, you just saved a tree" or "Good job—less air pollution next week!"

things that are themselves recycled. This is easy to do for some types of products like household paper products. The Natural Resources Defense Council (NRDC) estimates that if every household switched one package of regular napkins for a package of napkins made from 100 percent postconsumer recycled paper, one million trees would be saved (even more if you switched to cloth). Companies like Seventh Generation make household paper products from 100 percent recycled paper, and kitchen and trash bags from 55 to 80 percent recycled plastics.

### Recycling Tips

- Think about recycling before you even buy a product. Choose packages that are recyclable over ones that are not.
- Don't forget about household items like metal hangers, electronics, printer cartridges—all may be recycled. Some communities have annual pickup days for items like these. Ask your local government or community association.

## KEEPING IT GREEN IN BABY'S BACKYARD

If Baby is lucky enough to have a front or backyard, it will be a place for her to play and relax and get to know the natural world. If you use pesticides, harsh weed killers, or chemical fertilizers to maintain your patch of planet, it's time to rethink your methods. Organic lawn care and safer pest control techniques will keep harmful chemicals away from Baby and out of the surrounding waterways and animal habitats. *The Organic Lawn Care Manual* by Paul Tukey has a wealth of information for homeowners who want a healthy, safe, and beautiful lawn. And don't forget to keep harsh chemicals off your porch, driveway, and deck, too, because rainwater will carry these chemicals onto your lawn eventually.

- Once you find out your community's recycling rules, post them near your recycling bins or label your bins with exactly what's allowed to go in them.
- Try not to contaminate your recyclables with other garbage. It increases the costs of the recycling program and reduces the benefits.

# Energy and Water: Waste Not, Want Not

Certain aspects of greening your home provide clear and immediate benefits for Baby, like reducing your use of household chemicals, using more natural baby gear, and serving organic foods. Now let's turn to something with a more indirect but still crucial effect on Baby's well-being: energy and water conservation. When you make an effort to conserve energy and water, the benefits may not be as immediately evident. But if you look at the big picture (and your utility bills), the upside will become clear. Making an effort to use and waste less electricity and water benefits the planet in the long term, and that's good for Baby, too.

Electricity and water flow into your home with such ease that it's easy to forget how precious they are. Most of our electricity comes from the burning of the fossil fuels coal and oil, both nonrenewable resources in finite supply. The generation of our electricity at fossil-fuel-burning power plants releases carbon dioxide, nitrogen, nitrous oxides, and sulfur oxides into the atmosphere. Coal-burning power plants also emit ash and mercury. The pollution from power plants contributes to global climate change and acid rain, and threatens wildlife and their habitats.

Water, though technically renewable because it falls from the sky as rain and snow, is actually in short supply because we use it faster than it replenishes. Plus, water use is closely tied to energy use and water pollution:

- The treatment and pumping of the water that goes into our homes requires fifty-six billion kilowatt-hours of power annually—that's enough to power five million homes for a whole year.[6]
- Using too much water increases water pollution because sewage and waste treatment systems may become overloaded.
- Taking too much water out of the water supply changes the flow of rivers and streams, and can affect the health and survival of wildlife.

American households use about seventy gallons of water a day per person, and it's estimated that up to 10 percent of household water is wasted—water just running down the drain and leaking from the plumbing.[7] Your family can conserve water by fixing leaks and installing water-saving features like high-efficiency toilets (HET toilets) and low-flow showerheads. If all households used these water-saving features, Americans could save more than five billion gallons of water a day.[8] You'll also save lots of water simply by being smarter about how you use it.

With Baby around you're probably using more energy and water than you used to. If you (or a caregiver) stay in your home with Baby each day, chances are your air-conditioning or heat are on a lot. You may have more lights on around the house. There are more dishes to do.

And way more laundry. Some of the household changes you can make to conserve water and electricity do take time and money and equipment, such as installing low-flow showerheads, insulating the water heater, replacing old windows, and fixing leaky plumbing. But so many other changes are just a matter of being more conscious and changing your habits, for example, turning off the lights when you leave a room, un-plugging appliances when they aren't in use, and washing more of your laundry with cold water instead of hot.

## ROOM-BY-ROOM ENERGY AND WATER CONSERVATION TIPS

### Kitchen

Nowhere else do you have so many appliances in one place and so many opportunities to conserve:

- When you buy new kitchen appliances choose ones with the Energy Star label.
- Make sure the appliances you already have are working in the most efficient way. If they are more than ten or fifteen years old you may want to consider just buying new. Standards for energy efficiency have changed considerably since the early 1990s, and older appliances may be draining your wallet.
- Refrigerators use the most energy of any kitchen appliance. For efficiency, keep yours set to 37 to 40 degrees Fahrenheit—cold enough to keep the food safe, not so cold that you're wasting energy.
- Check to see if your refrigerator is leaking cold air. The door gasket should be tight enough to hold a dollar bill when the door is closed.
- The dishwasher is more efficient than hand washing if you skip any prerinsing, run it only when it's full, and air dry your dishes whenever possible.
- If you hand wash your dishes, fill the sink with soapy hot water instead of letting the water run while you wash.

## The Living Rooms: Baby's Room, Family Room, Office, and Playroom

Small changes in the rooms where you do most of your living can create big savings:

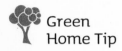

- Wherever you can, switch to energy-efficient compact fluorescent lamp (CFL) lightbulbs instead of incandescent bulbs. CFLs use 75 percent less energy and last six to ten times longer than incandescent bulbs.[9] They're so common nowadays that you'll find them anywhere lightbulbs are sold.
- Turn off the lights when you leave a room. Lighting accounts for more than ten percent of your home's energy use.[10] Every little savings can help.
- Open your blinds to let sunlight in whenever possible, especially in cold weather. On really hot days, keep them shut to keep out the warm rays of sun.
- Plug appliances like stereo and computer equipment into a power strip, and then turn the strip off when the equipment is not in use. If you don't use a power strip, unplug the equipment when you aren't using it.

### Bathroom

Toilet flushing accounts for more than one quarter of your home's water use, and pretty soon you'll have another family member using the potty. Take steps to make your bathroom more efficient:

- If you have a pre-1994 toilet, consider getting a new one with the EPA's WaterSense certification. It's a relatively inexpensive home improvement, and it could mean 60 percent less water use.
- Fix a leaking toilet to save up to two hundred gallons a day. To see if your toilet leaks, put a drop or two of food coloring into the bowl. If there's a leak, the color will show up in the tank after a minute or so.

- Don't run the water while bathing or brushing teeth. The average open faucet sends two gallons down the drain each minute.
- If you have to run the bath for a minute before the water heats up, catch this water in a bucket and use it to water the plants or grass in your yard.
- Consider replacing pre-1994 showerheads with low-flow showerheads instead.

## Laundry Room

You have to do the laundry—lots and lots of laundry! Do it better:

- Do more of your laundry in cold water. If you do 80 percent of your laundry in cold, you could save one hundred dollars per year in power bills. And switching just two of your hot loads to cold each week reduces your home's $CO_2$ emissions by five hundred pounds per year. Use hot water only for diapers, towels, sheets, and anything that Baby has pooped on. Hot water kills dust mites, mold, mildew, and bacteria.
- The washing machine is most energy and water efficient when it's run full.
- Instead of using your clothes dryer, hang things outside in the sun or in the laundry room to dry.
- If you're in the market for a new washer, choose an energy-efficient one with the government's Energy Star label. Efficient washers can save up to seven thousand gallons of water a year and can cut your utility bills by fifty dollars a year, on average.[9] (The Energy Star program doesn't qualify clothes dryers because all of them are about the same in terms of efficiency.)

## Behind the Scenes

Venture into your garage, crawl space, basement, or utility closet for even more energy and water savings. A few of these ideas take no effort and no time, but others are more of a commitment:

- If you have a programmable thermostat, use the programming feature to reduce your energy use by setting specific temperatures for sleeping and for hours when nobody is in your home.
- The U.S. Department of Energy recommends keeping your house at 68 degrees when you're home in the winter and at 60 degrees when you are away. In the summer, crank it up to 78 degrees when you're home, 85 degrees when you're away.[10]
- Use fans to circulate the air in your home instead of cranking up the A/C.
- Save on the energy it takes to heat your water by insulating your hot water heater and your plumbing.

A NOTE FROM DR. BOB

## A New Baby Doesn't Mean New Thermostat Settings

Many new parents believe that they must keep the house warmer when they have a new baby. This isn't true. Healthy full-term babies are perfectly capable of keeping themselves warm, within reason. You can add a layer of clothing if you feel your baby is a little cool. And let baby be mostly naked during hot weather. You'll know if your baby is too cold (cold hands and feet) or too hot (sweaty head) by feel. Using a heater unnecessarily will dry the air and cause Baby's nose to become irritated and stuffy. Of course, use common sense. You'll need the heater during the winter and the air conditioner during the summer to some extent. Just don't use them more simply because you now have a baby. Adjusting the thermostat by just two degrees in the winter and two degrees in the summer could save two thousand pounds of $CO_2$ emissions in one year.

- Check for plumbing leaks: Check your water meter and then use no water for the next two hours. If the meter doesn't read exactly the same amount after the two hours, you have a leak.
- Set your water heater temperature to 120 degrees. (This is also an important safety precaution to avoid scalding Baby with too-hot water from a faucet.)
- Make sure your attic or crawl space is properly insulated and sealed, especially during the winter.
- Properly maintain your air-conditioning unit(s) according to manufacturer instructions, e.g., change or clean the filters as directed.

## Outside

Up to 30 percent of your household water use may be outside in the yard, garden, and driveway.[8]

- Don't hose down your sidewalks, deck, or patio. Sweep with a broom instead.
- Let your grass grow a little taller—three inches is optimal for helping the soil to retain water.
- Don't overwater your yard. In the summer, water every three to five days (if there's no soaking rain), and in the winter, every ten to fourteen days.
- Keep your plants mulched to help the soil retain moisture.

### Green Home Tip

Planting trees around your home, particularly on the southern and western sides and around air-conditioning units, can save you energy. Trees also absorb carbon dioxide, so they help offset your family's carbon emissions.

# Taking It Home . . .

Going green is, in a sense, about cleaning up your family's lifestyle in order to help clean up the planet. Why not start at home where Baby benefits, too?

- *Clean green:* Keeping your house clean naturally is a good way to keep some toxic chemicals away from Baby—chemicals that can irritate her lungs and skin. Besides avoiding the really bad stuff, such as chemical drain cleaners and anything else labeled as poison, you can also minimize the impact of your cleaning by choosing products with more natural ingredients and reducing your use of disposable cleaning supplies like paper towels and wipes. If you want to go all the way into the green, make your own simple cleaning solutions, and use rags instead of paper products.

- *Reduce, reuse, recycle:* Cut the volume of garbage your family is sending to landfills or incinerators by taking steps like reducing your consumption of disposable items, giving your outgrown baby things to someone else to reuse, and recycling materials whenever you can.

- *Conservation and efficiency at home:* Water and electricity are both so easy to come by, it's easy to forget how precious they are and how overuse and waste is hurting the environment. Take steps in every room of the house (and outside, too) to cut your water and energy waste, and conserve these natural resources.

## PART FOUR

# More
# Happy
# Habits

# 10

# Check, Please

## A Checklist for Baby and Toddler Wellness

Y ou have learned all about going green for yourself, your baby, and your planet. We've focused on nutrition, exercise, relaxation, and organic environmentally friendly living. When looking at the whole child you can't forget about basic healthy habits to complete the picture of a healthy baby and toddler. This chapter provides a checklist of the health-promoting preventive steps that will help keep Baby healthy today and in the future. With practical tips for how to incorporate some of these healthy lifestyle changes into busy lives, this chapter will help you understand all the main aspects of prevention for babies and toddlers up to age two: healthy behaviors, active lifestyle, stress management, good hygiene, plenty of sleep, and preventive medical services.

Picture the healthy lifestyle you want your child to have five, ten, even twenty years into the future. Healthy habits don't just happen overnight. They're called habits because they need to be behaviors you do over and over, without really thinking. During the first two years you make all such choices *for* Baby. As Baby grows into the preschool years and beyond, she will begin to decide which habits and lifestyle choices she'll happily comply with—such as picking the right foods, finding opportunities for physical activity, and brushing her teeth—so that she will learn and develop to make those same healthy choices when she's older. We'll show you all the best habits you can start that will hopefully rub off on your growing baby.

As we see it, Baby's health, now and for years to come, is supported by five pillars:

1. A healthy and green diet
2. Daily physical activity
3. Healthy responses to stress and strong emotional health
4. Good hygiene
5. Sufficient sleep

Let's take a closer look at each of these pillars.

# Pillar 1—a Healthy and Green Diet

We've given you a lot of information about what a healthy and green diet for Baby looks like and tips for getting Baby to eat well. What we haven't discussed yet is how to manage the people who are going to influence her diet and her development of healthy eating habits: you and her other caregivers.

### BABY'S NUTRITION ROLE MODEL: YOU

As Baby's Mama you select and prepare the best foods possible to help her thrive and develop in a healthy way. Your influence goes far beyond that, however. Let's say, for purposes of this discussion, that you give Baby only the healthiest all-natural foods, but you don't really like to eat fruits and vegetables, and you grab fast food or convenience store snacks when you get hungry. How long do you think it will be before Baby abandons her carrot sticks and heads for your french fries? Faster than you can say, "junk food." You are not only Baby's grocery shopper and chef, but you're also her nutrition role model, starting long before you suspect that she notices what you're eating.

Baby wants to be just like you, so that puts you in a delicate position. Think about your own food choices and whether or not you'd be happy if Baby made the same choices for herself. That means, if you expect Baby to sit at the table to eat, don't eat standing at the kitchen counter. If you want her to know that healthy snacks are things like fruit and yogurt, don't reach for junky snack foods yourself. At mealtime, serve yourself vegetables and show her that you enjoy them. Look at this time as an opportunity to clean up your eating habits if you're not on the right track already. You'll both be healthier for it.

## BABYSITTERS AND DAY CARE

If Baby spends time with a babysitter or day care provider, that person will play a major role in her nutrition—not something to take lightly. Your provider may be choosing foods for Baby and eating meals in front of her, too. Your responsibility as the Mama is to work with Baby's caregivers to ensure that her nutrition isn't compromised when she's in someone else's care.

No matter who is taking care of Baby, whether it's her doting grandma or someone you've hired to do the job, don't assume the person knows how or what to feed her. Discuss Baby's eating routines and include the following in the conversation:

- Show the caregiver how Baby tells you that she's hungry and how she indicates that she's full.
- Give the caregiver an idea of how much you expect Baby will eat and let her know that it's OK to leave leftovers.
- Be specific about what Baby should be eating and drinking. during the day, and tell your caregiver when to give Baby her bottles or drinks.

Next, consider which foods will be served to Baby while she's in her care. If Baby is at a day care or child care center, ask to see a menu or list of meals and snacks that will be served. Some child care centers qualify for government reimbursement for meals and snacks. These centers will follow basic guidelines for which kinds of foods to provide, but this is no guarantee that the food will be particularly healthy. For example, freezer chicken nuggets and french fries could technically fall under "chicken" and "potato" on a suggested menu, but they aren't necessarily the foods you want your toddler eating on a daily basis.

When you're looking at the day care menu, remember the basics of good nutrition: Baby needs some whole grains and dairy foods (or other calcium-rich foods), many fruits and vegetables, and good-quality proteins. If there are foods that you prefer your child not eat, be direct. Here are some recommendations:

- Ask the provider not to serve your child processed meats like hot dogs and bologna.
- Place limits on how much juice or milk you want Baby to drink each day.
- Tell your provider how often, if at all, Baby is allowed to have "treats" like cookies or other sweets.
- If you can, get the menu before the week begins so you can compensate for any shortfalls by adjusting Baby's menu at home. For example, if you know that Baby didn't have enough vegetables during the day, you can be sure to serve more at dinner.

Unless your day care provider is particularly passionate about organic foods, chances are the day care's standard offerings will not be organic. If you want Baby to eat organic foods, you may just have to pack them for her. Some providers will be glad to purchase some of the specific foods you request for your child. Or, they will allow you to bring food to leave in the facility—a box of HAPPYBABY meals for the freezer or a jar of organic applesauce or a box of all-natural crackers, for example. If you have decided to provide some or all of Baby's foods at day care, refer to the list on page 194 for the main foods that should be organic, and then don't make yourself nuts about the rest.

Let the day care provide the foods that tend to be lower in pesticides and contaminants—conventional bananas and oranges, for example.

If Baby has a nanny or babysitter in your home, you have a little more control over Baby's menu, but you still have to be proactive about communicating it. Here are some ideas:

- Post a list of meal and snack ideas for Baby on your fridge. At the beginning, when Baby is just starting solid foods, this is a nice way to keep track of which foods she's tried so she doesn't get too many new foods served to her at once. When Baby is older and eating a larger variety of foods, this list helps babysitters choose from several options instead of repeating the same meals over and over.
- Devote a shelf in the refrigerator to Baby's meals to make it easy for your sitter to identify which foods are for her. You can wrap up the leftovers from dinner and put them on Baby's shelf for her to have for lunch the next day. Any fruit or vegetables that you prepare for Baby can go there, too.

Overall, view Baby's caregivers as your partners in her care and nutrition. If you keep the lines of communication open and respectfully let them know what your wishes are you can help Baby achieve a healthy and wholesome diet, even when you're not around.

A NOTE FROM DR. BOB

## Post a List of Chokable Foods

Don't assume that every caregiver will have as much "food sense" as you do. A very useful safety precaution is to post a list of chokable foods (see page 169) so your caregiver can refer to it as needed.

# Pillar 2—an Active Lifestyle

Think about the unbelievable physical changes that you will see in Baby between birth and age two. She comes out as floppy as a doll, with no head control and arms and legs that flail about aimlessly. But in just twenty-four months she'll be running and climbing the stairs by herself. It's amazing! How does she go from lump to leap? Practice, practice practice. Sitting, crawling, walking, throwing a ball—these motions don't just occur magically when Baby reaches a particular stage of development. She has to practice moving through her world in order to learn how to do it and to gain the strength she needs to be successful. You're like her cruise ship director, making sure she has opportunities to participate in activities each day.

Physical activity provides Baby more than just the physical benefits that you'd expect. Let's take tummy time as an example. Spending time on her stomach helps strengthen Baby's neck and upper body, and it provides gentle pressure on the belly that can help relieve gas and discomfort. But it also helps her brain development and prepares her for future learning. Tummy time engages Baby's brain and helps to create connections throughout her nervous system. As Baby moves more, these connections grow, forming pathways like maps that her brain will use to learn new things in the future. More complex movements like crawling will develop even more complex brain maps. Being on her tummy also helps Baby develop spatial awareness because her brain and body have to figure out where she is in relation to other things around her.

Strength, endurance, *and* brainpower! Ready to run out to a gym class? Well, don't get Baby a fitness club membership just yet. An active lifestyle for a baby is pretty simple to create and doesn't require too many props or special facilities. While Baby is still an infant, here's what you need to do:

· First and foremost, give Baby safe surroundings to move around in and explore.

## Playpens Are a Thing of the Past

Research has shown that babies who spend more time in a play-pen actually develop more slowly—slower motor, intellectual, and social skills. I'll admit that it's nice to be able to set a mobile baby down for a few minutes in a totally secure area while you go to bathroom or take a shower, but playpens should be strictly limited to brief periods (if you even use one at all). Babies develop faster and better when they are engaged with you in your arms or free to move about an engaging play area. Taking a green look at this, skipping the purchase of a portable playpen not only saves you money but keeps one less large, bulky, plastic, and environmentally unfriendly item out of landfills. When your baby outgrows her playpen, be sure to pass it along to someone else whom you know is planning to buy one.

- Play games with Baby that have an element of movement, like peekaboo or patty-cake. Clap her hands and move her arms until she learns to do it herself.
- Don't restrict Baby's movement for a long period of time by keeping her in the stroller, car seat, or swing for too long. Be sure to move her around to different positions and let her lie on a blanket and swing her arms and kick her legs.

Once Baby is toddling around, by age two, she can engage in more of what you probably think of as physical activity:

- For about thirty minutes each day, engage her in some kind of structured activity. That means that you or another caregiver should play active games with Baby, such as duck, duck, goose; tag; or ring-around-the-rosy. Walking to a nearby destination with a push toy is a nice activity once Baby is about eighteen months old. A toddler gym class would work, too.

- In addition, aim for at least sixty minutes of unstructured activity each day, such as running around the yard or playing at a playground.
- Give Baby exposure to things like stairs and balls so she can learn physical skills like climbing and throwing.
- Plus, (there's more?!) your toddler shouldn't be still for more than sixty minutes at a time unless she's sleeping. If you have to make long car trips or shopping excursions, try to take breaks for stretching and running around. Don't let her sit in front of the television for extended periods of time, either.

(Source: National Association for Sport and Physical Education.)

A NOTE FROM DR. BOB

## Limit TV Time

Research has shown that the more TV or videos a baby or toddler watches, the higher the chance of having ADD and learning challenges as a child. It seems that TV really can "rot your brain," as my parents used to tell me when I was a kid. That type of prolonged, noninteractive input isn't good for a developing nervous system. One study even showed that a supposedly educational series of baby videos slowed down intellectual and motor development. Of course, you may find yourself needing a short break from time to time, and the TV is so convenient. Just please keep it to a minimum.

What if Baby is really skinny—does she need as much exercise as a heavier child? Absolutely. As adults, we tend to think about physical activity and exercise as being beneficial for weight management. But that limited view isn't right for adults, and it doesn't work for babies, either. A person's weight is only one factor in her overall health, and physical fitness is important for everyone.

At every age and stage of development there will be new skills for Baby to practice and master and things you can do to help her learn. Keep in mind that all babies develop on their own schedule. If your baby is more advanced in her development or moving through these stages more slowly, adapt these activities as needed.

| Approximate Age | New Activities to Try with Your Baby |
|---|---|
| Birth to 4 months | • Tummy time—lay Baby on a solid surface on her stomach for a few minutes at a time, several times a day, starting when Baby is a few weeks old. (Remember, though, always to put her to sleep on her back.) Get down on the floor with her so she can see you. Put a toy nearby so she has something to hold her interest.<br><br>• Once Baby can open and shut her hands, give her toys or objects to try to hold.<br><br>• Once she can support her head, hold her hands and pull her up to sitting from a lying-down position. |
| 4–7 months | • Give her toys to hold so she can perfect her grasp.<br><br>• Provide a safe place for her to lie on the floor, and practice rolling from back to front and front to back.<br><br>• Scatter toys or other objects around to give her things to reach for when she's playing on the floor or on a play mat.<br><br>• Show her hand motions like clapping and waving so she can start to learn how to do them herself.<br><br>• Help her practice sitting. At first she will be in a tripod position, supporting herself with her arms in front of her. Soon she'll be able to balance without her arms for moments at a time. Then she'll sit without support.<br><br>• When Baby is on your lap, pull her up to stand and let her bounce with her legs. |

| | |
|---|---|
| 7–12 months | • Give her palm-size objects to practice passing from one hand to the other.<br><br>• Give her plenty of floor time to practice crawling. Put toys just beyond her reach and encourage her to go get them.<br><br>• Gate off the first 2 steps of your staircase or find other steps for Baby to practice climbing on. (Always supervise this activity carefully.) She will probably be able to walk up and down by age 2.<br><br>• When Baby starts pulling herself up to stand, teach her how to get back down by bending her knees. (Some babies get stuck up there!)<br><br>• Make sure there are safe and sturdy things for her to hold on to as she's cruising around your home.<br><br>• Give Baby a sturdy push toy for practicing walking. Note: Skip the baby walker (the type a baby sits in). These toys actually don't help Baby learn to walk because they don't do a good job of strengthening all the muscles needed for walking. Plus, they are a safety hazard. |
| 10–18 months | • Let her hold on to you as she practices walking, and encourage her to let go, too.<br><br>• Babies love to dance. Put on music and dance together.<br><br>• Give Baby balls to bounce, throw, kick, and roll.<br><br>• Babies this age love riding toys. (Healthy Mama tip: suck in your abdominal muscles when pushing Baby on her riding toy—otherwise your back is vulnerable to injury.) |
| 18–24 months | • Now that Baby has mastered walking, find a large lightweight ball for her to practice kicking.<br><br>• Baby will now be able to carry objects while walking—give her palm-size toys or objects with handles to carry around.<br><br>• Chase Baby around the yard or playground. By the end of her second year she will start running! |

# CHILDHOOD OBESITY

## What Can You Do?

You've seen the reports in the newspaper and on the nightly news: too many of America's kids are at unhealthy weights. About 16 percent of children aged two to nineteen are obese—for this age group "obese" means that their body mass index, or BMI, is above the 95th percentile. Another 30 percent of American two- to nineteen-year-olds are overweight (with a BMI between the 85th and 95th percentiles).[1] The dangers of being obese can't be overstated, and we don't think it's alarmist to call the situation a public health crisis. Heavy children grow up with higher risks for health concerns like high blood pressure, type 2 diabetes, cardiovascular disease, and reproductive problems. Obese kids are more likely to experience depression and other psychological effects, too.

It's enough to make any parent nervous when she looks at her baby's double chin and sausage-link arms. But aren't babies supposed to be chubby? How do you know if there is a real cause for concern? Your pediatrician will track Baby's growth and monitor whether or not she's growing too fast or becoming too heavy. Babies start out with plenty of padding, but most will start to slim down as they crawl, walk, and run into their preschool years. Ideally, a baby under age two should have a weight-for-length between the 5th and 95th percentiles for her age and gender. If it's not in that range, your doctor may help you take a good look at what you're feeding Baby and how active a child she is so you can make some changes to help slow down her weight gain. Or maybe your doctor will advise you to wait until the next time Baby is weighed and measured to see if maybe her growth catches up to her weight. The tricky part of this story is that even if Baby is heavy for her age as an infant it doesn't necessarily mean she will become an overweight child. And normal weight babies can still become overweight kids.

Since it's hard to look at Baby's weight to determine if she'll be heavy later in life, rather than fixating on the number on the scale it makes more sense to learn how you can help raise her to be a healthy weight. First, consider some of the risk factors for becoming overweight:

- *You or Baby's other parent is obese.* Alternatively, if you are both a healthy weight, Baby is at a lower risk for becoming overweight later in life, even if she is heavy as a baby. Some of this may be due to genetics, but a lot of it is because Mom's and Dad's eating habits and lifestyle tend to rub off on their kids.
- *You tend to be a fast-food family.* Eating junk food, fast food, and soda increases a child's risk for becoming overweight.

- *She's not physically active.* For babies and toddlers, this means being sedentary for hours at a time (other than when sleeping) on a regular basis.
- *She was underweight at birth.* Some studies have shown that babies who are born very small and then experience very quick catch-up weight gain are at a higher risk for obesity.[2]

Luckily, some of these risk factors are changeable and, at least theoretically, within your control as a parent. If any of these areas describe you or your child, make some changes. Here are more ways to prevent future weight problems for Baby:

- *Breast-feed.* Breast-feeding may give your child an advantage in the weight department, though it's not entirely due to the composition of the milk itself. When breast-fed babies are full they pull off the breast and stop eating. But when a bottle-fed baby is full, parents may miss the cues because they are too focused on emptying the bottle. The result is that sometimes bottle-fed babies are overfed.
- *Don't rush solids.* Waiting to start solid foods until six months may help prevent weight problems.[3]
- *Feed her right.* Offer only healthy foods to Baby. Don't introduce her to sugary or junky foods. See chapters 4–6 for details about a healthy diet for Baby.
- *Follow her lead.* Pay attention to Baby's cues when you are feeding her breast milk, formula, or solids. When she stops accepting the spoon or milk, unless she simply has to burp, it probably means she is full. Allow Baby to decide when the feeding is over. Not only will you avoid overfeeding Baby, but you'll help her learn how to listen to her body and respond to her own hunger and fullness cues.
- *Calcium-fortify her.* Some studies suggest that calcium, specifically from dairy foods, lowers the risk of overweight and reduces body fat in older children.[4,5] Is it something in those foods that helps the body stay a healthy weight, or is it simply that little kids who drink milk are less likely to drink soda or too much juice? We don't know. Either way, serve Baby good calcium sources and dairy foods on a regular basis. (See page 206 for a list.)
- *Encourage physical movement.* Getting kids to move more may be the most effective strategy in reducing overweight. Start some healthy habits at a young age, such as outdoor play, dancing to music, and ball play.
- *Help her sleep.* Babies who get fewer than twelve hours of sleep (versus more than thirteen) per day have a higher risk of being overweight by their third birthday.[6] See page 363 for some tips on helping Baby get more shut-eye.
- *Be a healthy role model.* Eat healthy foods and lead an active life. Baby will imitate these healthy habits.

# Pillar 3—Dealing with Stress and Emotions

Babies are pretty happy-go-lucky creatures, but there are still things that stress them out and they have emotions that they will learn to process. Baby may feel stress when she hears a loud startling noise, when she's taken out of a nice warm bath, or when a stranger comes into the room. As her Mama you want Baby to be happy, but you can't completely eliminate her stress. The best you can do is help teach her how to handle the stress she is sure to encounter.

How Baby handles stress, her ability to deal with her emotions, and how she relates to others all contribute to her mental and physical health as she gets older. These aspects of her personality are the products of both nature (genetic factors) and nurture (her environment and upbringing). Genes definitely play a role in this: if anxiety or depression or serious mental illness is common in your family, there's a chance your baby is at a higher risk for them, too. Even if that's the case, though, it's not a foregone conclusion that Baby will inherit all of your mental health or emotional issues. And since you can't change your genes anyway, focus instead on creating a healthy environment for Baby and interacting with her in a way that promotes mental and emotional health.

## DE-STRESS YOUR HOME

Baby comes out of the nice warm, safe womb and is thrust into this crazy world. Your home should be her refuge from that craziness. Aim to make home a place of peace and comfort. For example, create consistent routines so Baby knows what to expect from day to day. Turn off the TV, and enjoy some peace and quiet. Shield Baby from fighting and other potentially frightening interactions. This doesn't mean you can never be in a bad mood, argue with your spouse, or turn up the volume on the stereo. Just aim to minimize stress by providing consistency and routines in a calm and joyful home.

You should also model healthy reactions to stress so Baby sees that it isn't necessary to freak out over things that aren't serious problems. You know, don't cry over spilt milk. Literally.

Of course, there's stress, and then there's STRESS. Serious problems in your household place Baby at higher risk for mental health problems and need to be addressed. We're talking about gross mistreatment by one of her caregivers, exposure to violence, caregivers who are abusing drugs or alcohol, poverty conditions, or a parent whose own mental health problems are left untreated. If any of these are factors in your baby's life, now is the time to get help.

## BECOME ATTACHED

Baby's emotional and social development may be most significantly influenced by her attachment, or bond, to one very special person in her life: her Mama. Baby's attachment to you develops over time, from the moment your eyes meet after birth. As Baby lets you know what she needs and how she feels, your sensitivity and responsiveness teach Baby to trust your care and develop a secure attachment to you. This strong and healthy attachment in turn helps Baby manage the stress of new or scary situations. Researchers have looked at babies who have responsive Mamas and found that when they are in stressful situations their levels of stress hormones and heart rates don't increase as much as other babies'.[7] In other words, they are better at handling the stress. They are also able to recover faster from the stressful event.

Having a secure attachment to you will also help Baby develop confidence as she explores her world. She may even become a more resilient child because of your bond. Here are some ways to form a strong attachment with Baby:

- Get plenty of physical contact with Baby, especially in the early months. Breast-feeding, baby-wearing, and cosleeping are all ways to connect and grow your bond.
- Pay attention to the little things. When you observe Baby in different situations you can learn how to read her cues and figure out how to respond to her.

- When Baby's in distress, show empathy in your response. Show her that you understand that she's upset and that you are concerned. Comfort her through actions such as hugging and through a gentle and soothing tone of voice.
- Don't be too rigid. Babies are unpredictable, and it might be hard to be responsive to Baby's needs if you're not able to go with the flow.
- If you have to be away from Baby to return to a career or to manage other responsibilities, you can still develop a strong attachment because it's the quality of your interactions that really matters. When you are able to be with her put aside your to-do list, reduce distractions and be "tuned in."

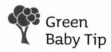

A NOTE FROM DR. BOB

# Attachment Research

If you peruse any parenting section of a bookstore, you will notice a wide variety of styles and advice on raising kids. Very little of this advice is based in research—it's mostly just one author's opinion. So what does research say about parenting? It's very clear—virtually every research study done in the past forty years on infant and child development shows that a more responsive, attached, and interactive parenting approach creates smarter, emotionally healthier, and better-adjusted children.[8] A stricter, less interactive parenting style that focuses more on fostering independence and self-reliance for a baby results in slower motor and intellectual development, and less stable emotional health as an older child.

If this is true, why don't all parents take the attachment route? It does take more work, more time, and more energy to be an attached parent. We believe it's well worth the investment, though.

By the time Baby is six to eight months old, her brain can experience a broad range of emotions like happiness, fear, and frustration. The next step is figuring out what to do with all of those feelings, or developing what's called emotional intelligence.

Baby will learn that her emotions are valid when you are empathetic—when you smile when Baby laughs or act concerned when she cries. She'll also learn how to figure out what others are feeling and how to respond by reading your face and body language. For example, if a stranger offers to hold her and you act nervous, she's likely to protest being held. If, on the other hand, you give her a comforting smile and act relaxed, she knows not to be afraid. One of the ways we communicate with our babies before they can talk to us is through this interpretation and mirroring of emotions.

As Baby approaches and passes her first birthday she will be increasingly aware of her surroundings and will often have a clear personal agenda. This can lead to frustration and disappointment sometimes. By eighteen months you may even start to see some real temper tantrums. As she begins to experience these kinds of emotions, don't try to fix every situation for Baby or allow her to get away with things just because you fear that saying no will make her unhappy. Instead, show her that you understand how she's feeling and then help her learn to express and deal with her unpleasant feelings. They are a part of life!

# Pillar 4—Good Hygiene

Most Mamas we know want to keep Baby clean but don't necessarily want to be obsessive about it. On the other hand, after bringing Baby home from the hospital, some Mamas want to spray hand sanitizer all over anyone who crosses their threshold. Have they crossed over into the obsessive place? Well, perhaps, but it's not crazy to want to protect newborns from germs. Young babies don't have fully developed immune systems, so they can get sick easily. If they do get sick, it can be very scary. A high fever during the first two months buys you a visit to the hospital. So, for the first few months of Baby's life really paying attention to hygiene—yours, mostly—is of the utmost importance. Keep that hand soap flowing. A little obsession at this stage is not only understandable but warranted.

Once Baby is past the newborn stage (the first two months of life), her immune system will be better able to handle exposure to many germs. She may catch minor illnesses, like colds or stomach bugs, but she will be able to recover fully with basic treatment. Exposure to some germs may even help her immune system get stronger as it works to fight them off. Vaccinations will be available to protect her against more serious illnesses, for example, measles, meningitis, and the flu.

At this point you can breathe a little sigh of relief. But just a little one. You can't throw hygiene out the window by any means, but once Baby can pick things up and move around, being obsessive about cleanliness will only frustrate you. Babies and toddlers are going to come in contact with dirt and germs. They put everything in their mouths, including their hands, which they are absolutely incapable of keeping to themselves. Even in your relatively clean home Baby will probably find dirty messes to get into. To keep Baby healthy without going nuts about being "clean," focus on these three personal hygiene essentials: washing everyone's hands often, bathing Baby occasionally, and cleaning her teeth daily.

## WASH EVERYONE'S HANDS

Most illnesses are spread by people touching their nose or mouth after touching something contaminated with bacteria or a virus. Washing hands may be the single most important thing you can do to keep the germs at bay. Simple hand washing with basic soap and water is especially important for preventing diarrhea, the flu, and other respiratory infections.

Get in the habit, if you aren't already, of washing your hands when you walk in the door after being outside. Also wash your hands before feeding Baby, after all diaper changes, after you use the bathroom, after touching animals, and before touching food. Wash Baby's hands, too—before and after she eats, after she touches something that could be germy or dirty, and when she gets home from the park or other hands-on place. This is not only for removing germs but also to help Baby develop the habit. They learn early. One eleven-month-old baby we know rubs his hands together as if he's washing them whenever his Mama announces that it's time to eat a meal.

I know you've been washing your hands all your life, but make sure you are doing it correctly.

- Moisten hands with warm water, lather with soap, and rub them together for at least twenty seconds—if you need help timing it, sing two rounds of "Happy Birthday" silently. Then rinse and dry off.
- Choose basic hand soap instead of antibacterial varieties. Antibacterial soaps are contributing to the problems we've seen with antibiotic-resistant bacteria. Besides, plain soap is actually just as effective at killing germs as antibacterial soaps. Try all-natural soaps with plant-based ingredients. like the Natural Moisturizing Body Bar (unscented) from Tom's of Maine (www.tomsofmaine.com) or the liquid hand soaps by Pangea Organics (www.pangeaorganics.com), Nature's Gate (www.naturesgate.com), or EO Products (www.eoproducts.com).
- If you're on the go or if there's no soap for washing your hands, an alcohol-based hand sanitizer is a good substitute. Find one that is at least 60 percent alcohol so that it is potent enough to kill bacteria and viruses. EO Products makes a nice one that contains only all-natural ingredients—no added chemicals or synthetic fragrances. Pour some into your hands and rub them together until dry. Don't use these on Baby's hands, though, and keep your sanitizer safely out of her reach (be careful when you keep one in your diaper bag, for example). Ingesting it can actually cause alcohol poisoning.
- If you prefer a non-alcohol-based hand sanitizer, try the plant-based one by CleanWell (www.cleanwelltoday.com). Their

## At What Age Can You Take a Baby Outside and Around Town?

As you learned in the previous chapter, you don't need to obsess about keeping Baby away from every last germ. But you do want to prevent the most common and troublesome illnesses as best you can. When can you take Baby outside and around town? Babies don't get sick simply by going outside or walking around with you. They get sick by being held or touched by sick people, or by being directly coughed or sneezed on. So, you can actually take Baby out the day she is born if you want to. Just don't pass her around to everyone. For the first few months of life it's prudent to screen all visitors for any symptoms of illness, such as sore throat, fever, or runny nose. Make all visitors wash their hands. Keep Baby to yourself when you go out; wearing her in a baby sling is a great way to keep well-meaning baby lovers from coming up and asking to hold her.

sanitizer spray gets rave reviews from eco-conscious moms, and the company claims that its main ingredient, made with the herb thyme, kills 99.99 percent of germs. It's available at Target and on www.Amazon.com, or search the CleanWell web site for stores in your area.

## BATHE BABY . . . AT LEAST OCCASIONALLY

The sight and scent of a clean baby is certainly delightful, and baths are of course part of any healthy baby's hygiene routine. Newborns aren't particularly dirty creatures, so bathing every few days (or even once a week) is fine. Later, depending on how messy Baby gets, you may want to bathe her more often (but don't bathe more than once a day because it will dry out the natural oils on Baby's skin). It may make sense to bathe Baby less often in the winter, when she's covered from head to toe in clothes and doesn't get sweaty. Then, during the spring and summer, daily baths may be a necessity if Baby is getting dirty outside and is covered in sunscreen all the time.

Bathe Baby in a safe place where it's least likely that she'll slip—such as a small infant tub or oversize basin on the floor. If you're using a sink, be cautious about the faucet—if it were turned on accidentally it could burn Baby. Some Mamas prefer placing an infant tub on the counter. Never ever leave Baby unattended in the sink or on the counter. Once Baby can sit without support, you can put her in a larger bathtub and give her some bath toys, too. You can make Baby's bath part of her bedtime routine or do it at another time of day. More bath tips:

- Make the water warm enough, not too hot. Ninety degrees is recommended.
- Keep the door to your bathroom shut to keep in the warm air. You can also dampen a washcloth with warm water and lay it on her chest during her bath.
- Wash her hair last because a wet head makes her feel cold.
- Never ever leave Baby unattended in the bath or turn your attention away from her. It takes only a moment for a baby to inhale some water or turn on the hot water.
- Give Baby age-appropriate toys to make bath time fun, but skip the spraying bath toys that hold water—mildew grows quickly in these.

When it's not bath night, wash Baby's face before bed and use a wet washcloth to clean her diaper area or any other parts that need it. These modified sponge baths work well, even for older babies.

## BASIC BABY GROOMING

### Nail Care

Baby's nails should be smoothed with a baby nail file or trimmed with infant nail clippers. During the first few months her arms will flail about, and she can scratch herself with long nails. Once she is able to grab things on purpose, like your nose or, say, your nipple, you will want those nails to be short! When using the clippers be very careful not to cut Baby's skin. To avoid mishaps, choose a well-lit place and a time when she is calm. Gently pull the pad of her finger back to separate the nail from the skin, and don't cut the nail so short—leave a little of the white part of the nail. It may make sense to cut Baby's nails when she's sleeping. If you do cut her skin (it's bound to happen at least once), don't beat yourself up. Get a gauze pad and apply gentle pressure to the bleeding fingertip for a while. Don't put a bandage on it because it will likely fall off and Baby could choke on it.

### Baby Acne

Shortly after Baby is born you may notice that she looks downright adolescent. The little pimples that appear on her face, chest, and back are totally normal and due to hormones. They don't really have anything to do with hygiene and will most likely go away on their own so just wash baby's face as usual. And resist the urge to pick at them (we know you want to!). Picking can damage Baby's delicate skin or cause infection.

### Cradle Cap

This flaky, scaly rash on baby's scalp can show up anytime in the first few months. It's caused by hormones that Baby got from you before birth. These hormones make the sebaceous glands on baby's scalp create grease that traps dead skin cells that would otherwise just fall off as new skin cells are formed. The resulting rash is, well, icky looking and is hard to get off. Rest assured that it doesn't bother baby—it's not itchy or uncomfortable. And it doesn't mean you aren't washing her well enough. Like baby acne, it has nothing to do with cleanliness. You can continue to use a mild baby shampoo during a cradle cap outbreak. You can also buy a baby shampoo with tea tree oil (like California Baby's Tea Tree & Lavender Shampoo and Body Wash, www.californiababy .com) for a natural way to be rid of cradle cap. If Baby is older than six months, you can even try a little dandruff shampoo. Be careful not to get it in her eyes. You can also rub a little olive oil onto the rash and wait several minutes for the flaky patches to soften. Then brush the scalp with a comb or brush or use a washcloth to try to loosen and remove the scales. If Baby still has cradle cap after she's eight months old, be sure to point it out to your pediatrician.

## CLEAN HER TEETH DAILY

Baby's teeth started to form during your second trimester of pregnancy, so even if you can't see them in Baby's mouth it doesn't mean they aren't there. This means good oral health needs to start early. People may tell you, "Relax, they're just baby teeth. Aren't they going to fall out in a few years anyway?" Well, unfortunately it doesn't work that way. Baby teeth can decay and cause pain. Plus, baby teeth are important for learning to chew and to speak properly. To encourage a healthy mouth:

- Never put Baby to bed with a bottle of milk because the milk sugars can sit on her teeth and cause decay, referred to as baby bottle rot. Yuck.
- For babies with no teeth: Before bed, wipe Baby's gums with a wet washcloth to remove any sugars left her in mouth. This helps you and her both to develop the brushing habit early.
- For babies with teeth: Use either water or fluoride-free tooth-paste until Baby is old enough to learn to spit out the tooth-paste (after age three for most kids). Swallowing too much fluoride can cause white spots to form on Baby's permanent teeth, which are developing beneath the surface. Our favorite toothpastes contain few, if any, artificial ingredients and are perfectly safe for Baby to swallow. Try JASON Natural Cosmet-ics Earth's Best toddler toothpaste (www.jason-natural.com),

A NOTE FROM DR. BOB

## What's in Your Toothpaste?

I was curious one day about what was in my kids' cartoon character colored, sparkly toothpaste. I was shocked! Saccharin and food coloring. I was grinding some very questionable ingredients into my children's teeth every night. I was probably doing more harm than good. Be sure to use a natural toothpaste for your kids. In fact, until a child is old enough to use fluoride toothpaste and spit it out, you really don't need to use any at all.

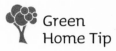

**Green Home Tip**

Don't leave the water running when brushing Baby's teeth. An open faucet sends two gallons down the drain every minute.

Weleda Children's Tooth Gel (www.usa.weleda.com) or Burt's Bees Doctor Burt's Children's Toothpaste.

- Open the tap. Fluoride, found in most municipal tap water, helps protect Baby's teeth from decay. Formula-fed babies will get fluoride from the formula itself, but if Baby is breast-fed, use tap water to mix Baby's cereal, and starting at around six months, give Baby tap water to drink. It's OK if you use a water filter, as most filters sold for residential use don't remove the fluoride. If your water isn't fluoridated, ask your pediatrician or dentist about a supplement of this important mineral for your breast-fed baby (see page 93 for more info).

# Pillar 5—a Good Night's Sleep

Perhaps you don't really think of sleep as being a healthy habit, but it is, just like eating right or washing hands. And it's key for Baby's overall health. She needs sufficient rest to grow and develop properly. Plus, not getting enough sleep is associated with tantrums, behavior prob-

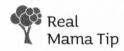

**Real Mama Tip**

"Using a supersoft baby toothbrush as a teething aid when those back teeth come in not only feels good but it's a sneaky way to get them used to the feel of brushing. Logan is twenty months now and has fabulous dental hygiene habits!"

—*Taryn, Frederick, Maryland*

lems, and poor school performance in older children, as well as be-coming overweight. And let's be honest, Baby not getting enough sleep is also associated with grumpy moods in Mamas and dads.

Of course we know that for some babies sleep does come naturally, so it's not a habit that most of you have to work at developing. These babies drift off to sleep easily when they are tired and are able to stay asleep until they have had enough rest. If you're the lucky Mama of one of these sleepy dreamers, count your blessings! Other babies need a little help figuring it out. They require rocking, back rubbing, stroller rides, moving swings, earnest prayers, cosleeping, conapping, etc.

As you well know, there are whole books devoted to the topic of sleep. We're not going to do an exhaustive (or exhausting) review of the many methods touted for getting your child to sleep through the night or take longer naps. It's virtually impossible for someone to tell you an absolute right way to encourage better sleep because every baby and every family is different, and what works for one child may not be right for another. Regardless of which sleep theory you subscribe to, we think these tips will help you foster healthy sleep habits in Baby so you both can get through the exhausting first two years:

## UNDERSTAND THAT YOU ARE FORMING HABITS

After Baby is about three months old the how and the where of her sleep will slowly become ingrained as habits. For example, if she's rocked to sleep for every nap and at bedtime, she's going to get used to that. If she's learned to fall asleep on her own, great! If you've nursed Baby down to sleep every night, and it's working well, that's just fine. Realize, though, that whatever habits you are creating now, Baby will become used to and insist on for the next year or two. So if you were hoping for a more independent sleeper, you'd want to try some less parent-involved bedtime routines by the time Baby is three months old.

## PUT BABY DOWN DROWSY BUT AWAKE

From about six weeks on, you can try to get Baby used to being put down when she is drowsy but still awake. The key here is learning to read Baby's tired signs and soothing her to sleep as soon as you see them. For some babies, the sleep sweet spot is a yawn. For others it's the first time they rub their eyes. Babies get overtired really quickly and then have a hard time falling asleep—if you miss the signs and wait even ten to fifteen minutes, you could be in for a tough time getting her to go down.

## HAVE REALISTIC EXPECTATIONS

There may come a time when you feel as though all of your friends' babies sleep through the night and you're the only exhausted basket case. You're not. It might take Baby a long time to figure out how to sleep the whole night. And even then, there will be bumps in the road, such as illness, changing patterns, nightmares, potty training—the list could go on and on. The early years are exhausting, but you'll make it through. Plus—and this may sound like hogwash to you if you're currently up all night with a young baby—one day you may miss the special quiet moments you and Baby shared while everyone else was sleeping.

Be realistic about Baby's schedule, too. Type A Mamas sometimes try to get Baby on a schedule right away because they want their days to be as predictable as possible, but a natural predictable pattern won't emerge until Baby is at least four or five months old, if not older. Even then, schedules work best when they follow Baby's natural rhythms. If you try to impose an unnatural sleep schedule on a baby, it will likely backfire.

## DON'T OVERSTIMULATE BABY
## WHEN IT'S TIME FOR SLEEP

In the middle of the night, if you attend to Baby for feeding, changing, or soothing, try not to interact with her too much. Don't turn on the light or jostle her. This isn't the time for tickling. Rub her back or

# Where Should Baby Sleep?

The simple answer is, wherever you and Baby sleep best. The American Academy of Pediatrics now recommends that babies (especially if breast-feeding) sleep in the same room as the parents.[9] For reasons that aren't clear, sharing your room with Baby decreases the chances of sudden infant death syndrome (SIDS). It's likely that your proximity to baby (sound, smell, and touch) stimulates and regulates Baby's breathing and heart functions. Room sharing also facilitates nursing in the early months. Once Baby is sleeping longer stretches, you can decide where you and Baby get the best night's sleep.

replace the pacifier, and then leave her alone to try to go back to sleep. You can listen at the door and go back in to soothe again as needed. If you are cosleeping—having Baby sleep in your bed with you, keep any stimulation or verbal interaction to a minimum as you nurse or snuggle Baby back to sleep.

## BE CONSISTENT WITH YOUR BEDTIME AND NAPTIME ROUTINES

Before you think Baby is old enough to need one, start a bedtime and naptime routine. For naps, it can be something as simple as rocking in a chair with her for a minute while singing her a song. A typical bedtime routine may look something like this: bath, breast or bottle, a book, and then into bed. Have all of Baby's in-home caregivers do it the same way so she'll always know when it's time for sleep.

## GIVE BABY A "LOVEY"

A cuddly object can ease Baby's transition from your arms to her bed. Once Baby can roll in both directions and can grasp a toy and move it around, you can give her something to cuddle. The lovey you choose should be relatively small—not big enough that it could cover her face. Find a small stuffed animal, a little blanket, or other soft toy. Choose something that is made of natural fibers and is machine washable, if possible. (For more on choosing safe toys, see chapter 8.) Get Baby used to associating this object with comfort by holding it close to her while you are snuggling or nursing. You can also sleep with the object for a couple of nights so it takes on your scent. If you find something that helps to soothe Baby, buy a few more in case one gets lost!

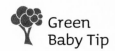

### Green Baby Tip

Baby's comfort blanket or stuffed animal is going to end up in her mouth, and she'll likely bury her head in it for snuggle time, so choose one made with natural and organic fibers like those by Under the Nile (www.underthenile.com), for example.

## ADOPT A WAIT-AND-SEE POLICY

Don't rush to every fuss you hear coming from Baby's room. But wait, you're thinking, you just told us to be responsive to Baby's needs! Yes, but just because Baby makes some noise doesn't mean that she needs you. In fact, you may unnecessarily wake Baby by moving in too soon. If Baby is awake, a little fuss might become a wail once Baby sees you come into her room and then leave again. It's normal for babies to wake up to fuss, gnaw on their fingers or pacifier, or babble during the night or midway through a nap. Unless she's crying out in distress, let her be for five or ten minutes to see if she falls back asleep on her own. Use your intuition to decide if Baby's fussing has turned into real crying that warrants responding to.

## SEND BABY TO BED EARLY

Most sleep experts agree that a bedtime between 7 p.m. and 8 p.m. is ideal for babies, toddlers, and preschoolers. After birth, Baby will be up and down around the clock and won't have a bedtime. Then, after one to two months, you'll probably notice that she goes down for a longer stretch of sleep at some point in the evening, usually kind of late—ten or eleven o'clock. For all intents and purposes, that's her bedtime. If you are attentive to her need for sleep, you will probably notice that slowly as she gets older, likely by six or seven months old, this natural bedtime (i.e., the time she gets tired and then sleeps for a long stretch) will move earlier and earlier until it settles between 7 p.m. and 8 p.m. If this doesn't naturally occur for your baby, try to establish this as Baby's bedtime by the time she's seven or eight months old.

## BALANCE BABY'S NEED FOR STILLNESS WITH YOUR NEED FOR MOTION

Some sleep books can make you feel that if you let Baby sleep in a swing, the stroller, or the car, it will ruin her. It is true that still sleep is better sleep. It's better for helping Baby learn how to fall and stay asleep on her own, and it's better for the quality of the sleep Baby will get. But in the real world, sometimes an on-the-go nap is necessary. Strike a balance: Commit to giving Baby at least one motion-free nap each day. You may have to rearrange your schedule to do it, but it's worth the sacrifice. Then, if you're out and about the rest of the day and Baby is sleeping in the car or stroller, so be it.

## BALANCE BABY'S NEED FOR CONSISTENCY WITH HER NEED FOR FLEXIBILITY

Sometimes we see parents who go to extremes when it comes to sleep. There are the ones who are completely laissez-faire and never impose any kind of structure on Baby. On the other end of the spectrum are the parents who are so vigilant about their sleep rules and routines that they can become overly rigid. Try to find whatever middle ground feels right to you. Establish consistent routines because they are healthy for Baby, but don't get so uptight about sleeping and schedules that you make yourself and your baby miserable.

# An Ounce of Prevention

The five pillars that we've discussed above are lifestyle behaviors that you and Baby can practice to put Baby on the path to good health. To complete the picture of good health for Baby, let's go over the things you need professionals to do for you: preventive medical services like checkups and vaccinations.

## WELL CHILD CHECKUPS

Ideally, Baby should have a medical "home"—a primary doctor or medical provider who sees her when she's well and when she's sick. Children with a medical home tend to have fewer visits to the emergency room for routine health problems, and their doctors may be better at spotting concerns early. Regular checkups with one provider also help you as a parent because you get to develop a relationship with that person, and you will feel comfortable asking questions and trusting the doctor's advice. If your baby doesn't have one provider whom she sees regularly for well child checkups and sick visits, ask around in your community for referrals and interview the ones you are interested in using. Most pediatricians are available for short appointments designed so you can meet them, ask questions, and decide if their practice is right for your family.

At Baby's well child checkups her pediatrician will track her growth and development and assess her health in order to catch and treat any problems early. There will be recommended screenings, assessments, and vaccines at certain ages.

Although your family's well child checkup schedule may be different, depending on your insurance coverage and your doctor's practice, here is a typical schedule of well child checkup care for the first two years.

(Source: Consensus statement by AAP and Bright Futures, "Recommendations for Preventive Pediatric Health Care," 2008.)

## At Birth

- Measurements such as length, weight, head circumference
- Newborn hearing screen
- Developmental assessment
- Newborn metabolic screenings (these vary depending on the state where you live)
- General physical examination
- Guidance about what's going on at Baby's age and stage

## At One Month, Two Months, Four Months, Six Months, Nine Months

- Measurements such as length, weight, head circumference
- Developmental milestone check
- General physical examination
- Behavioral and social assessment
- Guidance about what's going on at Baby's age and stage

## At Twelve Months

Same as for previous checkups, plus:

- Iron status screening—test Baby's level hemoglobin in her blood to check for anemia
- Lead screening test to check exposure to lead
- Guidance about caring for Baby's teeth
- Tuberculin test for exposure to tuberculosis (this will be done every 1 to 3 years)

## At Fifteen Months, Eighteen Months, Twenty-four Months

Same as previous checkups, plus:

- Autism screening—the doctor will pay particular attention to language and social development to catch any such problems as early as possible.

## DENTAL CHECKUPS

Just like medical checkups, dental checkups are helpful in monitoring Baby's development and for catching any problems. At your first visit to the dentist you will learn about proper brushing technique and other practices for keeping Baby's mouth healthy. At subsequent visits Baby will have her teeth cleaned thoroughly and the dentist will look for signs of decay.

The dentists at the American Dental Association recommend that Baby see a dentist sometime after her teeth start to come in, preferably around her first birthday. You may find that this early visit isn't covered by your insurance or even available at your dentist's practice. At the latest, we recommend a visit to the dentist by age two. Then follow your dentist's recommendation for follow-up—we take our kids every six months.

## TREATING COMMON ILLNESSES RESPONSIBLY AND NATURALLY

Part of raising Baby green is to make responsible health care choices and limit medications as best as you can. Of course, there will be times when a medical treatment is necessary. Here is a brief guide to how Dr. Bob likes to combine traditional with natural medicine in his practice.

- *Limit antibiotics.* Doctors are now being more and more careful with antibiotics because we are seeing more and more resistance in various germs. Common colds, coughs, and flus don't need antibiotics unless there is a moderate to severe bacterial complication. Find a doctor that uses antibiotics responsibly.
- *Ear infections.* It's almost inevitable that your child will get at least one ear infection. A new policy from the American Academy of Pediatrics states that mild ear infections should not be treated with antibiotics.[10] A wait-and-see approach is OK. If

## Garlic Drops for Ear Infections

Instead of doing nothing for an ear infection (while waiting to see if it worsens), I've had great success with mullein garlic oil ear drops (available online—Herb Pharm, www.herb-pharm.com, is a good brand). Put three drops in the infected ear three times daily until well. The oil helps with the pain, and the garlic is a good antibiotic.

fever persists for a few days or the child gets worse, treatment may then be warranted.

- *Colds and coughs:* The latest word on over-the-counter cold and cough medicines is that they shouldn't be used in children under four years of age (due to possible side effects). There are some natural ways you can help your child through, with steam, nasal suction, honey to quiet a cough (only for kids one year and older), vapor rubs, and herbal remedies such as Sinupret (www.sinupretforkids.com).
- *Sinus infections:* This is another area that has been overtreated with antibiotics. The AAP has also declared that children's sinus infections shouldn't be treated with antibiotics unless severe (several days of fever, headache, and feeling sick). A green nose alone isn't enough to warrant antibiotics. Sinupret's blend of five herbs is a great way to help support the sinuses instead of relying on antibiotics.
- *Immune boosting during an illness:* A natural regimen that I've found very effective for me, my children, and my patients is to begin Vitamin C and echinacea at the first sign of any illness. Vitamin C comes in various baby-friendly forms, such as pow-

ders and liquids, that are easily searchable online. Suggested dosing for Vitamin C:

- Babies 6 to 23 months—150 mg twice daily
- Kids 2 through 5—250 mg twice daily
- Children 6 through 11—500 mg twice daily
- Teens and adults—1000 mg twice daily

Echinacea is an herb that can temporarily boost the immune system's response to illness. Although some well-publicized research that came out a few years ago tried to debunk Echinacea's usefulness, the researchers "conveniently" used infant dosing in this adult study—no wonder they didn't get results! Suggested dosing for echinacea:

- Infants 6 to 23 months—follow instructions on the bottle of echinacea drops (I like Herb Pharm's Children's Orange Flavored echinacea drops at www.herb-pharm .com—these are the best tasting ones I've found). Give double the recommended drops twice daily for the first two days, then the regular dose twice daily until well.
- Children 2 to 5 years—take about 500 mg twice daily for two days, then 250 mg twice daily until well. If using Herb Pharm drops, see dosing for infants.
- Kids 6 to 11—take 1000 mg twice daily for two days, then 500 mg twice daily until well. I like Nature's Way brand of capsules (www.naturesway.com).
- Teens and adults—take 2000 mg twice daily for two days, then 1000 mg twice daily until well.

These immune boosters are a great way for Mama and Baby to get through an illness more easily.

- *Teething pain:* Try not to overdo the acetaminophen or ibuprofen. Various herbal and homeopathic teething gels and dissolving tablets can be somewhat effective. Look for ones with chamomilla and/or belladonna. You can find various examples (such as OralSoothe—www.NativeRemedies.com) by searching online. Rubbing a tiny amount of clove oil onto the gums can help, too. Also, give baby something to chew on, like a natural maple wooden teething ring or safe plastic teething toy (discussed on page 302).

- *Fever:* Don't be too quick to calm a fever. Fever is one way that the body fights off infections. It's OK to let a moderate temperature of 101 or 102 ride for a while, as long as your child isn't too miserable.

## VACCINES

Vaccines are a routine part of your baby's checkups. They have become more controversial, however, as the number of vaccines given to babies has increased from three different vaccines given in about eight total doses in the 1980s to twelve different vaccines given in about fifty total doses throughout childhood. Parents worry about the various germ and chemical ingredients in vaccines and wonder if there has been enough safety research. Of course, a thorough discussion on vaccines is beyond the scope of this book. For a complete look at vaccines and their diseases, check out *The Vaccine Book* by Dr. Robert Sears at TheVaccineBook.com.

We will, however, offer a few comments about vaccines from a green perspective. Every vaccine contains some chemicals, some more than others. This book has been all about avoiding chemical exposures. Vaccines, however, are very important. But should parents just turn a blind eye to vaccine chemicals and consider them a necessary part of their baby's medical care? That's the dilemma. Babies need the disease protection, but careful parents worry about the formaldehyde, aluminum, mercury (now only in most flu shots), and other chemicals, as well as various animal and human tissues and blood products used in manufacturing.

Many of the diseases these vaccines protect against can be very serious, not only to an infant or child but to our country as a whole. However, we are sensitive to some parents' desire to be more careful with vaccines. Some parents who want to vaccinate differently discuss with their pediatricians ways to spread the shots out a little and to delay some vaccines they feel are not as important. In *The Vaccine Book*, Dr. Bob offers various ways that parents can vaccinate their baby while spreading the shots out and choosing certain brands that limit the chemicals as much as possible.

# Taking It Home . . .

As Baby grows, support her overall health with five pillars of a healthy lifestyle:

1. *A healthy and green diet.* We have given you a plethora of green feeding tips throughout this book. It's up to you as the Mama (or dad) to provide Baby with the foods she needs to stay healthy, to set a good example (eat those french fries only when she's not looking!), and to work with Baby's caregivers to help Baby eat well when you're not around.
2. *Physical activity and exercise.* Give Baby safe and frequent opportunities to practice physical skills and be active.
3. *Stress management and emotional health.* You do all you can to help Baby to be happy, but stress and disappointment are inevitable, even for infants and toddlers. By modeling healthy reactions to stress, providing a calm, consistent, and safe environment, and being attentive and responsive to Baby's needs you'll help put her on the path to resilience, security, and positive relationships with others.
4. *Good hygiene.* There's no need to keep Baby in a sterile bubble. Basic good hygiene is all you need. Proper hand washing, occasional bathing, and regular toothbrushing keeps babies safe from most germs.
5. *Sleep.* It's not selfish to want Baby to get a good night's sleep. Sufficient sleep will help Baby's mood and overall health. With consistency, compassion, and realistic expectations, you and Baby will find sleep solutions that work for the whole family.

As you're fostering Baby's healthy lifestyle at home, medical practitioners will help you take care of the other important preventive care

Baby needs to protect her health. Regular well child checkups are recommended (and closer to age two, dental checkups, too). Vaccines, though controversial, are an important piece of Baby's preventive care, and they protect her from disease outbreaks. We encourage you to read more about them and speak to your pediatrician about a vaccination schedule that feels right for your family. And for the less serious common childhood illnesses, like colds and coughs, home remedies and natural treatments are helpful, especially when Baby is too young for many over-the-counter medications.

# Notes

**Chapter 1**

1. Environmental Working Group, "Body Burden—The Pollution in Newborns." July 14, 2005. Available: http://archive.ewg.org/reports/bodyburden2/execsumm.php

2. Office of Environmental Health Hazard Assessment, Proposition 65 List. Available: http://www.oehha.org/Prop65/prop65_list/Newlist.html

3. Lunder, S., and Jacob, A., "Fire Retardants in Toddlers and Their Mothers," September 2008. Available: http://www.ewg.org/reports/pbdesintoddlers

4. Buka, I., Koranteng, S., Osornio-Vargas, AR, "The Effects of Air Pollution on the Health of Children." *Paediatr Child Health*. 2006 Oct;11(8):513–6.

5. Salam, M., et al., "Early Life Environmental Risk Factors for Asthma: Findings From the Children's Health Study." *Environmental Health Perspectives Online*, Dec. 9, 2003. Available: http://www.ehponline.org/docs/2003/6662/abstract.html

6. Delfino, R. J., "Epidemiologic Evidence for Asthma and Exposure to Air Toxics: Linkages Between Occupational, Indoor, and Community Air Pollution Research." *Environ Health Perspect*. 2002 Aug;110 Suppl 4:573–89. Review.

7. Miller, R., et al., Polycyclic Aromatic Hydrocarbons, Environmental Tobacco Smoke, and Respiratory Symptoms in an Inner-City Birth Cohort, *CHEST*, Vol 126:4, October 2004.

8. Folstein, S., Rosen-Sheidley, B., "Genetics of Autism: Complex Aetiology for a Heterogeneous Disorder." *Nature Reviews/Genetics* 2:943–955, 2001.

9. Steffenberg, S., Gillberg, C., Hellgren, L., et al., "A Twin Study of Autism in Denmark, Finland, Iceland, Norway, and Sweden." *J Child Psychology and Psychiatry* 30:405–416, 1989.

10. Roberts, E. M., et al., Maternal Residence Near Agricultural Pesticide Applications and Autism Spectrum Disorders Among Children in the California Central Valley. *Environmental Health Perspectives*. 2007 Oct;115(10).

11. Desmond, M., Wilson, G., Melnick, J., et al., "Congenital Rubella Encephalitis." Course and Early Sequelae. *J Pediatrics* 71:311–331, 1967.

12. Institute of Medicine, *Immunization Safety Review*. "Vaccines and Autism." Washington: National Academy Press; 2004.

13. Work Group for Safe Markets, "Baby's Toxic Bottle: BPA Leaching from Popular Baby Bottles." Available: http://www.chej.org/documents/BabysToxicBottleFinal.pdf

14. Swan, S. H., Environmental Phthalate Exposure in Relation to Reproductive Outcomes and Other Health Endpoints in Humans. *Environmental Research*, 2008 Oct;108(2): 177–184.

15. Committee on Developmental Toxicology, Board on Environmental Studies and Toxicology, and National Research Council, *Scientific Frontiers in Developmental Toxicology and Risk Assessment* (The National Academies Press, 2000).

16. Branchi, I., Alleva, E., Costa, L. G., "Effects of Perinatal Exposure to a Polybrominated Diphenyl Ether (PBDE 99) on Mouse Neurobehavioural Development." *Neurotoxicology*. 2002 Sep;23(3):375–84.

17. Stewart, P. W., et al., Cognitive Development in Preschool Children Prenatally Exposed to PCBs and MeHg. *Neurotoxicology and Teratology*, 2003 Jan-Feb;Vol 25(No 1): 11–22.

18. Environmental Protective Agency, "Municipal Solid Waste in the US" (2007). Available: http://www.epa.gov/epawaste/nonhaz/municipal/pubs/msw07-fs.pdf

19. Steinway, D., "Trashing Superfund: The Role of Municipal Solid Waste in CERCLA Cases," November 1999. Available: http://library.findlaw.com/1999/Nov/1/130490.html

20. Governmental Accounting Office, "Freshwater Supply: States' Views of How Federal Agencies Could Help Them Meet the Challenges of Expected Shortages" (GAO-03–514). Available: http://www.gao.gov/new.items/d03514.pdf

21. California Energy Commission, "California's Water-Energy Relationship," 2005. Available: www.energy.ca.gov

22. Environmental Working Group, "A National Assessment of Tap Water Quality," December 20, 2005. Available: http://www.ewg.org/tapwater/findings.php

23. Environmental Protection Agency, "Climate Change: Greenhouse Gas Emissions" (2008). Available: http://www.epa.gov/climatechange/emissions/ind_home.html

24. Curl, C. L., Fenske, R. A., Elgethun, K., "Organophosphorus Pesticide Exposure of Urban and Suburban Preschool Children with Organic and Conventional Diets." *Environ Health Perspect*. 2003 Mar;111(3):377–82.

25. According to Scorecard (www.scorecard.org)

26. Bell, E. M., Hertz-Picciotto, I., Beaumont, J., "A Case-Control Study of Pesticides and Fetal Death Due to Congenital Anomalies." *Epidemiology*. 12(2):148–156, March 2001.

27. Cohen, M., "Environmental Toxins and Health: The Health Impact of Pesticides." *Australian Family Physician*, Vol 38, No 12, December 2007, 1003–6. Available: http://www.racgp.org.au/afp/200712/200712Cohen2.pdf

28. Daniels, J. L., et al., "Pesticides and Childhood Cancers." *Environmental Health Perspectives* 105, 10 (1997): 1068–1077. Available: http://www.ehponline.org/members/1997/105-10/daniels-full.html

29. Hansen, M. J., et al., "Potential Public Health Impacts of the Use of Recombinant Bovine Somatotropin in Dairy Production": Prepared for a Scientific Review by the Joint Expert Committee on Food Additives, September 1997. Available: http://www.consumersunion.org/pub/core_food_safety/002272.html

30. Orlando, E. F., et al., "Endocrine-Disrupting Effects of Cattle Feedlot Effluent on an Aquatic Sentinel Species, the Fathead Minnow." Environmental Health Perspectives, Vol. 112, 2004.

31. Sierra Club, "Abuse of Antibiotics at Factory Farms Threatens the Effectiveness of Drugs Used to Treat Disease in Humans." Available: http://www.sierraclub.org/factoryfarms/factsheets/antibiotics.asp

32. Pimentel, D., et al., "Environmental, Energetic, and Economic Comparisons of Organic and Conventional Farming Systems." *BioScience*, 2005 July;55(7): 573–582.

33. 2002 University of Missouri study, "Oranges Have 30% More Vitamin C." American Chemical Society (2002, June 3). Research at Great Lakes Meeting Shows More Vitamin C in Organic Oranges than Conventional Oranges." *ScienceDaily*. Available: http://www.sciencedaily.com/releases/2002/06/020603071017.htm

34. Worthington, V., "Effect of Agricultural Methods on Nutritional Quality: A Comparison of Organic with Conventional Crops." *Alternative Therapies*, Volume 4, 1998, pages 58–69.

35. Davis, D. R., et al., Changes in USDA Food Composition Data for 43 Garden Crops, 1950 to 1999. *J Am Coll Nutr*. 2004;23: 669–682.

36. Rule, D. C., Broughton, K. S., Shellito, S. M., "Comparison of Muscle Fatty Acid Profiles and Cholesterol Concentrations of Bison, Beef Cattle, Elk, and Chicken." *J Anim Sci* (2002);80:1202–11.

37. Ellis, K. A., et al., Comparing the Fatty Acid Composition of Organic and Conventional Milk. *J. Dairy Sci.* 89: 1938–1950.

38. Theuer, R. C., "Do Organic Fruits and Vegetables Taste Better than Conventional Produce?" Available: www.organic-center.org

## Chapter 2

1. Oken, E., et al., "Television, Walking, and Diet: Associations with Postpartum Weight Retention. *Am J Prev Med* 32(4), 2007.

2. Dewey, K., et al., "A Randomized Study of the Effects of Aerobic Exercise by Lactating Women on Breast Milk Volume and Composition." *N Engl J Med* 1994; 330(7):449–53.

3. Lovelady, C., et al., "Lactation Performance of Exercising Women." *Am J Clin Nutr* 1990; 52:103–09.

4. Heinig, M., et al., "Lactation and Postpartum Weight Loss." *Mechanisms Regulating Lactation and Infant Nutrient Utilization* 1992; 30: 397–400.

5. Dewey, K. and McCrory, M., "Effects of Dieting and Physical Activity on Pregnancy and Lactation." *Am J Clin Nutr* 1994; 59(Suppl):446S–59S.

6. Mezzacappa, E. S., "Breastfeeding and Maternal Stress Response and Health" (Review). *Nutr Rev*. 2004 Jul; 62(7 Pt 1): 261–8.

7. Kimata, H., "Laughter Elevates the Levels of Breast-milk Melatonin." *Journal of Psychosomatic Research*, Volume 62, Issue 6, Pages 699–702.

8. Field, et al., Cortisol Decreases and Serotonin and Dopamine Increase Following Massage Therapy. *International Journal of Neuroscience*, 2005;115:1397–1413.

9. Starbucks, 2006 Corporate Social Responsibility report. Available: http://www.starbucks.com/aboutus/FY06_CSR_AR.pdf

10. Bell, Silvia M., and Ainsworth, Mary D. S., "Infant Crying and Maternal Responsiveness." *Child Development*, 43(1972):1171–1190.

11. Freeman, M. P. , "Omega-3 Fatty Acids and Perinatal Depression: A Review of the Literature and Recommendations for Future Research." *Prostaglandins Leukot Essent Fatty Acids*. 2006 Oct-Nov;75(4–5):291–7.

## Chapter 3

1. Gartner, L. M, et al., "Breastfeeding and the Use of Human Milk." *Pediatrics*. 2005 Feb;115(2):496–506.

2. Saarinen, U. M., et al., "Iron Absorption in Infants: High Bioavailability of Breast Milk Iron as Indicated by the Extrinsic Tag Method of Iron Absorption and by the Concentration of Serum Ferritin." *J Pediatr*. 1977 Jul;91(1):36–9.

3. Chantry, C. J., Howard, C. R., Auinger, P., "Full Breastfeeding Duration and Associated Decrease in Respiratory Tract Infection in US Children." *Pediatrics*. 2006 Feb;117(2):425–32.

4. van Odijk, J., et al., "Breastfeeding and Allergic Disease: A Multidisciplinary Review of the Literature (1966–2001) on the Mode of Early Feeding in Infancy and Its Impact on Later Atopic Manifestations." *Allergy*. Sep 2003; 58 (9): 833–843

5. Gdalevich, M., Mimouni, D., Mimouni, M., "Breast-feeding and the Risk of Bronchial Asthma in Childhood: A Systematic Review with Meta-analysis of Prospective Studies." *J Pediatr* 2001 Aug;139(2):261–6

6. Scariati, P. D., et al., "A Longitudinal Analysis of Infant Morbidity and the Extent of Breastfeeding in the United States." *Pediatrics* 1997 Jun;99(6):E5

7. Quigley, M. A., et al., "How Protective is Breast Feeding Against Diarrhoeal Disease in Infants in 1990s England? A Case-control Study." *Arch Dis Child*. 2006 Mar;91(3):245–50

8. Coppa, G. V., et al., "Human Milk Oligosaccharides Inhibit the Adhesion to Caco-2 Cells of Diarrheal Pathogens: Escherichia Coli, Vibrio Cholerae, and Salmonella Fyris." *Pediatr Res*. 2006 Mar;59(3):377–82.

9. Baker, D., et al., "Inequality in Infant Morbidity: Causes and Consequences in England in the 1990s." *J Epidemiol Community Health* 1998 Jul;52(7):451–8

10. Heacock, H. J., "Influence of Breast vs. Formula Milk in Physiologic Gastroesophageal Reflux in Healthy Newborn Infants." *J. Pediatr Gastroenterol Nutr*, 1992 January; 14(1): 41–6

11. Chatzimichael, A., et al., "The Role of Breastfeeding and Passive Smoking on the Development of Severe Bronchiolitis in Infants." *Minerva Pediatr*. 2007 Jun;59(3):199–206.

12. Owen, C. G., et al., "Does Breastfeeding Influence Risk of Type 2 Diabetes in Later Life? A Quantitative Analysis of Published Evidence." *Am J Clin Nutr*. 2006 Nov;84(5):1043–54.

13. Weyermann, M., Rothenbacher, D., Brenner, H., "Duration of Breastfeeding and Risk of Overweight in Childhood: A Prospective Birth Cohort Study from Germany." *Int J Obes*. 2006 Aug;30(8):1281–7.

14. Harder, T., et al., "Duration of Breastfeeding and Risk of Overweight: A Meta-analysis." *Am J Epidemiol* 2005;162: 397–403.

15. Britton, J. R., Britton, H. L., and Gronwaldt, V., "Breastfeeding, Sensitivity, and Attachment." *Pediatrics* Vol. 118 No. 5 November 2006, pp. e1436–e1443

16. Kac, G., et al., "Breastfeeding and Postpartum Weight Retention in a Cohort of Brazilian Women." *American Journal of Clinical Nutrition*. Mar 2004; 79 (3) : 487–493

17. Groer, M. W., "Differences Between Exclusive Breastfeeders, Formula-feeders, and Controls: A Study of Stress, Mood, and Endocrine Variables." *Biol Res Nurs*. 2005 Oct;7(2):106–17.

18. Beral, V., et al., "Breast Cancer and Breastfeeding: Collaborative Reanalysis of Individual Data from 47 Epidemiological Studies in 30 Countries, Including 50,302 Women with Breast Cancer and 96,973 Women Without the Disease." *Lancet*, Jul 20 2002; 360 (9328): 187–195.

19. Siskind, V., et al., "Breastfeeding, Menopause, and Epithelial Ovarian Cancer. *Epidemiology* 1997 Mar;8(2):188–91.

20. Howard, C. R., et al., "Randomized Clinical Trial of Pacifier Use and Bottle-feeding or Cupfeeding and their Effect on Breastfeeding." *Pediatrics*. 2003 March;111(3): 511–518.

21. Howard, C. R., et al., "The Effects of Early Pacifier Use on Breastfeeding Duration." *Pediatrics*. 1999 March; 103(3):e33.

22. Aarts, C., et al., "Breastfeeding Patterns in Relation to Thumb Sucking and Pacifier Use." *Pediatrics* Vol. 104 No. 4 October 1999, p. e50.

23. Cesar Gomes, V., et al., "Pacifier Use and Short Breastfeeding Duration: Cause, Consequence, or Coincidence?" *Pediatrics* Vol. 99 No. 3 March 1997, pp. 445–453.

24. Environmental Working Group, "Babies at Risk: BPA in Dangerous Levels in Liquid Formula." Available: http://www.ewg.org/node/27257

25. Food & Drug Administration, "Melamine Contamination in China." (Updated January 5, 2009) Available: http://www.fda.gov/oc/opacom/hottopics/melamine.html

26. Environmental Working Group, "A National Assessment of Tap Water Quality." December 20, 2005. Available: http://www.ewg.org/tapwater/findings.php

27. Natural Resources Defense Council, "What's on Tap? Grading Drinking Water in U.S. Cities", June 2003. Available: http://www.nrdc.org/water/drinking/uscities/contents.asp

## Chapter 4

1. World Wildlife Fund, "Meet the Amazing Atlantic Bluefin Tuna (Thunnus thynnus)" Available: www.panda.org/tuna.
2. Child & Family Research Institute (2008, March 11), "Typical North American Diet is Deficient in Omega-3 Fatty Acids." *ScienceDaily*. Available: www.sciencedaily.com/releases/2008/03/080307133659.htm
3. Otten, J. J., Hellwig, J. P., and Meyers, L. D., eds., *Dietary Reference Intakes: The Essential Guide to Nutrient Requirements* (Food and Nutrition Board of the Institute of Medicine, 2006)
4. United States Department of Agriculture, "My Pyramid for Pregancy and Breastfeeding." Available: www.mypyramid.gov
5. Kalkwarf, H. J., Specker, B.L., 1995, "Bone Mineral Loss During Lactation and Recovery After Weaning." *Obstet Gynecol*. 86:26–32.
6. Specker, B. L., Tsang, R. C., Ho, M. L., 1991, "Changes in Calcium Homeostasis Over the First Year Postpartum: Effect of Lactation and Weaning." *Obstet Gynecol*. 78:56–62.
7. Center for the Evaluation of Risks to Human Reproduction, National Toxicology Program, "Mercury." Available: http://cerhr.niehs.nih.gov/common/mercury.html
8. Blaylock, R., "Excitotoxins: The Taste that Kills." Health Press (1996)
9. Mohrbacher, N., and Stock, J., *The Breastfeeding Answer Book* (La Leche League International, 2003).
10. Greer, R., MD, "Effects of Early Nutritional Interventions on the Development of Atopic Disease in Infants and Children: The Role of Maternal Dietary Restriction, Breastfeeding, Timing of Introduction of Complementary Foods, and Hydrolyzed Formulas." *Pediatrics*, Vol. 121 No. 1 January 2008, pp. 183–191.
11. Rautava, S., Kalliomäki, M., Isolauri, E., "Probiotics During Pregnancy and Breast-feeding Might Confer Immunomodulatory Protection Against Atopic Disease in the Infant." *J Allergy Clin Immunol*. 2002 Jan;109(1):119–21.
12. Rooney, B. L., Schauberger, C. W., "Excess Pregnancy Weight Gain and Long-term Obesity: One Decade Later." *Obstet Gynecol*. 2002 Aug;100(2)

## Chapter 5

1. Natural Resources Defense Council, "What's on Tap? Grading Drinking Water in U.S. Cities," June 2003. Available: http://www.nrdc.org/water/drinking/uscities/contents.asp.
2. Branum, A. M., and Lukacs, S. L., "Food Allergy Among U.S. Children: Trends in Prevalence and Hospitalizations," NCHS Data Brief, Number 10, October 2008. Available: http://www.cdc.gov/nchs/data/databriefs/db10.htm
3. EPA, "Municipal Solid Waste in the US," 2007. Available: http://www.epa.gov/epawaste/nonhaz/municipal/pubs/msw07-fs.pdf
4. Favell, D. J., "A Comparison of the Vitamin C Content of Fresh and Frozen Vegetables." *Food Chemistry*. 1998 May;62(1):59–64.
5. Greer, F. R., and Shannon, M., "Infant Methemoglobinemia: The Role of Dietary Nitrate in Food and Water." *Pediatrics* 2005 September;116(3):784–786.
6. Bartoshuk, L. M. (1991), "Sweetness: History, Preference, and Genetic Variability." *Food Technology*. 45(11): 108–113.

## Chapter 6

1. USDA, "Pesticide Data Program—Annual Summary Calendar Year. 2004." Available: http://www.organic-center.org/reportfiles/Milk_Pesticides_FAQs.pdf

2. Ishida, B. K., Chapman, M. H., "A Comparison of Carotenoid Content and Total Antioxidant Activity in Catsup from Several Commercial Sources in the United States." *J Agric Food Chem.* 2004 Dec 29;52(26):8017–20. 2004.

3. Fox, M. K., et al., "Feeding Infants and Toddlers Study: What Foods are Infants and Toddlers Eating?" *J Am Diet Assoc.* 2004 Jan;104(1 Suppl 1):s22–30.

4. Blakeslee, S., "New Light Being Shed on Early Mechanisms of Coronary Disease," *New York Times*, March 27, 1990.

5. Roy, P. K., et al., "Lactose Intolerance." Available at: http://emedicine.medscape.com/article/187249-overview

6. Environmental Defense Fund, "Seafood Selector." Available: http://www.edf.org/page.cfm?tagID=1521

7. Robertson, J., and Fanning, C., 2004, *Omega 3 Polyunsaturated Fatty Acids in Organic and Conventional Milk* (University of Aberdeen).

8. Butchko, H. H., et al., "Aspartame: Review of Safety." *Regul Toxicol Pharmacol.* 2002;35:S1–S93.

9. Soffritti, M., et al.. "Life-span Exposure to Low Doses of Aspartame Beginning During Prenatal Life Increases Cancer Effects in Rats." *Environmental Health Perspectives* Volume 115, Number 9, September 2007

10. Humphries, P., Pretorius, E., Naude, H., Direct and Indirect Cellular Effects of Aspartame on the Brain. *European Journal of Clinical Nutrition*, 2008

11. FDA Office of Public Affairs, Artificial Sweeteners: No Calories . . . Sweet! *FDA Consumer* magazine. July–August 2006. Available: http://www.fda.gov/fdac/features/2006/406_sweeteners.html

12. Forshee, R. A., et al., "A Critical Examination of the Evidence Relating High Fructose Corn Syrup and Weight Gain." *Crit Rev Food Sci Nutr.* 2007;47(6):561–82.


## Chapter 7

1. Moreno, L. A., Rodríguez, G., "Dietary Risk Factors for Development of Childhood Obesity." *Curr Opin Clin Nutr Metab Care.* 2007 May;10(3):336–41. (Review)

2. Bellisle, F., "Effects of Diet on Behaviour and Cognition in Children." *Br J Nutr.* 2004 Oct;92 Suppl 2:S227–32. (Review)

3. McCann, D., et al., Food Additives and Hyperactive Behaviour in 3-year-old and 8/9-year-old Children in the Community: A Randomised, Double-blinded, Placebo-controlled Trial. *Lancet.* 2007 Nov 3;370(9598):1560–7.

4. *Neilson Consumer Insight Magazine*, "Eating Out in America: A New War Wages," May 2008 issue. Available: http://www.nielsen.com/consumer_insight/issue8/ci_topline_article_VII.html)

5. Jones, T. W., "Using Contemporary Archaeology and Applied Anthropology to Understand Food Loss in the American Food System" (USDA Food Loss Project). Available: http://www.communitycompost.org/info/usafood.pdf

6. www.reusablebags.com


## Chapter 8

1. Sauer, B., et al., "Resource and Environmental Profile Analysis of Children's Diaper Systems," *Environmental Toxicology and Chemistry*, Vol 13, No 6, pp 1003–1009, 1994.

2. Environmental Protection Agency, "Municipal Solid Waste in the United States, 2007." Available: http://www.epa.gov/osw/nonhaz/municipal/pubs/msw07-rpt.pdf

3. Lehrburger, C., Mullen, J., and Jones, C. V., *Diapers: Environmental Impacts and Lifecycle Analysis.* Philadelphia, PA: Report to The National Association of Diaper Services (NADS), 1991.

4. The Green Guide, Diapers Buying Guide. Available: http://www.thegreenguide.com/greenguide/buying-guide/diapers/environmental_impact

5. Anderson, R. C., and Anderson, J. H., "Acute Respiratory Effects of Diaper Emissions." *Archives of Environmental Health*, 1999 Sep-Oct;54(5):353–8.

6. Partsch, C. J., Aukamp, M., Sippell, W. G., "Scrotal Temperature is Increased in Disposable Plastic Lined Nappies." *Archives of Disease in Childhood*, 2000;83:364–368.

7. Lane, A. T., Rehder, P. A., Helm, K., "Evaluations of Diapers Containing Absorbent Gelling Material with Conventional Disposable Diapers in Newborn Infants." *Am J Dis Child.* 1990 Mar;144(3):315–8.

8. Kosemund, K., et al., "Safety Evaluation of Superabsorbent Baby Diapers." *Regul Toxicol Pharmacol.* 2008 Nov 1.

9. Swan, et al., "Decrease in Anogenital Distance Among Male Infants with Prenatal Phthalate Exposure." *Environmental Health Perspectives* Volume 113, Number 8, August 2005. Available: http://www.ehponline.org/docs/2005/113–8/ss.html

10. Main, K. M., et al., "Human Breast Milk Contamination with Phthalates and Alterations of Endogenous Reproductive Hormones in Infants Three Months of Age." *Environmental Health Perspectives Volume* 114, Number 2, February 2006. Available: http://www.ehponline.org/docs/2005/8075/abstract.html

11. Darbre, P. D., Harvey, P. W. , "Paraben Esters: Review of Recent Studies of Endocrine Toxicity, Absorption, Esterase and Human Exposure, and Discussion of Potential Human Health Risks." *J Appl Toxicol.* 2008 Jul;28(5):561–78. (Review)

12. Children's Health and Environmental Coalition, Sodium Laureth Sulfate Chemical Profile. Available: http://www.checnet.org/HEALTHEHOUSE/chemicals/chemicals-detail2.asp?Main_ID=285.

13. National Cancer Institute, Skin Cancer. Available: http://www.cancer.gov/cancertopics/types/skin

14. Natural Resources Defense Council, "Healthy Milk, Healthy Baby: Chemical Pollution and Mother's Milk." Available: http://www.nrdc.org/breastmilk/pbde.asp

15. Lunder, S., and Sharp, R., Mothers' Milk: "Record Levels of Toxic Flame Retardants Found in Amercian Mothers' Breast Milk, 2003." Available: http://www.ewg.org/files/MothersMilk_final.pdf

16. Lau, C., et al., "Perfluoroalkyl Acids: A Review of Monitoring and Toxicological Findings." *Toxicol Sci.* 2007 Oct;99(2):366–94. Epub 2007 May 22. Available: http://toxsci.oxfordjournals.org/cgi/reprint/kfm128v1.pdf

17. Organic Trade Association, "Cotton and the Environment." Available: http://www.ota.com/organic/environment/cotton_environment.html

18. Northwest Coalition for Alternatives to Pesticides, "Does Government Registration Mean Pesticides are Safe?" *Journal of Pesticide Reform*, Summer 1999, Vol 19, No 2. Available: http://www.pesticide.org/BasicRegistration.pdf


**Chapter 9**

1. Environmental Protection Agency, www.epa.gov

2. Natural Resources Defense Council, "A Shopper's Guide to Home Tissue Products. Available: http://www.nrdc.org/land/forests/gtissue.asp

3. Farrow, A., Taylor, H., Northstone, K., Golding, J., "Symptoms of Mothers and Infants Related to Total Volatile Organic Compounds in Household Products." *Arch Environ Health.* 2003 Oct;58(10):633–41.

4. Environmental Protection Agency, "Municipal Solid Waste Generation, Recycling, and Disposal in the United States: Facts and Figures for 2007." Available: http://www.epa.gov/osw/nonhaz/municipal/pubs/msw07-fs.pdf

5. Environmental Literacy Council. www.enviroliteracy.org

6. Environmental Protection Agency, "Energy and Water." Available: http://www.epa.gov/waterinfrastructure/bettermanagement_energy.html

7. American Water Works Association. www.drinktap.org

8. Environmental Protection Agency, "WaterSense." Available: http://www.epa.gov/watersense/water/simple.htm

9. www.energystar.gov

10. US Department of Energy, Office of Energy Efficiency and Renewable Energy. Available: http://www.eere.energy.gov/

**Chapter 10**

1. Ogden, C. L., Carroll, M. D., Flegal, K. M., "High Body Mass Index for Age Among US Children and Adolescents, 2003–2006." *JAMA*. 2008;299(20):2401–2405.

2. Ong, K. K., et al., "Association Between Postnatal Catch-up Growth and Obesity in Childhood: A Prospective Cohort Study." *BMJ*, 2000 Apr 8;320(7240):967–71.

3. Grummer-Strawn, L. M., Scanlon, K. S., Fein, S. B., "Infant Feeding and Feeding Transitions Furing the First Year of Life." *Pediatrics*. 2008 Oct;122 Suppl 2:S36–42.

4. Schrager, S., "Dietary Calcium Intake and Obesity." *Journal of the American Board of Family Practice*, Vol 18: 205–210 (2005).

5. Zemel, M. B., "The Role of Dairy Foods in Weight Management." *J Am Coll Nutr*. 2005 Dec;24(6 Suppl): 537S–46S.

6. Taveras, E. M., et al., "Short Sleep Duration in Infancy and Risk of Childhood Overweight." *Arch Pediatr Adolesc Med*. 2008 Apr;162(4):305–11.

7. Institute of Medicine, "From Neurons to Neighborhoods: The Science of Early Childhood Development" (2000). Available: http://www.nap.edu/catalog.php?record_id=9824#toc

8. Sunderland, M., *The Science of Parenting*. (DK Adult, May 2006)

9. American Academy of Pediatrics Task Force on Sudden Infant Death Syndrome, "The Changing Concept of Sudden Infant Death Syndrome: Diagnostic Coding Shifts, Controversies Regarding the Sleeping Environment, and New Variables to Consider in Reducing Risk." *Pediatrics* 2005 116: 1245–1255.

10. American Academy of Pediatrics Subcommittee on Management of Acute Otitis Media, "Diagnosis and Management of Otitis Media." *Pediatrics*. 2004 May; 113(5):1451–65.

# Green Resources
## Additional Resouces

### Green Living

- The Green Guide, www.thegreenguide.com—From National Geographic, a practical guide for everyday consumers who want to make eco-conscious choices.
- Green Your . . . , www.greenyour.com—A guide to green living full of informative facts and practical tips.
- *Green Living for Dummies* by Yvonne Jeffery, Liz Barclay, and Michael Grosvenor
- *It's Easy Being Green: A Handbook for Earth-Friendly Living* by Crissy Trask
- Environmental Literacy Council, www.enviroliteracy.org—An independent non-profit organization that seeks to provide environmental science information to teachers, this Web site features lots of basic background information about a plethora of eco-topics.
- Environmental Protection Agency's WaterSense program, www.epa.gov/watersense—The EPA's water conservation resource for the public.
- Care 2, www.care2.com—An online community focused on healthy and green living.

### Green Parenting

ORGANIZATIONS
- Healthy Child, Healthy World, www.healthychild.org—Non-profit organization created to "help millions of parents, educators, health professionals, and the general public take action to create healthy environments and embrace green, non-toxic steps."

BLOGS AND OTHER ONLINE RESOURCES
- General green parenting sites: Ecochildsplay.com, momgogreen.com, www.enviromom.com, www.greenbabyguide.com, www.growbabygreen.com, www.greenmomfinds.com
- www.organic-baby-resource.com—Web site that provides readers with "everything you've ever wanted to know about organic baby care."

- Inhabitots, www.inhabitots.com—A resource for parents interested in sustainable modern design for babies and children.

## General Healthy Parenting

- Ask Dr. Sears, www.askdrsears.com—A comprehensive pediatric health Web site from Dr. Bob and his brother Dr. Jim, and parents Dr. William and Martha Sears.
- *The Baby Book* by William Sears, MD and Martha Sears, RN
- *The Vaccine Book* by Dr. Bob Sears
- *The Happiest Baby/Toddler on the Block* books by Dr. Harvey Karp

## Green and Healthy Feeding

BOOKS
- *The Nursing Mother's Companion* by Kathleen Huggins, RN, MS
- *Child of Mine: Feeding with Love and Good Sense* and *How to Get Your Kid to Eat . . . But Not Too Much* both by Ellyn Satter
- *The Family Nutrition Book* by William Sears, MD and Martha Sears, RN
- *Super Baby Food* by Ruth Yaron
- *First Meals* and *Superfoods: For Babies and Children* by Annabel Karmel

ORGANIZATIONS
- La Leche League, www.llli.org—International breastfeeding organization; their Web site features information and on-line support for nursing moms. You may also search their Web site for local breastfeeding support groups in your area.
- Center for Science in the Public Interest, www.cspinet.org—Advocacy organization focused on nutrition and health. They publish the informative "Nutrition Action Health Letter" newsletter, available on their Web site.
- Sustainable Table, www.sustainabletable.org—Program that educates and advocates for local and sustainable food. Website features the "Eat Well Guide," an online directory of sustainable food products in the U.S. and Canada.
- Local Harvest, www.localharvest.org—An organic and local food organization that links consumers with local farmers and markets. Their Web site provides online directories for local foods and Community Supported Agriculture (CSA) cooperatives.
- The Organic Center, www.organic-center.org—A non-profit organization dedicated to organic farming and products. If you are interested in reading some science pertaining to organic foods, this site is a good place to start.

WEB SITES
- HappyBaby, www.happybabyfood.com—HappyBaby's Web site featuring information about the company's products along with serving suggestions, recipes, and feeding tips.
- Fresh Baby, www.freshbaby.com—Products and advice for making homemade babyfood and breastfeeding
- Kelly Mom, www.Kellymom.com—Breastfeeding and parenting information, tips, tools, and articles written by lactation consultants.
- Wholesome Baby Food, www.wholesomebabyfood.com—Baby food recipes, meal ideas, and nutrition information.
- The Six O'clock Scramble, http://thescramble.com—Each week this Web site's online newsletter provides a menu and 30-minute recipes for a week's worth of healthy and easy dinners.

- The Soft Landing, www.thesoftlanding.com—Online retailer of safe baby-feeding gear. Web site features a blog with news and opinion about feeding products.
- Smallbites, www.smallbitesonline.com—Resources, classes, and services for parents to learn "how to make healthy, safe and sustainable food choices"; Web site features recipes, tips, and a monthly newsletter.

HEALTHY BABY GEAR AND BABY CARE PRODUCTS
- To compare baby care products: The Good Guide, www.goodguide.com and Enviornmental Working Group's www.cosmeticsdatabase.com
- Information about toy safety: www.Healthytoys.org
- Product reviews and consumer advocacy for parents: SafeMama, safemama.com; Z Recommends, zrecommends.com
- *Guide to Natural Baby Care* by Mindy Pennybacker, Aisha Ikramuddin, Mothers & Others for a Livable Planet
- Cloth diaper retailers whose Web sites feature a great deal of how-to information about cloth diapering: Soft Cloth Bunz, www.softclothbunz.com and Green Mountain Diapers, www.greenmountaindiapers.com.

GREEN HOME INFORMATION
- *Green Housekeeping* by Ellen Sandbeck
- *Better Basics for the Home: Simple Solutions for Less Toxic Living* by Annie Berthold-Bond
- SafeLawns.org, www.safelawns.org—A non-profit organization devoted to eco-friendly lawn and grounds care.
- Eco Terric, www.eco-terric.com—Retailer of natural and organic home furnishings.
- Online bulletin boards for swapping and selling baby gear or other household items: Zwaggle—http://Zwaggle.com, Freepeats—http://Freepeats.org, Craigslist—www.Craigslist.org

PARENTING SUPPORT
- See Mommy Run, www.seemommyrun.com—Running and walking groups for Mamas nationwide
- La Leche League International, www.llli.org—Breast feeding support groups and online forums
- Parents Without Partners, www.parentswithoutpartners.org—Support groups and resources for single parents
- National Organization of Mothers with Twins Clubs, www.nomotc.org—Network of support groups for Mamas with multiples
- Mothers and More, www.mothersandmore.org—Network of support groups and resources for Mamas
- The Mommies Network, www.themommiesnetwork.org—Network of local support groups for Mamas
- The Dads Network, www.thedadsnetwork.org—Network of local support groups for Dad
- Mocha Moms, www.mochamoms.org—Support group for Mamas of color
- MOMS Club, www.momsclub.org—Support group for "at-home" Mamas
- Moms in Business Network, www.mibn.org—Support for employed Mamas
- Moxie Moms, www.moxie-moms.com—Support for "fitness and business focused" Mamas

CLASSES FOR MAMA AND BABY
- Fitness for Mama (bring Baby): Baby Boot Camp, www.babybootcamp.com; Stroller Strides, www.strollerstrides.com.
- Fitness for Baby: My Gym, www.my-gym.com, The Little Gym, www.thelittlegym.com
- Enrichment for Baby: Baby Signs, www.babysigns.com; Signing Smart, www.signingsmart.com; Kindermusik, www.kindermusik.com; Music Together, www.musictogether.com

# Acknowledgments

Amy would like to thank and acknowledge: Shazi and Jessica of HappyBaby for your amazing vision and for letting me be a part of it. Bob, for this opportunity to partner with you and for all your thoughtful work. Everyone at Harper Collins, especially Lisa Sharkey for your passion for all things green and support for this project and Amy Kaplan for your day-to-day guidance and feedback. Ryan Fischer-Harbage of the Fischer-Harbage Agency for finding a home for this book. Helen Bernstein at HappyBaby for your help and support. Allison Topilow, RD for reviewing nutrition content and for our weekly playdates. Diane Norwood, RD, for reviewing recipes. Linda Sheehan for the cloth diapering crash course. Adam Nathanson, Lauren Brand, Meghan Dube, Nikkole Vlacancich, Janelle Diamond, Emily Perlman, Suzy Isack, Sepi Djavaheri, Brittany Ekleberry, and Shara Glickman for your friendship and good humor over the past year. Emily Martinez for being such a loving and positive influence for my kids when I'm busy with work. Mom, Dad, Marcy, George, Bobu, and all my in-law sibs for your love and encouragement. A million thanks to Josh for taking it all on and doing it so amazingly well and to Jenny Lazarus, my sister and friend, for reviewing every chapter with such insight and providing invaluable "real-mom" feedback. And finally, thanks to Grandma for extolling the many wonders of vinegar and for instilling in me the values of conservation, good nutrition, and good food.

Dr. Bob would like to thank Amy for all her hard work and dedication to this book, Denise at Denise Marcil Literary Agency for her many years of advice and guidance (and many more to come!), Shazi and Jessica at HappyBaby for their vision and passion for helping families Go Green and Lisa and Amy at HarperCollins for being a real joy to work with.

# Index

colostrum, 60, 64, 66, 67

community-supported
    agriculture (CSA), 252

composting, 201

constipation, 154

consumption, 324–26

coping skills, 42–50

cotton, 305–6

cow's milk, 96, 101–2, 169, 207,
    208, 213, 217

cradle cap, 289, 361–62

cradle hold, 69

crib mattresses, 294–96

cribs, 292–94, 299

crop rotation, 29

C-section, and breast-feeding,
    67

cups:
    choosing, 103–4
    introducing, 165


dairy products, 102, 208–9, 251

day care, 343–45

DDT, 12

dead zones, 27

dehydration, 65

dental checkups, 371

depression, therapy for, 53

detergents, 313, 316

diaper bags, 278

diaper covers, 280

diaper creams, 279

diaper liners, rice paper, 284

diaper pails, 285

diaper rash, 283

diapers, 75, 276–86
    all-in-ones, 281
    cloth, 280–84, 286
    contoured, 281, 284

disposable, 276–80, 286
    fitted, 281
    gDiaper, 284–85
    homemade, 288
    pocket, 281
    prefolds, 280–81, 284

diaper service, 284

diaper wipes, 285, 286–88

dinner, 132–33, 246–49

disinfectants, 321

disposables, 325–26

distractibility, 80–81, 87

diswashing detergents, 313

drain cleaners, 313

dust, 300

dyes, 308, 313


ear infections, 371–72

eating habits, 230–72
    behavior management,
        233–36
    developing, 184–86, 189,
        232–44
    developmental skills, 148,
        238–39
    environment, 236–39
    equipment, 238, 240–41
    picky eaters, 146, 230, 232
    setting boundaries, 237–38
    toddler-friendly foods, 239,
        242, 244, 247–48
    of toddlers, 231–32

echinacea, 373

eczema, 289, 306

eggs, 108, 205, 207

electricity, 331–32

emotional intelligence, 356

energy conservation, 17, 331–37

energy levels, 142–43

engorgement, 88

Environmental Protection
    Agency (EPA), 23

essential oils, 319

ethylene vinyl acetate (EVA),
    302

exercise:
    with baby, 40
    and breast-feeding, 36–37
    bridges, 38
    buddy for, 39
    eco-friendly gear for, 40
    energy for, 41
    and hydration, 39
    indoor, 38
    Kegel, 36, 37
    and postpartum depression,
        52–53
    push-ups, 38
    regular, 45
    running errands, 37–38
    stretching, 38
    support bra for, 37
    time for, 39–40
    TV channels, 39
    walking lunges, 38–39
    walking with the stroller, 39

fabrics, 305–8

fats, dietary, 210–14
    artificial, 224
    in mother's diet, 110–12
    in solid foods, 187
    tips, 210, 214

feeding, see bottles; breast-
    feeding; formula

feeding charts, 159–62

fertilizers, 27

fever, 374

HEPA-filter vacuum, 296, 323

herbal medications, 122

hindmilk, 63, 77

home:
    clutter-free, 321
    energy and water
        conservation, 331–37
    stress-free, 353–54
    ventilation of, 300, 314
    waste reduction, 323–28

home products, 275–309,
        310–38
    cleaning, 311–23
    fabrics, 305–8
    furniture, 292–300
    playroom, 303–5
    recycling, 328–31
    toys, 300–305

honey, 137, 170, 222

household waste, 28, 323–28

hunger signals, 72

hydration, 39, 116, 143, 217

hydrogen peroxide, 321

hygiene, 356–63

illness and ailments, 371–74

immune system, 357, 372–73

infant probiotic powder, 93

intellectual development,
        11–12

iron, 78, 115, 143, 150, 188, 209

jaundice, 66–69

jealousy, 94

journaling, 44

juices, 166, 218

junk food, 221

junk mail, 325

Kegel exercise, 36, 37

kitchen, water conservation in,
        333

kitchen storage, 181

lactation consultant, 90

lactose intolerance, 208

La Leche League, 90

landfills, overflowing, 324

lanolin, 295

latch, 69, 71

laughter, 44

laundry room, 335

lawn care, 331, 337

lead, exposure to, 12, 297–98,
        303

lead testing, 298

learning, lifelong, 49–50

Leonard, Annie, *The Story of
        Stuff*, 324

letdown reflex, 63, 77

library usage, 325

lifestyle, green, 7–8

lightbulbs, 334

living in the moment, 48

living room, conservation in,
        334

low birth weight, causes of, 5

lower lip flip, 71

lunch, 132–33, 246

lung disease, and toxins, 9

magnesium, 143

mantras, 44

maple syrup, 222

massage, 45

mastitis, 77, 88, 92, 93

materialism, discouraging,
        324

mattresses, 119, 294–96, 299

meats:
    deli, 108
    ground, 205–6
    iron from, 209

medical checkups, 369–70

medicines, and lactation, 122

melamine, 97

melatonin, 44

mercury, 10, 12, 117, 212

mildew, 322

milk:
    alternatives, 102
    daily intake of, 102
    organic, 194–95, 213
    pesticides in, 194
    transitioning from formula
        to, 101–2

"milk drunk," 75

mind-body connection, 45–48

minerals, in mother's diet,
        115–16

miscarriage, causes of, 5

molasses, 222

mother's diet, 106–44
    and breast milk, 108–20
    convenience foods, 133–34
    dietary fats, 110–12
    and environmental toxins,
        118–19
    fish, 117–18
    fluids, 116
    foods to avoid in pregnancy,
        108
    and fussy baby, 138–40
    grocery list, 123–27
    menus, 129–33, 135–36
    nutrition FAQs, 136–43
    organic foods, 109–10

mother's diet (*cont.*)
servings, 127–29
snacks, 134–35
vitamins and minerals,
112–16
MSG (monosodium glutamate),
130
mulch, 337

nail care, 361
napkins, 326
natural gas, 17
natural products, 322
natural resources:
nonrenewable, 17–20
reducing strain on, 29
nature, 47
networking, 48, 49
neurotoxins, 109
neurotransmitters, 50
nipple confusion, 76
nipple pain, 90–94
nipples:
moisturizing, 91
plugged ducts, 91
washing, 90
yeast infection on, 93
nitrates, 27, 176
nontoxic products, 322
noodles, 200–201
nursing apparel, 95
nursing cover-ups, 92

oatmeal, 130
obesity, 351–52
oil, 17
olive oil, 289
omega-3 fats, 50–51, 96, 110–12,
210, 211–13, 216

orange skin, 166
organic farms:
animals raised on, 24–25, 27
conserving resources, 29
costs of, 26
local, 196
and nutrient content, 31
pollution-free, 27, 193
sustainability of, 29, 196,
205
organic foods, 6, 21–33,
192–96
cost of, 193–94
for mother, 109–10
nutrients in, 30–31, 193
packaged, 193
pesticide-free, 23–24, 193
shopping list, 194–95
what they are, 22–23
yummy, 30–33, 193
*see also* green feeding
osteoporosis, 206
out and about, 359
oven cleaners, 313
overbite, 103

pacifiers, 77, 103
paint, 297–98, 299, 303
paint/removers, 119
paper products, 316, 330
paper towels, 315, 317
parabens, 12, 120, 290
paraffin wax, 323
pasta, 51
"paying it forward," 29–30
PBDEs (flame retardants), 11,
13, 294, 2985
PCBs (polychlorinated
biphenyls), 8, 12

perchloroethylene, 12
perfume, 120, 121, 289
pesticides, 12, 23–24, 109–10,
193, 194
pet's toys, 303
PFCs (perfluorochemicals), 12,
296–97
phosphates, 27, 313
phthlalates, 11, 120, 290
physical activity, 346–52
phytochemicals, 31, 197, 199
pincer grasp, 162
plasticizers, 11
plastics:
BPA-free, 6
BPA in, 11, 12, 118, 174
buying less, 325
hand washing, 103
phthalate-free, 6
PVC free, 302, 303
playpens, 51, 347
playroom, 303–5, 334
polycarbonate, plastics made
from, 11
positive thinking, 43–44
postconsumer materials,
304–5
postpartum depression, 52–53
postpartum fitness, 35–40
prayer, 45
precautionary principle, 27
pregnancy, foods to avoid
during, 108
preservatives, 223
probiotics, 93, 98, 214–15
Project Peanut Butter, 304
protein, 142, 187, 204–6, 251
PVC (polyvinyl chloride), 11,
302–3